HEART &
SCALPEL

A HISTORY OF
CARDIAC SURGERY

HEART & SCALPEL

A HISTORY OF CARDIAC SURGERY

REVISED EDITION WITH BIBLIOGRAPHY

ROBERT RICHARDSON

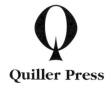

Quiller Press

First published in the UK under the title *The surgeon's heart*.
Copyright © 1969 Robert G Richardson.

Published in the USA under the title *The scalpel and the heart*.
Copyright © 1970 Robert G Richardson.

This edition published 2001
by Quiller Press Ltd.
46 Lillie Road,
London SW6 1TN.

Copyright © 1969, 1970 and 2001 Robert Richardson.
The moral right of the author has been asserted.

ISBN 1 899163 70 0

Designed by Jo Lee

Set in Garamond 10/13pt

Printed in Hong Kong through Colorcraft Ltd.

CONTENTS

PREFACE

This is the story of some very uncommon men who set out to achieve the seemingly impossible and in the end made a 'fantastic dream' come true. The story is based on their own writings – about 700 original articles and books form the direct references, and many more the indirect ones that gave the 'feel' of the times.

Except for mentioning the first cases of coronary artery bypass grafting and of coronary angioplasty, I have ended the story with the first heart transplants – as in the original edition. Much has happened since then, but it has consisted largely of widening the horizons with operations such as surgery for cardiac arrhythmias and excision of segments of the thickened ventricle in hypertrophic cardiomyopathy. Also much developmental work has been done in the attempt to produce a truly satisfactory artificial heart (as distinct from a strictly assist device) which will, I suspect, continue for quite a while into the future. But I stopped where I did because this book is a history and not a review of current progress in cardiac surgery – in the midst of events we lose perspective.

I have used the metric system for measurements except when the original author used the Imperial system, in which case the metric equivalent follows in parentheses.

The big difference in this new edition is the inclusion of the bibliographic sources, missing from the original. Sometimes the dates do not coincide with those given in the text; this is because publication took place at a later date than the event described. Sometimes, too, an author's initials are missing or the spelling of names varies slightly; in all cases I copied the details as given on the title page of the article or book. Lastly – and this applies mostly to the more modern references – the name of a senior author, as mentioned in the text, may not always be the first to be given.

The dates of birth and death in the Index of Personal Names are as complete as I can make them. When they eluded me I have simply put the date of the event with which that person is associated.

2001 RGR

1

PROLOGUE

The surgery of the heart is built on sure foundations. Although, to some, cardiac surgery may seem such a recent innovation that they are surprised it has a history at all before the Second World War. But it has, and a very varied and exciting one. It is difficult to say just when the story began, because in essence it follows the same broad lines as other branches of surgery[1]; however, mankind's emotions, traditions, and superstitions entered more strongly, and conditioned the mind unfavourably long before the scalpel first cut into the heart's muscle.

Surgery as we know it today began about a century-and-a-half ago with the discovery, first of anaesthesia in 1846 in America[2] and, second of antisepsis by Joseph Lister in the mid-1860s[3,4], which led on to asepsis. With an unconscious, anaesthetized patient, the surgeon could venture far into the human body and, within reason, take his time about it. Gone were the days when amputations, done in seconds, were the commonest operations, and the abdomen was almost forbidden territory. Admittedly, early anaesthesia with a mask and ether or chloroform left a lot to be desired, and the technique had a long way to go to reach the highly sophisticated specialty it is today. Nevertheless, pain had been conquered.

Unfortunately, before long, surgeons found they were up against another obstacle – infection. The increasing number of operations performed, and the ambition of the operators, made this a problem of the first order. What real advance had been achieved if half or more of the patients operated on died? When operating, most surgeons would wear an old morning coat, liberally caked with the pus and blood of their previous endeavours, and as like as not

1

would have come straight from the dissecting room without even bothering to wash their hands. A very few appreciated the need for cleanliness though, had they had been asked why, could have given no reason. Louis Pasteur was still in the process of discovering his microscopic organisms, which we know as bacteria[5].

When Lister heard of Pasteur's work he realized its importance to surgery, and he set about devising a way of killing the bacteria which infected surgical wounds. After much experimentation he decided on carbolic acid – carbolic acid dressings, carbolic acid soaking for the surgeon's hands and instruments, carbolic acid spraying over the operation site, carbolic acid by the gallon.

It worked. But it also had its disadvantages; for instance, at first when strong solutions were used they were prone to cause chemical burns, and in large wounds sufficient acid was occasionally absorbed into the blood stream to cause fatal poisoning. Also, the surgeon and his assistants sometimes developed dermatitis from contact with the carbolic. So, instead of trying to kill the bacteria, surgeons decided to work under conditions that excluded bacteria.

This step was taken in Germany in the 1880s and led eventually to the development of the aseptic ritual[6,7] – scrubbing-up; the wearing of sterilized gowns and gloves, of masks, caps, and rubber boots; the sterilization of instruments, dressings, drapes, and everything that would enter the operating field; ventilation of the theatre and similar measures.

But infection was merely brought under control; it had not been conquered, since, to this day, it remains an ever-present menace, especially for the unwary. And other problems by the score continued to confront the surgeon; he had to learn how to combat shock and haemorrhage, to learn that anaesthesia did not give him a licence to spend all day inside the patient, and to appreciate the need for delicate handling of the tissues. However, surgery was at last able to break out of the screaming, pus-laden agony of centuries.

Despite what seems to us the unbearable horror of long ago, patients lived to tell the tale, and surgeons managed to acquire the knowledge that enabled them to take full advantage of the breakthrough when it came. In the mid-1880s great strides were taken in understanding the structure and function of the human body; the microscope was coming into its own; in the latter part of the century the science of bacteriology was put on a sound footing by Robert Koch in Germany[8]; and the importance of pathology was really appreciated.

Slowly the nature of disease and the processes by which diseases evolved were becoming apparent; advances were made that enabled accurate diagnoses to be achieved. No longer was a diagnosis just a label to an illness. It implied a complete understanding of all its aspects. Progress in physics, chemistry, and other basic sciences led to improvements in diagnostic techniques and surgical methods. Experiments on animals showed the way to what might one day be possible on human beings.

In those early days of surgical freedom, the mainstream of advance was in 'general' surgery. Specialization as it is understood today had not yet split the subject into separate compartments. Surgeons had to be able to turn their hands to anything coming their way. Admittedly, some had special interests, and there was an element of specialization in subjects like ophthalmology, orthopaedics, obstetrics and gynaecology. But before long it became apparent that to achieve progress in certain fields surgeons had to concentrate their attention on their particular subject. So specialization gradually emerged.

Attention in the early days was focused on the three body cavities – the abdomen, the cranial cavity, and the chest. All are lined with membranes (the peritoneum encloses the abdominal organs; the dura mater covers the brain; and the pleura envelops the lungs), and surgeons believed that these membranes were effective barriers to the spread of infection from outside. It took a courageous man to cut through them unless the patient was already nearly dead; in fact cutting the peritoneum was reputed to produce a severe and frequently fatal peritonitis. But courageous surgeons there were, and outstanding among them was Theodor Billroth, a German, who became head of the surgical clinic in Vienna in 1867 at the age of 38. Billroth was a surgical giant in any company, and although he acquired a formidable list of successful 'first' operations, he is chiefly remembered as the founder of abdominal surgery. By his work he gave the lie to those who believed the peritoneum to be an enemy, and, particularly when asepsis arrived on the scene, he showed it to be a valuable ally because, when given a reasonable chance, it could put up a strong fight against infection and deal with most germs that gained entry by walling them off in a localized abscess.

One of the oldest of operations is trepanning, and it had remained virtually unchanged ever since prehistoric man chipped a circle of bone from the skull with a flint knife. As time passed, the instruments became more elaborate, but the reasons for its performance scarcely altered. It was used to let the devil out in cases of epilepsy, and later to relieve pressure on the brain when the skull was fractured. Infection and haemorrhage effectively protected the brain itself from intrusion. In the later years of the nineteenth century a number of surgeons laid the foundations of neurosurgery; but it was one man, Harvey Cushing, in America, who consolidated neurosurgery as a specialty in the opening decades of the 20th century.

The last body cavity to yield its secrets to the scalpel was the chest. One or two surgeons had ventured in before the days of anaesthesia but, generally speaking, the undertaking had been unprofitable. Chest surgery is dependent upon so many important considerations other than pure operative skill that its emergence as a specialty lagged far behind the others. Opening the chest was long believed to be tantamount to a sentence of death.

The physiology of respiration is extremely complex and had to be understood before any serious advance could be contemplated. The effect of opening the chest and letting air into the pleural cavity profoundly alters the mechanics of respiration, the immediate effect being for the lung on that side to collapse; there is also a variable degree of collapse of the opposite lung. If the hole is closed immediately the lung will gradually re-expand as the air is absorbed by the body or removed by the surgeon. But if the hole is big enough and remains open, air moves backward and forward from one lung to the other as the patient breathes (paradoxical respiration), instead of from lungs to outside atmosphere; and the heart, great vessels, and other structures lying between the two lungs in what is known as the mediastinum will flutter with the movements of breathing. The patient dies rapidly unless steps are taken to close the hole and remove the air. Should the hole into the pleural cavity act as a valve letting air in, but not out, the pressure inside the chest increases until respiration becomes impossible.

When air is present in the pleural cavity, the state is known as pneumo-thorax, and the two dangerous varieties are called open pneumothorax and tension pneumothorax, respectively. It will be appreciated that when a surgeon operates on the chest and enters the pleural cavity, he will create an open pneumothorax. However, it is possible for him to operate on structures, such as the heart, inside the chest without entering the pleural cavity. On many occasions this will be desirable, but on many others he has to open the cavity to have the best conditions for operating.

Before going further, it is advisable to digress for a moment and describe the anatomical arrangements of the lungs and pleurae and those of the heart and its surrounding membrane, the pericardium, which are basically similar. First of all, imagine a deflated balloon that has no outlet, then make a fist of the left hand and push this into the outside of the balloon so that the fist is completely surrounded by two layers of balloon except at the wrist. Over the fist and two layers of balloon lay the open right hand. The left fist now represents the lung (or the heart), and the wrist, the bronchus and blood vessels entering the lung (or the veins and great arteries entering and leaving the heart). The two layers of balloon are the pleurae (or pericardium); the space between them, which is potential not real, is the pleural cavity (or pericardial cavity); these two layers are lubricated and enable the lungs to move smoothly during respiration (or the heart to beat freely). The open right hand represents the chest wall in both instances.

Owing to negative pressure, considerable force is needed to separate the two layers of pleura, permitting an incision to be made through the chest wall, for instance to reach the heart, and if the pleura is not punctured the lung on that side will not collapse. But this calls for careful dissection and a knowledge of the detailed anatomy of the region because the pleura comes round between most of the heart and the chest wall.

What has all this got to do with cardiac surgery? The heart is inside the chest, and the problems of operating in there had to be overcome before a serious attack on the heart could even be contemplated. In particular, anaesthetists had to learn how to keep the lungs inflated when the pleural cavity *was* opened, suitable anaesthetics had to be discovered, the transfusion of blood had to be developed, and a great deal had to be learned about how the body reacted to the stresses of surgery.

Cardiac surgery was thus the last anatomical surgical specialty to emerge. It is the most intensely dramatic, due in part to the wide variety of intricate operations performed and the complicated apparatus needed, and in part to the symbolism of the heart, rooted deep within mankind.

2

THE CIRCULATION

From his earliest days mankind has viewed the heart with a superstitious awe; the organ has been considered the seat of life, of the soul, of the emotions, and of the intellect. Any damage to it was believed to be invariably lethal. (Although it may appear that the ancients, from Pythagoras onwards, were delving into the mysteries of anatomy and physiology, they were concerned with a far more esoteric, spiritual plane. For them, the Intellect, by means of which man discerns what lies beyond the earthly plane, resided in the Heart – not the anatomical heart, but the Heart that is the centre of the Soul. Consequently, the perplexities of the ancients over the location of the Intellect, the Soul and the Heart should not be taken at anatomical face value.) Old beliefs die hard and until the 16th century medical authority saw no reason to challenge these views, although gradually stripped of their metaphysical values.

Pythagoras and Hippocrates had both said that the brain was the seat of the intellect, but Aristotle disagreed. In fact he was quite contemptuous of the idea. His predecessors had been content with theory, he said, whereas he had carried out experiments in his never-ending search for facts, facts, and still more facts. He had shown that the brain was lacking in sensation. Its true function, he maintained (though where he obtained the experimental evidence is anyone's guess), was to cool the fire in the heart and so prevent overheating of the body. This the brain did by secreting a sort of water called pituita or phlegm.

The heart, according to Aristotle, was the source of the body's innate heat and the seat of sensation and thought. He arrived at this conclusion as a result of his embryological studies of hens' eggs. The first sign of life, he noted, was the small red pulsating spot of the heart, and it was his contention that organs appeared in their order of importance. He believed, and so later did Pliny the Elder, that the heart was so essential to life that it never suffered disease. How wrong they were! Essential to life it is, but heart disease in one form or another is the commonest cause of death in most countries today.

The real function of the heart, whatever else may be ascribed to it by the romantic poets, is to pump blood through the body. In an average man's lifetime, his heart beats well over 2600 million times and pumps something like 164 million litres of blood out of each of the two ventricles. The weight of this volume of fluid is about 152 000 tonnes. Expressed in another way, the work done by the heart in a lifetime is sufficient to raise more than 10 tonnes to a height of 10 miles (16km) – at least. And the organ weighs a mere 310 grams or thereabouts in the male.

Nowadays the facts of the circulation are commonplace knowledge. But they were not always so. In the third century BC the centre of medical learning was at Alexandria in Egypt, and it was there that the first real work on human anatomy and physiology was done, strange though some of the results may seem to us now. Only two names of any importance survive in this field, Herophilus and Erasistratus. Both men made considerable discoveries, but it was the ideas of Erasistratus that are of most interest to us.

The museum (or university) contained dissecting rooms, and in these Erasistratus lectured to students from all over the ancient world.

'We live because our bodies are pervaded by pneuma which is a most subtle vapour.' So his lecture on respiration might have started. 'The air we breathe enters our lungs from where it is taken to the heart which contracts and dilates because of a force inherent within it. In the heart the air is changed into this pneuma, or vital spirit, which is carried to all parts of the body by arteries. That part of the pneuma which reaches the cavities of the brain undergoes a further alteration into animal spirit which is taken to the structures of the body by the nerves, which are hollow. When we make a movement we do so because our muscles shorten by becoming distended with animal spirit.

'Further, the blood in our body is contained within the veins and at their terminations are innumerable communications with the arteries. When an artery is cut, the pneuma escapes first; its place is then taken by blood which enters from the veins and heart.'

Before his day the ideas on respiration and the function of the cardiovascular system were obscure, vague, and founded on speculation. The Greeks had a profound respect for the human body, and, anatomically speaking, what they could not see they did not bother about. In view of this, Erasistratus's theories were no mean achievement. What life is remains a mystery, and although we are gathering a great deal of knowledge about the function of the heart, the ultimate 'why' has yet to be discovered. Erasistratus was able to differentiate between veins and arteries, but was nothing less than honest in his perplexity over what they contained; for he admitted that he had never seen a corpse whose arteries bled when cut, yet somehow he had to explain that arteries bled when cut during life. He also realized that the two valves of exit from the heart prevented the return of blood.

And, although he might be said to have been thinking back to front, he considered that there were communications between the ends of the arteries and veins. It is probably wrong to credit him with being on the verge of discovering the circulation, but it was nevertheless a remarkable piece of deduction.

No further progress was made for nigh on 500 years. Medicine continued to be a popular subject, but only for argument. And there was indeed plenty to argue about, but no one did anything practical to advance learning. Disputation was more important than experience; the human mind alone was sufficient to seek out the truth, and imagination ran riot.

Then in the second century AD, Galen appeared on the scene during the reign of Marcus Aurelius, the last of the Five Good Emperors of Rome. Galen came to Rome from his native Pergamon, a Greek colonial city, at the age of 31; his brilliance was already evident, and despite the Romans' antagonism to foreigners he soon became respected for his drive and integrity and was appointed physician to the Emperor.

His object in life was to rationalize medicine, to rescue it from the metaphysical mess into which it had fallen. To this end his industry was enormous; he carried out experiments on animals to discover how different parts of the body functioned; he dissected every animal he could lay his hands on, but unfortunately this included very few human beings.

'Nature does nothing in vain,' Aristotle had said. Galen agreed with this and managed to give reasons for most of nature's actions. However, he had preconceived ideas about quite a lot of things, and this made him interpret some of his dissections inaccurately, and also he assumed that his findings in animals, such as the Barbary ape, applied to man. Add to this the fact that subsequent generations read mainly from inaccurate translations of inaccurate translations of his work, and it can well be imagined that some pretty erroneous ideas were perpetuated for the next 1500 or so years.

And what Galen said about medicine was gospel for all that time.

This came about because no one of sufficient calibre emerged to follow on with his work; the world of learning degenerated; the Christian Church was in the ascendant with all the troubles this caused. And Galen's medicine appealed to the Church. Galen was a monotheist; he worshipped Aesculapius, the god of medicine, and this was good since the Church was fighting against the plurality of Roman gods – it was convenient to forget that Aesculapius was a heathen god. Then again, Galen's belief that God had made everything with a purpose, and his proof of this, commended itself greatly to the Church. For these self-same reasons his work subsequently found favour with the Arabian school of medicine when the Mohammedans overran Alexandria and Spain but kept the light of Greek medicine flickering through the Dark Ages.

The theory of the function of the cardiovascular system that dominated for so many centuries such medical thought as there was, and became deeply imprinted on men's minds, can briefly be termed the ebb and flow theory.

Galen disagreed with Erasistratus over the content of arteries. He believed they contained blood which was 'thinner' than that in the veins; but he did agree that there was some sort of communication between the two types of vessel. He went astray, however, when he said that all vessels connected with the heart were arteries, and that the veins were all connected with the liver.

Air, Galen thought, was composed of many substances, one of which was our old friend pneuma; on this life depended. The inspired air was purified in the lungs and the pneuma separated out as a thin fluid which became mixed with blood and taken to the heart along what is now called the pulmonary artery. But this meant that it entered the right side of the heart. How then did it get into the left side? In two ways, according to Galen. The more important was through holes or pores in the dividing wall. These Galenic pores have achieved considerable notoriety, for they are non-existent, and the puzzle is whether Galen really believed in them or whether he invented them as a convenient way of justifying his theory. In all probability he believed in them and for the following reasons. The two sides of the heart are only completely separate in birds and mammals, and so from his dissection of lower animals Galen could have been led to believe that they were also separate in man, even if the holes were invisible. Secondly, at an early stage of its embryological development, communications exist between the atria and ventricles, and Galen had some knowledge of fetal anatomy. But perhaps more significantly these communications may persist as congenital abnormalities. The hole between the atria, known as the foramen ovale, normally does not close until after birth. If it remains open as a patent interatrial septum, it is compatible with survival into adult life and is one of the commoner congenital cardiac defects. Thus it is not difficult to realize how Galen may have drawn his wrong conclusions.

The second way in which Galen believed that blood entered the left side of the heart was through the pulmonary veins directly from the lungs. He devised an ingenious function for the pulmonary valve (which is situated at the exit from the right ventricle and prevents blood, which has been pumped out into the pulmonary artery on its way to the lungs, from re-entering the heart). This valve, he said, was closed during inspiration so that the blood in it would be forced into the pulmonary veins.

Galen maintained that when the heart contracted, blood was forced out, and when it relaxed, blood was sucked back in again – ebb and flow. In some strange way the valves between the atria and the ventricles (the mitral and the tricuspid) helped in this process. When the blood rushed out to the end of the body, the pneuma was removed. In the brain the pneuma determined the motor and sensory functions of the nervous system.

The blood on the right side of the heart received a contribution from the liver. When food was eaten it was converted to 'chyle' in the gut and carried to the liver where it became blood and endowed with 'natural spirit' which was responsible for carnal appetites and desires.

This theory of Galen's, obscure in parts and becoming more so as time passed, was the truth. It was heresy to challenge it and no one dared. At least not until the Renaissance.

The Renaissance was the turning point in medicine. Strange as it may seem, the turn in the practice of healing was back to Hippocrates. Men began wanting to see things as they were, to study with the evidence of their own senses and to get away from the dogma imposed upon them for so long. Hippocrates had observed for himself and built up a remarkably sound approach to disease, so what better starting point could there be for the Renaissance physician. Admittedly it was rather overdone, as the works of Hippocrates were still the standard texts in some medical schools even in the time of Laënnec, who invented the stethoscope, early in the 19th century.

In anatomy a start was made by artists who so desperately wanted to paint the body as it really was and not as the unlifelike stylized representations that were then the vogue. Most of them were content with dissecting muscles and superficial structures and studying the skeleton, but one was so fired with enthusiasm that he continued to study the anatomy of the whole body. This was Leonardo da Vinci[1]. But by a supreme calamity his drawings and notes were widely dispersed shortly after his death.

Many of his anatomical drawings found their way to the library at Windsor Castle, to be rediscovered in the 1890s. Only then did the full extent of his genius in anatomy become apparent. His earlier drawings of the heart were influenced by Galenic ideas on the subject; for instance, he showed only one 'auricle' (atrium) and indicated the presence of Galen's pores between the ventricles. But as his experience in dissection grew he was able to shake off these preconceived notions and reproduce the structures as he really saw them.

Leonardo's absorbing interest in mechanics is evident in many of his sketches, and in one he recorded his observations on the behaviour of three needles thrust into the heart through the chest wall of a living animal. The tip of the needle that entered the base of the heart moved downward with each contraction of the heart; the one in the middle of the ventricle also moved downward, but not so much; the one in the apex scarcely moved at all. The reason for this, although Leonardo did not say as much, is that the pericardium is firmly attached to the central tendon of the diaphragm, so serving to anchor the heart at its apex.

But perhaps his most remarkable studies so far as we are concerned centred around the haemodynamics in the region of the aortic valve. He first observed the characteristics of the flow of water in channels of changing width using special floats designed to be carried by currents at varying depths. Then he experimented in his laboratory with pipes and tanks and showed how the central flow from the end of a pipe travelled the farthest – the flow at the sides was slowed by the friction of the edges. His translation of his findings to the aortic region can only leave us gasping with admiration, since he gave detailed directions for the construction of an anatomical model – and there is no doubt that he himself made such a model. His drawings of this contain a number of apparently strange features that only research with modern techniques of cineangiography has proved correct. With this model he demonstrated the mechanism by which the aortic valve closed. It was not the central flow 'falling back' and slamming the valve cusps shut. Instead it was the slower flow at the sides curling round and more gently closing the upwardly curved cusps from the sides. The precise nature of the haemodynamics of the area is still obscure, but the inspired work of a man who lived 500 years ago could well prove to be correct. Yet, whether correct or not, it is an object lesson to all who today strive to perfect the surgical answer to disease of the aortic and other heart valves.

Even had Leonardo's notes not been lost to subsequent generations, it is most unlikely that they would have made an impact at the time. The whole concept of his studies was far too advanced to be acceptable or even understood. In the medical schools Galen's anatomy continued to be taught. When anything was found that did not conform with Galen's statements, the common explanation was that the body had changed since then. Yet sooner or later someone was bound to speak out for the truth. That someone was Andreas Vesalius.

Born in Belgium, Vesalius studied medicine in Paris and became professor of surgery and anatomy at Padua when only 23. In his dissections he found much that was at variance with accepted Galenic teaching, and because he did not hesitate to say so in his famous book, *De humani corporis fabrica*[2] he made many enemies, and the controversies of which he was the centre were heated and bitter. He was fortunate in having the illustrations for the book engraved by Jan Stephan van Calcar, a former pupil of Titian, who brought the subject vividly to life.

Galen's pores were shown in the first edition (1543), but in the second (1555) Vesalius was emphatic about their non-existence and said that blood could not pass between the ventricles. Two observations show that he was more concerned with structure than with function. He saw how organs were supplied with both arteries and veins, but considered this to be a convenient arrangement for the ebb and flow of the blood. He also noted the presence of valves in the veins.

The next step along the road towards understanding that the blood circulated was the discovery of the pulmonary or lesser circulation. This was made by Vesalius's successor at Padua, Realdus Columbus, although he did not publish his findings until 1557 when he was at Rome[3]. This part of the circulation had also been discovered independently by Michael Servetus of Navarre. Unfortunately, Servetus's book, *Christianismi restitutio*, led to his being condemned for heresy by John Calvin, and he was burned at the stake at Geneva.

Servetus came very close to the function of respiration when he wrote that in its course through the lungs, blood became crimson and was 'freed from fuliginous vapours by the acts of expiration.'

Another professor of anatomy at Padua was Fabricius ab Aquapendente, who studied the valves of the veins and realized that they were there to regulate the flow of blood[5]. What he failed to appreciate was their significance. This was grasped by his English pupil, William Harvey, who showed by years of patient, careful work that the blood circulated round the body; a discovery of tremendous importance in understanding how the body worked.

Harvey was born at Folkestone in 1578, and after his education at a school in Canterbury and at Caius College, Cambridge, he spent four years in Padua, where he obtained his MD in 1602. When he returned to England, he set up practice in London and soon became a Fellow of the College of Physicians. Then in 1618 he was appointed Physician Extraordinary to James I, and later Physician Ordinary to Charles I, who showed great interest in Harvey's work.

At the battle of Edgehill, during the Civil War, so the story goes, Harvey was responsible for the care of the two sons of King Charles and was reading to them not far from the scene of action until a stray cannon ball made them move farther away.

Harvey played a crafty game. He let his theory of the circulation become known little by little in his lectures and dissections; he was scrupulous in giving Galen credit where this was due, and where possible he cited Galen in support of his work. In this way he managed to forestall the anger and opposition of the out-and-out Galenists. Nevertheless, the publication in 1628 of his book *Exercitatio anatomica de motu cordis ex sanguinis in animalibus*[6], dedicated to King Charles, stirred up dissension; chief among his critics was Jean Riolan, professor of anatomy in Paris, another royal physician and an ardent Galenist to the end.

Harvey first demolished the established but erroneous views on the cardiovascular system. 'But, damme, there are no pores and it is not possible to show such,' was how he expressed himself on the subject of Galen's pores between the ventricles. Then he went on to show how the two ventricles beat together, as did the atria. He demonstrated that the heart expelled its blood during systole and filled passively during diastole. He confirmed that the blood passed from the right ventricle through the lungs and back into the left atrium. But it was the circulation round the body that was his primary concern.

He realized and showed by experiment that the purpose of the valves in the veins was to ensure a unidirectional flow of blood.

'It has been shown by reason and experiment,' he wrote, 'that blood by the beat of the ventricles flows through the lungs and heart and is pumped to the whole body. There it passes through pores in the flesh into the veins through which it returns from the periphery everywhere to the centre, from the smaller veins into the larger ones, finally coming to the vena cava and right atrium. This occurs in such an amount, with such an outflow through the arteries, and such a reflux through the veins, that it cannot be supplied by the food consumed. It is also much more than is needed for nourishment. It must therefore be concluded that the blood in the animal body moves around in a circle continuously, and that the action or function of the heart is to accomplish this by pumping. This is the only reason for the motion and beat of the heart.'

The only missing link was 'the pores in the flesh.' He knew that the capillaries must exist, but he had no means of finding them. For this a microscope was necessary, and during the same century this instrument became sufficiently developed for Marcello Malpighi to put the finishing touch to Harvey's work. Had he not done so, the truth about the circulation might well have become submerged once more in speculation and theory.

Malpighi was born and qualified in medicine at Bologna and held the chairs of anatomy there, at Pisa and at Messina. Three years before his death at the age of 66 in 1694, he became physician to Pope Innocent XII.

'And such is the wandering about of these vessels,' he wrote of the capillaries in the frog's lung to his friend, the mathematician Giovanni Borelli, in 1661[7], 'as they proceed on this side from the vein and on the other side from the artery, that the vessels no longer maintain a straight direction, but there appears a network made up of the continuations of the two vessels....Hence it was clear to the senses that the blood flowed away along tortuous vessels and was not poured into spaces, but was always contained within tubules, and that its dispersion is due to the multiple winding of the vessels.'

Thus, almost exactly 2000 years after their existence had first been suspected by Erasistratus, the reality of the capillaries was proved by Malpighi.

3

WOUNDS OF THE HEART

'A wound in the heart is mortal', said Hippocrates in one of his aphorisms[1]. And so for all intents and purposes it was, until quite recent times. Even today the surgeon's chances of success depend on the nature of the wound and the speed with which the patient is brought to him.

But before Hippocrates could be shown to be wrong, the medical profession had first to convince itself that the heart was not a mysterious organ that stopped working as soon as it was injured, and then, when surgery was sufficiently advanced, that operation had in fact something to offer. All this took a very long time indeed.

About 500 years after Hippocrates, at the beginning of the Christian era, Galen had ample opportunity for studying wounds. He had been a surgeon at the gladiatorial arena in his native Pergamon before coming to Rome, where he acted in a similar capacity at the shows put on by Marcus Aurelius and his son and successor as emperor, Commodus. At this time there was still a certain amount of fair play to the combats; they had not yet degenerated into the wholesale slaughter they eventually became. Nevertheless, death was more frequent than survival, and Galen must have seen every conceivable type of wound. As a result of his experience he drew attention to the immediacy of death if a ventricle were penetrated[2], an observation implying that he saw other chest wounds in which the heart was affected but death was not instantaneous.

Sacrificial rites were another Roman habit which gave Galen the chance of making the physiological observation that the heart would continue beating for a short time after its removal from the body. This is now a well-known fact and shows that the heart can beat independently of nervous control.

14

After Galen there was silence on the subject of heart wounds. Both Hippocrates and Galen had said they were lethal, and that was that – if anyone bothered to think about them at all.

When, in the Renaissance, men began to think for themselves again, a popular form of study was to take the writings of Hippocrates and comment on them. The first writer to introduce a note of doubt in a commentary on the aphorism about heart wounds was Hollerius, otherwise Jacques Houllier, a Parisian. As with many of the people whose writings contributed something to the history of cardiac surgery, we know little or nothing about him. This is a pity but not the tragedy it would be if it was the man's character or actions rather than his writings that had been the source of the contribution.

Writing in the early 1500s, Hollerius agreed that a wound of the heart was fatal if it was large, penetrated a ventricle, or injured one of the heart's arteries. But, he said, 'if it only affects the fleshy part, then I believe death is not inevitable.'[3] This was a step forward, but the writer did not produce any supporting evidence.

In cases of penetrating wounds, inflammation might block the hole and the patient might survive, but even though Hollerius mentioned this as a possibility, he viewed it with the greatest suspicion.

At that time there were some pretty far-fetched stories in circulation, one of which was that Galen had seen victims running around and shouting with their hearts hanging out. This was probably a distortion of Galen's observation on the continued beating of excised hearts. Hollerius just put it down to an old wives' tale.

The first person to produce conclusive evidence that a man could survive a heart wound was Barthélemy Cabrol of Montpellier. In a book of anatomical observations published in 1604[4], the year of his death, he recorded two postmortem examinations in which he found 'some wonderful things'. The first was a scar of two fingers' breadth in the base of the heart and 'what you could call a bump of the same size'. The other man's heart contained a scar in the same place the breadth of a myrtle leaf and 'deep enough'. He knew that these injuries could not have been the cause of death because in both cases the men had been criminals who had 'finished their lives in a noose'.

In view of this, Cabrol said he agreed with his contemporary, Jean Fernel, the greatest French physician of the Renaissance, in thinking that if death did not occur immediately it was possible for a man 'to survive a solution of the continuity of the heart for a long time.'

But the medical profession in general still believed that Hippocrates was right, and the reason for this was admirably expressed in the words of Paulus Zacchias that 'wounds of the heart were necessarily fatal because this, the most noble organ of the body, was unable to endure a solution of its continuity.'[5]

This statement appeared in the most important book on medical jurisprudence of the 17th century, and as its author was physician to Popes Innocent X and Alexander VII, the opinions carried a lot of weight. However, Zacchias went on to quote the famous Italian anatomist and pupil of Vesalius, Fallopius, as having said that a wound of the heart could only be survived by a miracle, since the heart could never heal as it was too hard, always in motion, and 'of an inflammatory heat'. This Fallopius did because he must have felt in need of moral support for his account of just such a 'miracle', which he related with considerable interest and gusto.

There was a mad priest who first of all cut off his penis and testicles and then jabbed himself with a stout needle many times below the left breast. The postmortem examination showed that all these wounds had penetrated the heart, yet the amazing thing to Zacchias was that this priest of Fallopius's had gone on living for five or six days.

The following years saw one or two accounts of healed wounds found in the hearts of animals, notably by William Harvey, who, with the permission of King Charles I, was allowed to study the deer in the royal parks[6], and by a gentleman named Idonis Wolf who in 1640 recorded another instance, also in a deer[7].

All this achieved was to make people wonder why some heart wounds were rapidly fatal and others were not; no one really believed that a man could survive for any length of time. Naturally enough, the theories put forward were entirely speculative, as practical experience was non-existent, but the general opinion was that if the wound only involved the substance of the muscle of the heart and did not penetrate the ventricles, the patient might live for as long as a day or two.

Other factors considered to affect the outcome were the obliquity and site of the wound: wounds of the right ventricle were believed to be more serious than those of the left; and wounds sustained when the heart was contracting in systole were more serious than when it was relaxing in diastole. For those days, this last was a tolerable supposition as it would have seemed reasonable for more damage to be sustained if the heart's muscle was actively contracting at the moment of injury. The snag was that no-one could tell just what stage of its cycle the heart was in at that precise moment – still, it was a nice point for debate.

But even while these desultory discussions were going on, doctors were beginning to realize the importance of pathology. The effect of disease could only be studied superficially during life, but a dead body could be dissected and the abnormal findings compared with the symptoms and signs before death.

The first major work along these lines was the collection of all known postmortems up to 1679 made by Théophile Bonet, a Swiss, and published in his book, the *Sepulchretum*[8,9]. This was an incredibly industrious compilation which filled Bonet's many leisure hours while physician to the Duc de Longueville. Alas! it was little more than a collection of some 3000 necropsies, as the level of medical knowledge at the time was insufficient for Bonet to group the cases adequately, and often he failed to use his own judgment by blindly accepting the original opinions. However, he did notice that if the pericardial cavity filled with blood, the pressure would stop the heart beating.

One day, about half-way through the next century, Giovanni Morgagni, professor of anatomy at Padua, was discussing the deficiencies of the *Sepulchretum* with a student, when he decided that the best answer was to do the job himself. So, for the next 20 years he meticulously recorded, in the form of letters to the student, all his postmortem examinations correlating the findings with the symptoms during life. The 70 letters were published in 1761 as a book, *De sedibus et causis morborum per anatomen indagatis*[10] (*The seats and causes of disease investigated by anatomy*[11]), which set the foundation of modern pathology. For the first time doctors were now able to form a mental picture of what was going on inside the bodies of their patients.

In one of the letters Morgagni implied – it cannot be put any more strongly – that most deaths from wounds of the heart occurred because of pressure of blood in the pericardial sac. But he was still puzzled as to why some patients survived longer than others. He was, however, groping in the right direction, because in the majority of straightforward stab wounds involving only the heart muscle, blood is pumped out through the slit-like wound into the pericardial cavity with each beat. Here it collects (because by no means all of it passes out into the chest through the wound in the pericardium) until the pressure built up in the pericardial cavity becomes too great and the heart is unable to relax.

The term 'Herztamponade' to describe this happening was coined by the Berlin surgeon, Edmund Rose, more than 100 years later in 1884[12]. The effect this had on surgical thinking was profound. The mere giving of a name to the condition gave it also a reality; here was something concrete that the mind could grasp; a previously uncertain state of affairs could be expressed in one word, and as a result surgeons began to realize the real nature of the problem of heart wounds and to feel they could do something about them.

In addition there had also been a change in outlook which made Rose's article a timely publication. Bonet's and Morgagni's observations had fallen on unreceptive ears, but when Rose wrote his paper explaining the condition and recording 23 case histories of ruptured and wounded hearts, with a mortality rate of 31 percent in 16 of them, it was widely accepted that a heart wound was not invariably fatal. This was largely owing to the work of Georg Fischer of Hanover, who, in 1868, had published a detailed analysis of 452 wounds of the heart and pericardium alone. Fischer had gathered the cases from the literature and had found that in 10 percent of heart wounds and 30 percent of pericardial wounds, the patients had survived[13].

Eight years previously, in 1860, an American doctor by the name of Galusha B Balch from North Lawrence, New York, had performed the postmortem on a patient with a fascinating case history. His report had no influence on the development of cardiac surgery, but it did highlight the amazing resilience of the heart in an extraordinary sequence of events. The patient was John Kelly. In 1840, when John was about 14 years old, he was accidentally shot, the bullet entering through his right shoulder. Three physicians probed the wound and located the bullet in the direction of the chest and lying near the inner end of the clavicle. As there was little bleeding and as John did not seem to be unduly disturbed by the wound, the physicians decided it would be inadvisable to remove the bullet – probably a wise decision considering that anaesthesia had not yet been discovered and because of the danger of entering the chest. The worthy physicians cannot be blamed for the future meanderings of that leaden bullet.

John grew into an apparently fit young man until, five years later, he developed severe pneumonia of the right upper lung. He recovered from this but subsequently the action of his heart was noted as tumultuous; 'at times the beating of his heart could be seen and heard at a distance of ten or twelve feet' (3·0-3·6m). Some years later valvular disease of the heart was diagnosed. Then, in the summer of 1860, he caught a cold which led to pneumonia again, and he died on June 14.

At the postmortem examination Dr Balch found the heart to be soft, flabby, and two or three times its natural size. The pericardium was adherent to the heart, more especially on the right side. When Dr Balch dissected the heart, he discovered the old bullet embedded in the wall of the right ventricle, but there was no scar or any other evidence of its passage[14].

The first bout of pneumonia was possibly directly due to, or aggravated by, the migration of the bullet; but by the time the second and fatal attack occurred, the heart had been weakened by its unwelcome intruder and could not cope with the strain put upon it by the lung infection.

We can now return to the main stream of events and to the first occasion when a surgeon deliberately operated on an injured heart: after a public house brawl, a 31-year-old man, Mr JE, missed a needle he usually kept in the left side of his coat. Next day he took himself to St Bartholomew's Hospital, London, although we are not told whether he suspected where the needle might have gone. At all events no wound or entry point was found, and JE returned to work.

Nine days later, on October 28, 1872, he felt distressed, and when he turned up at the hospital this time he was admitted. The surgeon, George Callender, an early supporter of Lister's principles, decided to make an incision between the ribs over the point where he thought the needle might be. His first shot was unsuccessful, but at the second attempt he withdrew a needle nearly two inches (5cm) long which had stuck in the heart close to the apex. JE made an uneventful recovery[15].

(*Plus ça change, plus c'est la même chose.* In 1966, a carpenter, James Upton, fell against a wooden plank. He felt a twinge of pain in his chest, but apart from that was unaware of any untoward injury. Three days later the pain returned and he decided something should be done about it. At the Beth Israel Hospital in Newark, New Jersey, an x-ray showed a needle in his heart muscle only 2mm from a coronary artery. Upton then recalled that for some strange reason he always kept a three-inch (7·5cm) sewing needle in his lapel. With all the then-modern conveniences it took the surgeons, David Schechter and Lawrence Gilbert, three hours of hard searching labour to find and remove the needle. They considered the case unusual because of the lack of bleeding and of gross symptoms[16].)

Although a step forward, Callender's earlier operation had not involved actual surgery on the heart itself. There was still a long way to go before this came about, and the next stage in the story concerns experimental work.

In 1882 the ill-starred Danizig surgeon, Block, whose first name is now unknown, found it simple and quick – a matter of three or four minutes – to insert sutures into the hearts of rabbits, and he suggested that it would be a practical proposition to repair wounds in human hearts[17]. But Block had ideas far ahead of his time, for the next year, encouraged by his experiments with lung surgery on animals, he operated on a young female relative who was supposed to have tuberculosis in the upper parts of both lungs. He was intending to remove the diseased tissues, a thing never before attempted, but the woman died on the operating table. Postmortem examination revealed that she had not, after all, been suffering from tuberculosis, and Block, utterly distraught, ended a potentially brilliant career by committing suicide.

At about this time we can find evidence of growing resistance to the idea of operating on the heart, and it is not really difficult to understand why this should have been so. To all intents and purposes the inside of the chest was forbidden territory; Block's effort showed just how dangerous it was even to attempt surgery on a lung. The physiology of respiration was still a mystery, and the notions about what happened when the chest was opened were extremely confused. Anaesthesia had scarcely progressed at all.

In the closing two decades of the 19th century, chest surgery consisted of nothing more than operations on the chest wall (which did not interfere with respiration) and the drainage of empyema. Empyema is a collection of pus inside the pleural cavity resulting usually either from an ordinary infection or from tuberculosis. Apart from its toxic effects, the pus could collect in such quantity that it interfered with breathing by compressing the lung, and if it did resolve with such medical treatment as was available, the patient was often left a respiratory cripple. In the early 1870s, physicians decided it would be a good thing to drain the pus away, but such was their fear of entering the chest that they only inserted tiny tubes, which were not much use, and completely ineffective if the pus was thick. Gradually they became more courageous and agreed to allow surgeons to remove a few ribs and, in chronic cases, some of the pleura which had become thickened in protest at the unwanted pus. Thus, towards the end of the century, the principle of the free evacuation of pus became firmly established.

An important contribution to the success, and one which was to become indispensable whenever it was necessary to drain fluid from the chest, was made in 1876 by Gotthard Bülau, a physician of Hamburg, who introduced subaqueous drainage[18]. In this, a drainage tube from the chest is carried below the level of water in a bottle under the bed, and thus air is prevented from entering the pleural cavity. Bülau was well aware of the dangers of open pneumothorax, and so much emphasis did he put upon them that for a number of years surgeons were reluctant to attempt any form of chest surgery.

So it is not surprising that, in the 1880s, when some people were talking about suturing heart wounds, wisdom should dictate caution. But there is a world of difference between advising cautious progress and being downright negative. Unfortunately, the impression left behind is that except for a few dedicated enthusiasts, the medical profession saw no future at all in heart surgery. The heart was an organ for the physician, its diseases were medical ones, and the surgeon had no business prying into it with his scalpel. But there was also an element of superstitious fear in their attitude.

Two remarks by the great Billroth were a godsend to those who, for whatever reason, wanted to see the infant science strangled at birth. Regrettably, because the remarks were catchy and repeatable, they were seized upon eagerly and have been quoted, misquoted, taken out of context, and misdated in innumerable publications ever since. Owing to the authority they have been invested with – an authority Billroth himself almost certainly never intended – it is worth while looking more closely into their origins.

Writing in the 1864 edition of his influential surgical textbook[19], Billroth had said that he only included the operation of incising the pericardium in cases of suppurative pericarditis for the sake of completeness despite the fact that (as we shall see in the next chapter) his former teacher, Bernhard von Langenbeck, had twice performed the operation successfully. He went on: 'I believe the operation is the next best thing to a frivolity and approaches what some surgeons might regard as a prostitution of the art of surgery.' But he concluded that future generations might think differently.

How the antagonists loved that bit about prostitution, and it was so easy to ignore the concluding sentence, and even to imply that the opinion referred to all cardiac surgery. To make matters worse, this section of the textbook was not revised with each succeeding edition and the original date of writing was not stated. So, when this sort of ammunition was needed, doctors went to their library shelves, took down the latest edition which by then was dated 1882, and Billroth's remark has been given this date most commonly ever since. The lack of revision is emphasized by the fact that Billroth's name at the foot of the chapter was followed by 'Professor of Surgery, Zurich', a post which he left in 1867 to go to Vienna.

The second of Billroth's remarks was made early in the 1880s: 'Any surgeon who wishes to preserve the respect of his colleagues would never attempt to suture the heart'. Without knowledge of his thoughts, this can be interpreted as wise advice, coming as it did about the time of Block's first experimental operation.

Nevertheless, this remark was spoken, not written, and the date has varied between 1881 and 1893 (the year before Billroth's death). The most authoritative dating was given many years later in 1925 by von Eiselsberg, at that time professor of surgery at Vienna. He said that as far as he could remember it was made by Billroth at a meeting of the Vienna Medical Society before he, von Eiselsberg, became Billroth's assistant, approximately in 1880 or 1881[20].

The reason why these two statements achieved such an influence was that they were made by the man who had built up abdominal surgery almost single-handed, and achieved a formidable list of 'first' operations both inside and outside the abdomen. He was one of the greatest surgeons of that or any other time. To lesser men, when Billroth had spoken, there was nothing left to be said. But not to Billroth himself, for in the Preface to the ninth edition of his textbook[21] (1880), he wrote:

'The practice of my profession, social duties, and my work as a teacher, have so absorbed my time during the past ten years that I have not followed the advance of medical science as closely as one should who was to present the results of recent workers to a new generation of students.'

So anyone considering a surgical attack on the heart had the weight of an adverse professional opinion to contend with. But there were still men who were prepared to plough the difficult furrow of research and experimentation in the hope that one day other men would be able to operate safely within the chest. And there were still men with the courage to grasp at surgical opportunity when they believed it justified, regardless of possible censure by their colleagues.

Representing the former in the context of heart wounds was an Italian, Simplicio del Vecchio, who had made wounds in dog hearts and successfully sutured them. He showed one of these dogs, which he had operated on 40 days previously, to a congress in 1894[22]. He also gave thoroughly practical details of how a surgeon should set about suturing a wound in a human heart.

The first of the latter body of men was Henry Dalton of St Louis, Missouri. Eugen L, a young man of 22, had been stabbed in the left side of his chest on

September 6, 1891. Dalton examined him in hospital and noted the wound, half an inch (1·25cm) long, and one-and-a-half inches (3·75cm) above the nipple. He found no increase in dullness over the heart or chest, which implied that at that stage there was no significant bleeding or effect on the lungs.

Ten hours later the situation was very different; the whole of the left chest gave a dull note when Dalton percussed it – the certain cause for this was blood filling the pleural cavity. So Eugen was taken to theatre, where the dressing was removed. Immediately blood and air gushed from the wound and continued to do so with each breath.

Dalton had no choice. As soon as Eugen was anaesthetized he made an incision eight inches (20cm) long over the left fourth rib and removed six inches (15cm) of its length. He then found the source of the bleeding – one of the arteries which runs between the ribs (an intercostal artery) had been injured. This he tied and then proceeded to swab the pleural cavity dry so that he could see what other damage had been done.

To his dismay he found a wound, two inches long, of the pericardium. But nothing daunted, he inserted a finger and felt the heart for any sign of injury. By great good fortune it was undamaged. So with a long needle holder and catgut, he sewed up the wound in the pericardium. This gave him the greatest difficulty, as the heart was beating at 140 to the minute, but at last he finished and closed the incision in the chest wall. Confident that he had stopped the bleeding, he inserted no drain. Eugen's recovery was uninterrupted and rapid[23].

Although Dalton had done all the situation demanded and would undoubtedly have sutured the heart had this been necessary, the fact remains that it was not. The barrier was still to be crossed.

Four years later, on September 4, 1895, in Norway, a 24-year-old man was stabbed between the fourth and fifth ribs on his left side. As a wounded animal runs away to hide, so the man made his way home – much-needed testimony to the remarkable resilience of the heart muscle – only to be discovered about an hour later lying in a pool of blood. He was rushed to hospital and into the operating theatre, by which time the bleeding had stopped.

The surgeon entered the chest by removing the fourth and part of the third ribs. Inside he found a wound an inch (2·5cm) long in the left ventricle. The lung, swelling up into his incision with each breath, caused considerable difficulty, but he managed to insert his stitches into the heart and to tie off one of the branches of a coronary artery that had been cut. During the operation an injection of saline solution was given hypodermically, which improved the patient's condition.

Alas! two-and-a-half days later the man died. Postmortem examination showed that the wound in the heart had begun to heal, but that death had been due to a large branch of a coronary artery having been damaged in the original stabbing. The surgeon whose magnificent effort merited success was Axel

Cappelen[24]. Nevertheless, he had lighted a beacon of hope.

In March of the next year, Guido Farina of Rome also had the misfortune to lose a patient whose wound he had sutured. The 30-year-old man was admitted to the Spedale della Consalazione where, after removing the fifth rib and costal cartilage, Farina found a wound 7mm long in the right ventricle; it had penetrated the wall to enter the cavity of the heart. Farina closed this wound with three main sutures and two of lesser importance.

All went well until the fifth day after operation when a right-sided bronchopneumonia developed which, three days later, killed the patient. Farina's bad luck was worse than Cappelen's, since the wound in the chest wall was healing well and at the postmortem he found the heart wound had healed perfectly.

The medical world was not to learn of these details for 12 or more years, although they knew of the bare facts from a three-line statement made at a congress in Rome later that year by one of Farina's friends, Dr Durante[25], and from Farina's own terse communication in which he explained his apparent reticence[26]. At the postmortem he had begged the judicial authorities to let him keep the heart for further study, but was refused. This so piqued him that 'I have not published any communication on this interesting case'.

Nevertheless, he relented after a fashion and later wrote to Sir John Bland-Sutton, the well-known London surgeon, describing the details. In 1908 Sir John quoted the letter in a lecture he gave on the treatment of injuries of the heart[27].

Even though the details were not published at the time, the tide was turning, and in September, 1896, success came to Ludwig Rehn of Frankfurt am Main[28,29]. His patient was a 22-year-old man who had been discharged from the army a short while previously with, of all things 'advanced heart disease'. In a drunken brawl he had received a wound 1·5cm long in the right ventricle. Bleeding and difficulty with breathing were severe, but Rehn managed to close the wound with three sutures; he then packed the pericardial cavity with iodoform gauze as a double precaution against infection and a renewal of haemorrhage. During his convalescence the patient suffered a setback when he developed pus in the pleural cavity, but in the end he made a complete recovery and was known to be living 10 years later.

This great achievement was not Ludwig Rehn's only claim to fame. In the previous year he had made a very astute observation connecting a high incidence of cancer of the urinary bladder among workers in the dye industry with their use of aniline. Except for the discovery by Percivall Pott in 1775[30] that cancer of the scrotum in chimney sweeps was due to the irritating effect of soot, this was the first time that anyone had shown that cancer could have an occupational origin.

We might think that, with Rehn's triumph, resistance to the surgical treatment of heart wounds would have finally been overcome. True, he had crossed the barrier, and as time went by the operation was attempted more and more frequently and with a gradually increasing rate of success. It was like the first four-minute mile – once it had been achieved, everyone seemed to be doing it. By 1909 an American had been able to collect, from the literature, reports of 159 cases although about 60 percent of the patients had died, mostly from supervening infection[31]. But in the very year of victory, an influential book was published which contained the following oft-quoted passage:

'Surgery of the heart has probably reached the limits set by Nature to all surgery: no new method, and no new discovery, can overcome the natural difficulties that attend a wound of the heart. It is true that "heart suture" has been vaguely proposed as a possible procedure, and has been done on animals; but I cannot find that it has ever been attempted in practice.'

The author was Stephen Paget, a man prominent in British surgical circles of the time, and his book was called *The surgery of the chest*[32]. Although published in 1896 it had taken some time to write; yet when Paget heard of Cappelen's operation, he did not think it worth while going back and amending the quoted paragraph, he simply commented on a later page, 'I think .... that suture of a wound is at least not impossible.'

His attitude is rather surprising, since he cited a case which showed in a striking fashion that the heart could be manhandled and the surgeon get away with it. The surgeon was Stelzner, a German, who in 1887[33] reported his operation on a 24-year-old man who had tried to commit suicide by stabbing himself in the heart with a needle. After opening the chest, Stelzner first plugged a wound in the pleura with gauze, but as the patient struggled for breath, the gauze vanished into the pleural cavity and could not be found. He then incised the pericardium, and, taking hold of the heart at its apex between his thumb and forefinger, he tried to push out the needle, lodged in the wall of the right ventricle, from behind. The eye of the needle appeared and was steadied with a fingernail, but before it could be grasped it slipped in again. Stelzner decided he had had enough and closed the chest; the patient recovered and with perfect health.

How then did Paget view the problem of wounds of the heart? 'Happily,' he wrote, 'these cases are rare; a needle wound is likely to do well after operation; a knife wound or bullet would give little room for hope, but if it be not at once fatal, the surgeon may be able even here to avert death.' And the way in which the surgeon could do this was to prescribe absolute and perfect rest of body and mind, a light diet, and in some cases morphine. Paget advised venesection (bloodletting) when the patient was restless, excited, or 'heavily oppressed' and the external haemorrhage not profuse. And he concluded that the pericardium might be tapped or a small incision made in it, if the heart was compressed.

On this last point credit must be given where credit is due, because incision of the pericardium with stitching of the heart wound only when necessary became accepted practice at the end of the Second World War. Paget was undoubtedly right for some wounds, yet if his advice were to be followed slavishly many lives would be lost unnecessarily. Without the benefit of blood transfusions, intravenous fluid replacement, and all the other paraphernalia of modern surgery, the best chance of success lay in suturing heart wounds.

The tenor of Paget's book provides a clue to his attitude – and his attitude was that of the establishment. Specialization within surgery had not yet arrived; in fact, its desirability was hotly debated and there were many people at the top of the profession who considered – with Paget – that surgery had reached the limits imposed by the human body. They were thus 'general' surgeons approaching specialist problems by recourse to the principles of 'general' surgery. They failed to realize that new principles were needed. Paget's own statement after reviewing the chief landmarks in the history of heart surgery, 'tradition and imagination stood in the way of it for centuries: . . . . we shall see again the same conflict between authority and clinical facts', might well apply to his own views.

Of chest surgery as a whole, he wrote, 'It is sometimes said that surgeons fifty years hence will think as little of our results as we think of the methods of fifty years ago. So far as regards the surgery of the chest, this is utterly untrue. Fifty years ago it had risen above the horizon, it is now nearly at its zenith. Indeed it is possible that we may see its upward movement checked.'

Paget saw no future in Bülau's method of subaqueous drainage and believed Tuffier's successful resection of a lung apex in 1891[34] to have been a freak. By recording, yet ignoring the significance of the advances that had already been made, Paget implied that his book represented the ultimate pinnacle of thoracic surgery. However, there were other men who saw clearly the possibilities of cardiac surgery and were already laying the foundations.

One of these was the Frenchman, Théodore Tuffier, a truly great surgeon. Born at Belleme in 1857, he qualified in Paris in 1885, and later became professor of surgery there and of experimental surgery at the Sorbonne. Although his interests were wide – he wrote a book on the experimental surgery of the kidney in 1889[35] – his first love was thoracic surgery and, appreciating the need for good operating conditions in this branch of surgery, he also carried out research into anaesthetic techniques. During the First World War he played an active part as a surgeon at the battlefront, being eventually made Inspector General of the army surgical services. He was the first person to evacuate casualties by air.

Back in 1895, a discovery had been made which had far-reaching effects in medicine and surgery, opening up an entirely fresh field of diagnosis and study of disease, and leading to a new form of treatment. The discovery was of x-rays and the man who made it Wilhelm Conrad Röntgen, the professor of physics at the University of Würtzburg[36]. The speed with which x-rays found a place in surgery was quite amazing and it was not long before radio-opaque foreign bodies such as bullets were being located with their help[37]. The first time they were used for a bullet in the heart was in 1903. An under-officer of the spahis was wounded by an Arab on March 15 of that year, and as he failed to make progress he was brought to Paris where Tuffier x-rayed him. The bullet appeared to lie in the left atrium and to move with the atrium during the heart-beat. On October 10, Tuffier operated; he went in under the first rib, removing a part of the second to improve the access. There was some doubt as to the exact position of the bullet, but it seemed to be inside the pericardial cavity and bound to the atrium by adhesions. These were freed with difficulty and the bullet was removed. Tuffier drained the wound and the under-officer went on to make a good recovery[38].

So, by the dawn years of the 20th century the heart had given itself into the hands of the surgeon, but only for the treatment of wounds which man himself had caused. After holding sway for more than 2000 years, one of Hippocrates's aphorisms was proved untrue. In Paget's words, chest surgery had risen above the horizon, but he too was wrong; it was in no way near its zenith. In truth, its day was still scarcely born.

4

THE PERICARDIUM

Man learned about wounds and developed ways of treating them before he learned about diseases, so it was reasonable for the heart to show itself amenable to surgery through operations for wounds. But today the treatment of wounds is only a small part of the cardiac surgeon's work; in fact the wheel has turned full circle and in an emergency any surgeon should be able to cope adequately, referring the patient to a specialist later for definitive treatment. This is not as strange as it may seem. The cases we discussed in the last chapter were dealt with by surgeons who had already made up their minds to operate should the occasion arise. There were many other stabbed patients who were not operated on. Today the principles of chest surgery have been incorporated into general surgery, thus accounting for the changed situation.

Diseases of the heart were quite another matter. Surgeons had to convince the physicians that so-called medical conditions could be helped by the knife, and this was far from easy. Long before the heart was seriously considered as a 'surgical' organ, a dent was made in the physicians' attitude by an attack on the pericardium, the membranous sac enclosing the heart. When fluid collected in this sac and thus had a deleterious physical effect on the heart's action, it was reasonable to expect that physical – that is, surgical – methods should be proposed to relieve the condition, even though this would not necessarily affect the underlying reason for the presence of the fluid. Even so, only one or two adventurous souls attempted to do anything about it before the second half of the 19th century.

Pericarditis, or inflammation of the pericardium, may be acute or chronic,

27

and dry (which need not concern us any more), wet, or fibroid (to which we shall return later). In wet pericarditis the fluid that collects may be clear (serous), pus-laden (suppurative) or bloody (haemorrhagic). There are many causes, some of which are rare and some only a relatively unimportant manifestation of other serious diseases. For our purposes serous pericarditis is usually due to tuberculosis or to a cause which cannot be discovered (so-called acute benign pericarditis or idiopathic pericarditis); suppurative pericarditis is usually due to infection with one of the common pus-forming organisms (such as the staphylococcus), and the heart is virtually surrounded by an abscess; and haemorrhagic pericarditis is usually due to injury, tuberculosis, or malignant disease.

Before getting down to business the problem of operating for pericardial effusion was discussed, and the first man to voice an opinion was Jean Riolan, the ardent Galenistical professor of anatomy in Paris, who objected to Harvey's theory of the circulation. In 1649 he asked the rhetorical question:

'When copious humour [fluid] collects and the heart is embarrassed, if hydrogues [medicines given to get rid of the fluid] have no effect, is it not lawful to open the sternum with a trephine at a thumb's interval above the xiphoid cartilage?'[1] His idea was then to tap the fluid with a trocar and cannula.

There is no record to say whether or not he attempted to find the answer.

The next person to offer advice was Jean Baptiste de Senac, who again had no takers. de Senac, physician to Louis XV of France, in 1749 wrote a most important treatise on diseases of the heart[2], in which he noted the frequent association of pericarditis and pleurisy. Discussing the treatment of pericarditis, he referred to Riolan's idea, but got it wrong because he misinterpreted the instructions. Instead of a thumb's breadth up the breastbone from the small cartilage at its bottom end, he thought Riolan had advised a thumb's breadth to the *side* of the bone. This would have endangered the internal mammary artery on that side (one of these pair of arteries runs down inside the chest wall on each side of the sternum). To avoid this and also the heart beating on to the point of the instrument, he recommended plunging a trocar into the space between the third and fourth ribs, two thumbs' breadth from the sternum on the left side and that it should be pointed toward the xiphoid cartilage along the rib space. He believed the disturbing effect of the fluid on the heart's action was a greater danger than any risk of haemorrhage from this form of treatment, but as he himself admitted, he had no cases to guide him.

In another part of his book he described for the first time a case of patent interventricular septum – a hole in the heart of congenital origin between the two ventricles – and quite correctly attributed the blueness of the skin to the unnatural mixing of venous and arterial blood.

The first practical attempts to deal with pericardial effusion were made by a Spaniard, Francisco Romero of Barcelona[3]. Remembering de Senac's observation about the commonness with which a pericardial effusion is accompanied by a pleural effusion – though the converse does not apply – and being very well aware of the difficulty of making an accurate diagnosis, he craftily designed a technique which would meet either contingency.

Romero placed his incision in the space between the fifth and sixth ribs, and then probed the outside of the pericardium with a blunt probe. If he found a pericardial effusion, he picked up the sac with forceps and opened it with curved scissors. After fluid had gushed out, he inserted a gauze drain for three days to draw off the remaining fluid and any that had collected in the meantime; the wound was then allowed to close naturally. A point on which Romero laid great stress was that no air should be allowed to enter, though how he achieved this he did not make clear. Two of the first three patients on whom he operated recovered, which was no mean achievement for those days.

At about the same time, in the second decade of the 19th century, a Scandinavian named Michael Skielderup read a paper to his medical society[4] describing his technique which was basically the same as Riolan had proposed the best part of 200 years earlier. He drained the effusion through a trephine hole made in the breastbone on a level with the fifth rib cartilage. By adopting this route, he said, he avoided the possible dangers of damage to the pleura, lung, or internal mammary artery should a lateral incision be used. The pain of boring through the sternum without an anaesthetic must have been excruciating, and it is small wonder the method was abandoned.

So far we have largely been dealing with men who had an idea which was sometimes put into practice, recorded in a publication, and then more or less forgotten about. The surgeon who pursued a practical approach throughout his career whenever the need arose was Baron Dominique Jean Larrey, Surgeon-in-Chief to Napoleon's Imperial Guard[5] and, on two occasions, Surgeon-in-Chief to the *Grande Armée*: on the Russian Campaign of 1812-13 and from half-way through the Waterloo Campaign.

Perhaps his greatest claim to fame was his invention of the flying ambulance – light, two-wheeled vehicles designed for the rescue of wounded soldiers on the field of battle[6]. Yet this was only the first aspect of his unending struggle to care for the wounded, since he developed a complete system of casualty evacuation back to a base hospital which survives, in principle, to our own day. When operating, often on the battlefield, he would treat the casualties in order of need, regardless of rank or allegiance, a practice not always appreciated by the French officers[7]. At the battle of Borodino, in 1812, he performed 200 amputations in 24 hours, a feat impossible today and not least because of a revolution in methods of treatment[8].

In 1810, during a two-year lull between campaigns, Larrey had operated on a case of suppurative pericarditis for the first time[9]. On March 18 of that year, Bernard Saint-Ogne, a 30-year-old foot soldier, stabbed himself in the left breast after being accused of a crime he did not commit. A lobe of the lung was injured and Larrey treated his patient with embrocations of camphorated oil. On the seventh day the pain increased, so, in keeping with current methods, the chest was scarified as a form of counterirritation. (This amounts to taking the patent's mind off the pain by giving him something else to think about.) By the ninth day the pain was becoming severe so vesicants (blister-producing agents) were applied – another type of counterirritation. But Saint-Ogne's condition was rapidly deteriorating and his extremities had become oedematous (waterlogged).

Examination disclosed fluid in the pericardial cavity and, with virtually nothing to lose, Larrey decided to operate. He went in between the fifth and sixth ribs on the left; when he opened the pericardium a yellow serous fluid shot out in jets with each heart-beat – in all, about two-and-a-half to three pounds of the fluid was collected. And, as Larrey said, the patient was in terrible agony. Nevertheless, he improved, as his heart was freed of the constricting influence of the fluid; but alas! the wound became infected and 10 days later signs of cardiac compression again appeared. Nothing daunted, Larrey operated for the second time, using a bistoury, a special form of scalpel, and released three to four ounces of sero-purulent matter. Saint-Ogne improved once more, and was doing well until Larrey's instructions regarding diet were disobeyed. Vomiting and 'dysenteric flux' were the penalty, and Saint-Ogne died just over two months after his suicide attempt.

In the second volume of his five-volume account of his surgical experiences in military camps and hospitals which Larrey wrote between 1829 and 1836, he mentioned six other cases of wounds of the heart and pericardium[10]. One of these was a 24-year-old soldier wounded in the chest in February, 1824. Before operating, Larrey carried out a number of experiments on cadavers to see whether, from the story the soldier gave him, it was possible for the pericardium to have been wounded. He concluded that it was.

The first stage of the operation was débridement of the wound, a technique which is now standard practice, but was not always so. The essence of the procedure is the surgical removal of all foreign material and all dead and dying tissue with, where appropriate, incision of the deep layers of fascia to prevent tension (the original and strict meaning of the word) and to allow drainage to take place freely. Its importance had originally been appreciated by Leonardo Botallo[11], an Italian who became physician to King Charles IX of France in the 16th century, but had been ignored until Desault[12], Larrey's teacher, reintroduced it at the end of the 18th century. Larrey applied the lesson to great effect during the Napoleonic wars, but débridement lapsed once more into obscurity until the late 1890s.

After Larrey had débrided the soldier's wound, he inserted a gum-elastic catheter into the pericardial cavity to drain off the blood-stained fluid.

Everything went well, and the man recovered.

The Larreys of this world are few and far between, and it was not until the second half of the century that, despite other occasional successes, treatment of pericardial effusions by surgical means came to be accepted.

However, one of these other successes concerned a 25-year-old German postman, Mathias Huser. On his rounds in October, 1843, he felt hot· and jumped in a river to cool off. Not surprisingly, he caught a chill and developed a pericardial effusion. In the March of the following year the effusion became purulent. All manner of medical measures were tried, but Mathias was going steadily downhill. Then at the beginning of July, Friedrich Joseph Hilsmann was called in. On the 20th, in the patient's own home, he operated. He used a bistoury to make the incision between the fourth and fifth ribs on the left side, and then an instrument known as a Richter's fistula knife to incise the pericardium. Pus shot out in squirts, so Hilsmann enlarged the opening to one inch (2.5cm) in length and managed to collect four 'water-glasses' full of pus. Immediately Mathias said he felt much easier. A long metal drain was inserted, the wound closed with stitches, and the dressings bound tight. Thereafter there was hourly improvement and eventually seven more glasses were filled with fluid. By the end of September, Mathias was completely recovered and back at work.

The medical world did not learn of this operation until 1875 when the surgeon's son, Friedrich Alexander Hilsmann, with understandable pride, used it as the basis for his inaugural thesis at the University of Kiel[13].

Two other successful operations for suppurative pericarditis were both performed by Bernhard von Langenbeck, the professor of surgery at Berlin[14]. (Note the date of publication – 1888.) The first, in 1850, was the result of a duel in which a bullet had smashed five of the man's ribs. Langenbeck incised the pericardium with a scalpel and healing was uneventful. In the second case, Langenbeck used a trocar and cannula to drain off the purulent fluid. He concluded that incision of the pericardium was simple and not dangerous.

This was the opinion with which Billroth disagreed and led to his remark about the operation being a prostitution of the art of surgery. But it should be remembered that Billroth was writing in a textbook of general surgery and his views reflected those held in Germany at the time, although in France and Russia many lives had been saved by incising the pericardium. What does seem strange is that the Germans should have felt as they did about the operation, because von Langenbeck was a most influential surgeon and had personally trained most of the best surgeons at that time. He was the founder of the German Society of Surgery and of a well-known German surgical journal, *Archiv für Klinische Chirurgie*. Perhaps his fellow countrymen were in awe of the man and believed they could not approach his extraordinary skill as an operator.

When we enter the second half of the 19th century, we find the difficulties of diagnosing pericardial disease – known to Romero – causing very great confusion. There was first of all the problem of deciding whether there was fluid in the pericardial cavity at all, and having made the decision, whether it was serous or purulent. When the pericarditis was of the fibroid variety, constricting the heart's action, the difficulties were compounded by an inability to sort out the symptoms due to the constriction and those due to the underlying disease. All this confusion seriously retarded progress in finding suitable treatments. The only satisfactory way to deal with the situation is to take the different forms of pericarditis separately – a solution only possible with the benefit of hindsight.

Owing largely to the work of Siegmund Rosenstein of Leiden, John Roberts of Philadelphia, Samuel West in England, and Edmond Delorme in France, surgeons came to realize that adequate incision was the treatment of choice for suppurative pericarditis. But it was a uphill struggle because Georges Dieulafoy of Toulouse, the doyen of the 'aspirationists', brought all his considerable influence to bear in favour of sucking the purulent fluid out through a needle. (We will consider his arguments later when we come to discuss serous pericarditis; suffice it to say at the moment that he seemed unaware of the difficulty, indeed often the impossibility, of sucking thick pus out through a narrow-bore needle.)

Rosenstein's case was a really important advance[15]. A 10-year-old boy was admitted to hospital on January 16, 1879, and purulent pericarditis was diagnosed. After twice puncturing the pericardium, Rosenstein realized the utter uselessness of the technique; there could be no hope unless he laid open the pericardial sac and drained it properly. This he did on the night of January 29-30, releasing a considerable quantity of pus. The boy then went on to make a satisfactory recovery.

The second nail in the coffin of aspiration was hammered home by Samuel West, who 'freely laid open' the pericardium of a boy of 17. When West read his paper to the Pathological Society in London in 1883[16], he reported that the youth had made a complete recovery in five weeks.

On the other side of the Atlantic, John Roberts, writing in 1881[17], said that he had been advocating incision and drainage since 1876, despite the opposition he had encountered. The surgeon should not, he emphasized, wait until the last moment to operate, but should do so promptly when signs of embarrassment of the heart were evident.

Some of these surgeons were not quite as explicit as they might have been in their writings. For instance, although Samuel West talked of freely laying open the pericardium, in the title of his paper he used the word 'tapping', which would imply aspiration. Perhaps he was worried about the reception the revolutionary technique would receive and so played down the impact in the belief that it would thus not seem so vastly different to the general practice.

More attention was, however, paid to serous than to suppurative pericardial effusion, and in the second half of the 19th century arguments raged over the relative merits of aspiration and incision, with Georges Dieulafoy in the van of the aspirationists.

Dieulafoy was great character with a tremendous personality; into the bargain he was handsome and debonair, with the ability to present a case to his colleagues in such a way as to excite their unstinted admiration. But he was always kind and considerate to his patients, putting their own interests and comfort before all else. Perhaps for this reason he never worried overmuch about scientific speculation; the human approach was what mattered most to him. He was a natural speaker and actor who put over his beliefs with fire and intensity, so it is scarcely surprising that his championing of aspiration – for pleural effusions as well as pericardial – influenced many who might otherwise have had doubts about its general applicability.

In his aspiration technique he used a needle, 0·5-1mm in diameter, connected by tubing to a glass aspirator (a bottle) in which a vacuum was created. For pericardial effusions the needle was inserted in the space between the fourth and fifth ribs on the left side, 5 or 6cm beyond the edge of the breastbone. He preferred this method to the use of a trocar and cannula, which, he said, was 'full of uncertainty and danger', and to incision with a bistoury which was 'a difficult and little-practised operation'[18].

It is fairly evident that he had made his mind up at an early stage about the merits of aspiration. In a communication on November 2, 1869, he first proposed applying the technique, which he had been using successfully in other areas, to the pericardium, and on April 7, 1870, it was put into practice by M. Ponroy on 21-year-old James R after other treatment had failed.

Slowly, however, the dangers and inadequacies of aspiration in other hands were realized, although our old friend Stephen Paget was still recommending it in 1896. In the previous year the Parisians, Edmond Delorme and Mignon[19], introduced the procedure, named after them, in which a vertical pericardotomy (incision in the pericardial sac) was performed after removing the fifth and sixth rib cartilages on the left side. This operation gave complete evacuation of the fluid and held the field for many years. In 1920, the British surgeon, Sir Charles Ballance, said that aspiration should be banished from surgery as it was neither simple nor safe[20].

But times changed, methods of diagnosis improved, techniques advanced, and antibiotics were discovered. It is now quite legitimate to aspirate some of the fluid for diagnostic purposes, and to continue aspirating as part of the treatment to remove all the fluid. Surgical incision is, however, still necessary when aspiration fails. Nevertheless, aspiration remains a dangerous undertaking unless carefully performed; the needle may well tear a coronary artery or the muscle of the heart. Sometimes, even, the heart may stop beating.

What all this really amounts to is that when one is in full possession of the facts and knows precisely what is going on, it is possible to succeed with manoeuvres that in earlier times would have been extremely dangerous.

And now we come to fibroid pericarditis. If serous and purulent pericarditis caused confusion, it was as nothing to that surrounding the group of conditions comprising fibroid percarditis.

Basically there are two main conditions with which we are concerned: constrictive pericarditis and pericardial adhesions. Constrictive pericarditis is a chronic condition usually due to tuberculosis; the pericardial membrane becomes thicker and thicker until the heart is eventually encased in a rigid bag and cannot relax properly to fill with blood. The heart therefore fails in its function. In pericardial adhesions, which are rare, the outer layer of the pericardium becomes stuck to surrounding structures; the precise effect of this on the heart is uncertain. Adhesions of one layer of the pericardium to the other within the pericardial cavity are of no importance in themselves, but at the end of the 19th century they were believed to be so. Heart disease was then improperly understood and the adhesions were blamed for symptoms which were, in fact, due to underlying conditions, such as disease of the heart muscle or pericardial fibrosis and thickening. The true state of affairs did not emerge until the 1930s. The results of the early operations were adversely affected by a failure to appreciate the real pathology and what the surgeon was really trying to achieve with the operation. Once again, to make the story comprehensible, we must make use of modern knowledge to unravel the tangled mess of those days.

The first suggestions that these forms of pericardial disease might be treated surgically came from France, when Edmond Weill[21] and Edmond Delorme[22] independently in 1895 proposed the removal of the thickened pericardium in constrictive pericarditis. Weill believed that there were occasions when it would be perfectly legitimate to try to liberate at least a part of the heart, such as the more readily accessible apex and anterior aspect. When, however, the disease was obviously due to tuberculosis, he thought it might be preferable just to incise the pericardium and so weaken the virulence of the tubercle bacillus by exposure to air. (This was indeed the belief in those days, and incision of the peritoneum was practised when the abdominal cavity filled with fluid due to tuberculous infection.)

Weill went on to admit that medical measures were no good for constrictive pericarditis unless they were treating the cause. He concluded: 'The day will come when we will depend on surgery to deliver the heart from the shell which strangles it.'

Delorme took a more active interest in the problem, although even he did not attempt the operation, known as decortication, on a live patient. He did, however, take an important step forward by showing that it was technically feasible on cadavers, provided the disease was not of long-standing. His recommendation was for early operation, and preferably in young people. He also said that the surgeon should free any adhesions he might find between the pericardium and the ribs or sternum; in other words, those he could reach easily.

Nevertheless, decortication seemed to be a formidable undertaking, and it was not until some years later that anyone put the idea into practice; and then it was for adhesive, not constrictive pericarditis, thus giving further demonstration of the confusion in surgeons' minds about the whole subject.

The operation took place at the Necker Hospital in Paris in August, 1910. A 16-year-old boy had been admitted with adhesive pericarditis and dilatation of his heart. The physicians on the staff had tried the effect of puncturing the pericardium, without success. So Paul Hallopeau[23] was asked to do a pericardotomy. He agreed, but once inside he decided to go further and remove the adherent pericardium from the front of the heart; and this he did, using only local anaesthesia. No one, apparently, believed the operation would be of any use at all; so it was a great surprise when the boy improved rapidly and was discharged from hospital, fit and well, three weeks later. Yet, despite this success, the operation did not catch on immediately, and it was the later work of Ludwig Rehn[24] and Ferdinand Sauerbruch[25] that drew attention to its value and was instrumental in getting it accepted.

The attack on adhesions began in 1902 when Ludolph Brauer, a Heidelberg physician, proposed an operation for chronic adhesive mediastino-pericarditis (which is just another way of saying that the pericardium is stuck to its surrounding structures); the name he coined for the technique was cardiolysis[26,27].

'When the pericardium is adherent,' he said, 'to the heart itself and to the rigid chest wall in front of it, removal of part of the chest wall will ease the intolerable burden the heart has to bear.'

Brauer was fortunate in having two co-operative surgical colleagues, and on April 1, 1902, Professor Petersen performed the first cardiolysis. He removed 7, 8 and 9cm, respectively, of the third, fourth and fifth ribs. On May 13, Otto Simon carried out a second cardiolysis; his resection was more extensive and included part of the sternum. He was also responsible for the third of these operations.

In successful cases there was a rapid reduction in the size of the heart, because it was able to pull against a yielding chest wall rather than the normal rigid one. But some of the early failures were due to inaccurate diagnosis of what was in fact constrictive pericarditis. In these cases cardiolysis could be of no help. Even so, the value of the operation is still in doubt today.

Although a physician, Brauer[28] made a significant contribution to chest surgery when he drew attention to the importance of leaving the periosteum (the membrane surrounding a bone) of the ribs intact during the operation of thoracostomy. At that time, thoracostomy, or removal of a number of ribs, was becoming a popular treatment for tuberculosis of the lungs. It allowed the chest wall to fall in over the diseased lung, thus resting it and giving it a fair chance to heal. By leaving the periosteum intact, the bone could regenerate and so preserve the stability of the chest wall.

Those who like their stories in watertight compartments would be advised to stop reading this chapter here, before two unpluggable leaks are mentioned. They can rest assured they will miss nothing, as the two episodes were of no lasting importance and are only mentioned to show yet again how perplexing was the whole situation.

Another physician, William Mackenzie, an Australian, was apparently unaware of Brauer's work, since in 1906 he recommended a similar operation. His paper[29] shows with a vengeance the strange reasoning and incorrect views of the time. He attributed adhesions of the pericardium to the anterior chest wall quite correctly to rheumatic disease, but went on to emphasize the constrictive effect of the same disease. We now know that rheumatic fever never causes constrictive pericarditis. Where he probably went astray was in confusing the late effects of rheumatic involvement (calcified, 'stony' plaques) with the tough fibrous, unyielding shell probably due to tuberculosis. Thus, on the evidence available, it would seem that in attempting to treat one disease, he was in fact advising the same operation for two different conditions; in one of these (the constrictive form) failure was inevitable. The net result, therefore, was Brauer's operation, independently discovered.

The resection Mackenzie advised, included as much as possible of the third, fourth and fifth rib cartilages on the left side, and even part of the sternum and sixth cartilage. Mackenzie's aims were to allow free cardiac action by enlarging the space available to the heart within the chest, and to remove the rigid chest wall to which the adhesions were attached.

Mackenzie said that the operation had first been performed about two years before his report, but the case was unsuitable since the heart had begun to fail some time previously – and the object of the exercise was to postpone failure! He also advocated a partial resection as a diagnostic measure, which at any rate was thinking directed along the right lines.

The aggressive attitude of physicians toward heart disease at this time was also shown by Alexander Morison of London, who suggested operating to relieve the cardiac pain associated with an enlarged heart in a 19-year-old youth with disease of the aortic valve[30].

'I therefore determined,' he wrote, 'to afford the enlarged heart more room to act in, while its power was still good, and asked Mr Stabb to secure free space for cardiac systole without the incarcerating barrier of hard rib, in the area of thoracic concussion.'

Ewen Stabb did just this on May 1, 1908, and the patient was pleased with the result.

The performance of this operation was the same as that of cardiolysis, but the underlying principles were utterly different. Nevertheless, as may well be imagined, the similarity led to terrible confusion – which is why the operation is mentioned here. The outcome was that the principles of Morison's operation were not generally accepted.

The present situation in the surgery of pericardial disease has been reached through a clearer understanding of the underlying causes and a greater ability to diagnose them accurately. The underlying disease must always be treated by medical on other appropriate measures, but when surgery becomes necessary a simplified scheme would be as follows:

Serous, suppurative and haemorhagic pericarditis call for aspiration in the first instance (this would have pleased Georges Dieulafoy). If this fails, surgical incision and free drainage are used. Constrictive pericarditis is treated by releasing the heart from its strangling shell. But the merits of treating adhesions of the pericardium to surrounding structures by cardiolysis remain unsettled

So, perhaps, with a sigh of relief, we can leave the historically disturbed waters of pericardial disease and turn our attentions to cardiac arrest. At least when the heart stops, treatment has only one clear-cut objective.

5

CARDIAC ARREST

A beating heart is indeed essential to life, but this does not mean that death and a stopped heart are synonymous. Most people in the civilized world today know that it is possible to start an arrested heart beating again. This of course raises the question, what is death? No one knows, and it is not really satisfactory to define it as the end of life. For what is life?

All that can be done is to recognize death when it occurs, and even that is not always easy. It is no longer the state which for centuries has been recognized as death – the death of the body with cessation of the vital functions of heartbeat and respiration. It must now be considered as death of the cells and the cessation of biochemical and enzymatic functions. Put simply, we can look on the heart as a pump and the lungs as bellows; provided both are still capable of performing their mechanical tasks, there is often a good chance that they can be helped to carry on working where they left off – provided again that the rest of the body is still alive.

Two points need to be appreciated here. First, the heart and the lungs in this context are a physiological unit. It is no good making the heart beat if the blood it is pumping is not oxygenated by the lungs. Second, action to restore the heart-beat must start quickly. Generally speaking, the brain cells die if deprived of oxygen for more than three or four minutes, although there are records of cases where the patient survived, apparently unharmed, after 10 or even 20 minutes of cardiac arrest.

How then does the doctor recognize death? Largely by commonsense, experience, and knowledge of the circumstances. The technique, beloved by novelists, of holding a mirror in front of the mouth and nose and watching for it to mist over is a non-starter. The pulse may be too faint to be felt and the doctor may hear no sound when he listens for several minutes with his stethoscope over the heart; in cases of extreme cooling – from exposure or in old people in winter, for example, or in cases of deep coma from drug overdose or hypersensitivity – the heart may still be weakly beating, though too faintly to be heard. The pupils may fail to react to light from causes other than death. Conversely, reflexes may still be present for an hour or so after death, particularly if the death is sudden. The only sure findings in the uncommon cases where there is real doubt are silent electrocardiograms and electroencephalograms. But these techniques for recording the electrical activity of the heart and brain are practical only in hospital. The doctor faced with a drowned person or the surgeon with a patient whose heart stops on the operating table does not call for an electroencephalogram to be taken before he does anything. He acts, and acts quickly, and only stops when common-sense and experience tell him that life is extinct.

Death is the one sure fact of life, and in death the heart is still. But doctors do not try to resuscitate every person who dies. Put simply again, resuscitation is attempted when the heart stops in a body that has no reason to die. Patients, apparently dead with a stopped heart from a heart attack, can now often be revived to live a useful life, if action is taken quickly enough – their pump stops from what might loosely be termed 'shock' but it is not so badly damaged that it cannot be made to start again.

The heart may stop when the patient is on the operating table for a variety of reasons, connected both with the surgery and the anaesthesia. Stimulation of the vagus nerve, for instance, by pressure on a certain area in the neck, and some drugs can stop the heart; so also can drowning, electric shock, and that complex clinical entity known as 'shock'. Very rarely emotional shock or some minor medical procedure (taking a blood sample, for instance) may be the cause of the heart standing still. In cases such as these there need be no other cause for the patient to die, and cardiac massage with artificial respiration may bring him back to life. Treatment for concomitant happenings such as haemorrhage or injuries in a 'shocked' patient is of course necessary, but the top priority is to get the pump and bellows working again.

Before the advent of anaesthetics, the treatment of an arrested heart was not even contemplated – the patient was dead, and that was that. The story of the introduction of anaesthesia is long, complicated, and bedevilled with arguments and litigation over priorities[1]. Suffice it to say that ether was accepted after an historic operation on October 16, 1846, at the Massachusetts General Hospital, Boston. The 'anaesthetist' was William Thomas Green Morton[2,3], a medical student and one-time dentist. The anaesthetic effect of chloroform, which is pertinent here, was discovered a little more than a year later by James Young Simpson, professor of obstetrics at Edinburgh University.

He first used the vapour early in November, 1847, for a woman in labour, and within the month had recorded 50 administrations in obstetrics and a variety of operations[4].

Chloroform soon became overwhelmingly the more popular anaesthetic in Great Britain and Europe, and only slightly less so in North America, a situation that persisted for nearly 40 years until the combined use of nitrous oxide (laughing gas) and ether, and the introduction of other agents displaced – but by no means entirely – the use of chloroform for most purposes.

But chloroform could stop the heart.

The first person to die was pretty 15-year-old Hannah Greener of Newcastle while having a toenail removed on January 28, 1848[5]. The case attracted a good deal of publicity, the more so because she had had a similar operation two weeks previously under ether; the coroner absolved the surgeon from blame and said that death was due to the chloroform. When Simpson heard of this, he leapt to the defence of his anaesthetic, denying that it could have been responsible[6].

Over the years more deaths were reported. Admittedly they also occurred when other anaesthetics were used, but much less frequently. It is difficult to give comparative figures, but the danger of chloroform was very soon realized, and the condition of 'chloroform syncope' became a popular subject of discussion in the medical journals.

How then can we account for the seemingly amazing preference for this agent over ether? On both sides of the Atlantic voices were raised in praise of ether. In 1850, WTG Morton took time off from his litigations over priority to write a book *On the physiological effects of sulphuric ether, and its superiority to chloroform*[7]. Although obviously biased, he made some well-balanced remarks. He realized that it was dangerous to use chloroform if the patient was weak from any cause, if the heart was unsound, or if the patient was old or frightened.

'There is no reason for diminution of confidence in the efficacy or perfect safety of sulphuric ether;' he wrote, 'while there is an unanswerable reason why chloroform should be abandoned.' Because of the risk of heart failure he considered it unjustifiable to use chloroform simply because it was more agreeable, more powerful, and cheaper.

In England, John Snow, one of the attendants on Queen Victoria during the birth of Prince Leopold in 1853, and the man who did more research than anyone else in those early days into the use of anaesthetic drugs, preferred ether. In *On chloroform and other anaesthetics: Their action and administration*[8], the book he left unfinished at his early death in 1858, he wrote:

'I believe that ether is altogether incapable of causing the sudden death by paralysis of the heart, which has caused the accidents which have happened during the administration of chloroform.' Yet in the last 11 years of his life he had given chloroform nearly 4000 times, and ether only 12. His personal choice was overruled by the wishes of the surgeons.

So, it seems, the dice were loaded in favour of chloroform mainly for reasons of convenience. It worked more quickly than ether and was more pleasant; it was less irritating to the air passages yet more powerful; it was non-inflammable and was considerably easier to administer. A towel, a handkerchief, a sponge, or even a nightcap was all the apparatus required, whereas ether called for inhalers and vapourizers.

Opinion was divided over the cause of the deaths from chloroform syncope. Snow and others who approached the subject scientifically maintained that death was due to heart failure brought on by too high a concentration of the vapour. They accordingly designed apparatus that would deliver measurable quantities of the vapour, and advised keeping a finger on the patient's pulse during the administration.

Others, including Simpson and later Joseph Lister, believed that the trouble came only during light anaesthesia and that respiratory failure was the cause of death. They were quite happy with giving chloroform on a cloth, but advised the anaesthetist to watch the patient's breathing.

Both sides had got things the wrong way round, but it took many years and innumerable committees and commissions to arrive at the truth. In 1890 it was proved that killing dogs with chloroform (ie, using too high a concentration) did not harm their hearts, and that death was due to respiratory failure[9,10]. As this did not give a satisfactory answer to those who believed in the heart-failure theory, research continued, and only in 1911 did the solution come when AG Levy[11], in London, showed that cardiac failure could occur suddenly in cats under light chloroform anaesthesia, and was usually due to a form of arrest known as ventricular fibrillation.

When the heart stops, it may do so completely (cardiac asystole) or it may fibrillate. The two conditions cannot be differentiated clinically; an electrocardiogram (if immediately available or already in place) or opening the chest and the pericardium and looking at the heart are the only satisfactory methods, although a knowledge of the circumstances may give the surgeon a clue as to which has happened. Fibrillation means that the ventricles are faintly twitching, but are performing no useful work. The condition was first recognized by Vesalius in his animal experiments and he described the sensation he felt when holding the fibrillating heart as like a 'bag of worms'[12]. Fibrillation may take as long as 15 minutes to fade completely, but unless the heart is electrically defibrillated within a minute of the onset, massage is needed until the apparatus arrives.

This digression has been necessary because the story of reviving the arrested heart started with chloroform syncope and continued with it for many years. The accounts of the first successful cases of resuscitation leave little doubt that the hearts had stopped – that the patients were, in fact, 'dead' and not suffering from respiratory arrest with a still-beating heart. Yet success was due to artificial *respiration*, and mouth-to-mouth respiration into the bargain. (We will return to this form of resuscitation later.) When faced with chloroform syncope the usual course of action was to fling the windows wide open; splash cold water on the patient's face; waft ammonia under the nose; give brandy; shake, rub, and press on the chest – in those days the natural and obvious things to do.

Then, on July 3, 1849, Charles Bleeck of Warminster was removing a breast from a strong stout woman of 42 – it took him four minutes. The anaesthetic was chloroform. But just as the last incision was completed the patient fell, out of the grasp of the 'athletic' woman who was supporting her, 'apparently dead upon the floor'. Dr Bleeck could find no pulse anywhere, and could hear not the slightest sound of the heart's action or of respiration. Cold water, ammonia, and so on were tried, to no avail. So, remembering how he revived newborn babies, he applied his mouth to the patient's with a single fold of handkerchief intervening. On the fourth inspiration she gave a convulsive gasp and the doctor 'had the delightful relief to see her revive'. With incredible sangfroid he went on to remove a diseased lymph node from the woman's axilla, at which 'she cried out a little'[13].

That same year Philippe Ricord, in France, unaware of Bleeck's success, revived two patients who were 'in that state of syncope which is the herald of death'. His method was similar and, reporting the first case, he wrote: 'The patient was saved, and we escaped with the fright'[14].

On the other side of the Atlantic on October 5, 1850, John Metcalf read a paper to the New York Academy of Medicine in which he described how a patient's pulse disappeared and his breathing stopped during chloroform anaesthesia. 'I at once applied my lips to those of the patient, holding his mouth open with my right hand and closing his nose with the left, and inflated the lungs slowly and gently, so as to imitate as much as possible a natural inspiration.' After 15 to 20 of these inspirations the patient gave a feeble gasp and an artery in the surgical wound began to spurt blood[15].

This was the first occasion on which mouth-to-mouth respiration was given without trying the 'usual' methods first. Metcalf, quite naturally, recommended that artificial resuscitation should be started *immediately* chloroform syncope was diagnosed, but for some reason the idea never caught on.

The first two of these cases were reported in the *Lancet*, yet in the next volume of the same journal we find great sympathy expressed for Edward Cock of Guy's Hospital who lost a patient from chloroform syncope. He tried brandy, ether, ammonia, cold air, cold water, shaking, rubbing, electricity, and artificial respiration, for which purpose he opened the larynx and inserted a tube[16].

Cases were reported with monotonous regularity thereafter, and when artificial respiration was applied it was usually by Silvester's method (an arm-lift chest-pressure technique introduced in 1858[17]; the patient has to be on his back and the jaw and tongue often fall backwards, obstructing the airway), and then after the other contemporary methods had failed.

The writers frequently noted that the accidents happened very soon after the administration of chloroform was started, and the clue to their inaction seems to have been that the deaths were 'appallingly sudden', 'as if struck by lightning'. The wretched doctors had the wind taken right out of their sails and were thus more able to discuss the mechanism of death after they had regained their equilibrium, than to take effective action when it was needed.

The person who first performed cardiac massage, albeit experimentally, was Moritz Schiff of Frankfurt am Main. This was only one facet of the vast amount of original physiological research he carried out, paying great attention to detail[18]; but as he seemed to like argument for argument's sake, much of his far-sighted work tended to be overlooked. In the early 1870s, while professor of physiology at Florence, he was investigating deaths in dogs caused by chloroform and ether and made the point that respiratory failure due to ether could be overcome by artificial respiration. But with chloroform, heart failure was likely to occur first; on these dogs he found resuscitation to be ineffective unless the chest was opened and the heart massaged.

'One makes', he said, 'rhythmic movements with the hand holding the whole heart.' But what is even more surprising is the modernness of his explanation. Success, he maintained, was due to the massage filling the heart's own arteries and not to the mechanical stimulation – the pump needs its fuel. He also drew attention to the value of compressing the abdominal aorta during massage, so as to ensure that as much of the heart's output as possible went to the brain where the oxygenated blood was so badly needed[19].

In 1882, during his experiments on suturing experimental heart wounds in rabbits, Block found he could make a heart start contracting after it had stopped by gently squeezing it[20].

Whether Paul Niehaus of Berne knew of this experimental work or whether it was just the counsel of despair is unknown, but whichever it was, he was the first surgeon to attempt cardiac massage on a human patient. This he did in 1880, although the case was not reported until 1903 when his assistant, Denis Zesas, made the facts public[21]. Maybe Niehaus thought it discreet to keep quiet at the time, but by 1903 other attempts had been made and Zesas felt it safe to put his chief's effort on record:

During the induction of chloroform anaesthesia before an operation for goitre in a 40-year-old man, the patient's heart stopped. After the contemporary methods had failed, Niehaus resected the ribs, laid bare the heart, and began rhythmical compression; the anaesthetist continued with artificial respiration. But though the heart twitched, Niehaus was unable to make it contract normally. The postmortem, carried out by Theodor Langhans, one of the early workers on immunity, revealed a normal heart.

Considering the general attitude towards any surgery on the heart, or indeed inside the chest, it is hardly surprising that for some years no one else had the temerity to emulate Niehaus. Cardiac puncture, instead, occupied the minds of those few who bothered to think at all constructively. Although in more recent times various drugs, such as atropine or adrenaline (epinephrine), have been injected directly into the heart muscle or a ventricular cavity, either as the sole method or as an adjunct to massage, in the early days simple puncture was the technique toyed with. In 1887, BA Watson of New Jersey carried out experiments with dogs in which puncture or, even better, letting out a little blood through a hollow needle, was successful. He believed that puncture actually stimulated the heart and that withdrawal of blood gave the distended heart a better chance of contracting[22]. But this was in dogs, and Paget, in his book (1896)[23] said that no results of a similar kind had been achieved in human surgery. He remarked that when Georg Fischer of Breslau had tried it in a case of chloroform syncope, the postmortem had shown the pericardial cavity to be full of blood. Evidently the unfortunate surgeon must have had the bad luck to hit a coronary vessel. Nevertheless, Paget concluded that in cases of cardiac arrest one might as well have a shot at puncture as do nothing.

Two years after Ludwig Rehn's successful suture of a heart wound when the tide was turning, at least in the minds of certain adventurous souls, cardiac massage was again attempted, this time by someone who had experience of operating inside the chest – Théodore Tuffier. In 1898, a 24-year-old man died suddenly five days after drainage of an appendix abscess. By chance Tuffier was in the ward; quickly he crossed to the patient's bed and tried the 'usual' methods of resuscitation. As soon as he realized these were in vain he called for a knife and made an incision in the third space between the ribs on the left. Through this wound he pressed on the pericardium with his index finger and rhythmically compressed the ventricular region for one or two minutes. The man's pulse and respiration returned and he opened his eyes, but the pulse could not be sustained, and after more attempts at massage the heart stopped forever[24].

As it turned out, Tuffier could not have succeeded; postmortem examination disclosed that death had been caused by a clot in the pulmonary artery – a problem we shall be dealing with in the next chapter. During the discussion of Tuffier's paper, Pierre Bazy said that in 1892 he had seen a colleague do the same thing for chloroform syncope. But nothing more is known about it.

Inspired by Tuffier's boldness which, in a sense, was a pointer to success, a number of other Frenchmen enthusiastically followed in their master's footsteps, but were unrewarded for their efforts.

The first clinically successful cardiac massage was performed by Kristian

Igelsrud of Tromsö, Norway. The date is uncertain but was probably sometime in 1901. Igelsrud did not publish details of the case; they only became known because he wrote to an American, William Williams Keen, who published the letter in 1904[25]. The patient was a woman of 43 with carcinoma of the uterus, the operation total hysterectomy, and the anaesthetic chloroform. Almost at the end of the operation the woman collapsed. Artificial respiration and other manoeuvres were carried out for three or four minutes; then Igelsrud courageously decided to remove part of the third and fourth ribs. He opened the pericardium and seized the heart between his thumb and middle and index fingers. For about a minute he squeezed quite strongly and rhythmically, and the heart began to beat by itself. After a further minute's massage, because the beat started to weaken, the patient made a complete recovery.

A year later, in 1902, Sir William Arbuthnot Lane, famous in many spheres of surgery but particularly in orthopaedics and for his 'no-touch' technique, achieved another success. The patient was a man of 65 undergoing abdominal operation for adhesion about the colon. (Quite what was really going on inside him is uncertain because Lane had a bee in his bonnet about chronic intestinal stasis, and believed that short-circuiting the intestine was the answer to many of mankind's ills. This man's illness may have been appendicitis, because a terse note in the report[26], said: 'The appendix being found unhealthy was removed.') In this case the anaesthetic was ether. When the heart stopped beating, artificial respiration by compression of the chest had no effect, so Lane 'introduced his hand through the abdominal incision and felt the heart through the diaphragm; it was quite motionless; he gave it a squeeze or two and felt it re-start beating.' Artificial respiration was continued for 12 minutes and the man went on to an uneventful convalescence.

Cardiac massage had arrived, but by no means all the attempts in the next few years were successful, one reason being that the surgeons did not persist long enough. This is understandable in view of their lack of comprehension and experience of the situation, and the undeveloped state of anaesthesia. Another reason was the tendency to overlook the importance of treating the associated respiratory failure. It was George Crile, a great 'physiological' surgeon of Cleveland, who emphasized that respiration must be established as well, and he also stated that vasomotor activity (the tone of the smaller vessels in the peripheral circulation) must be restored. To this end he devised and used (he must have been about the only person to do so) a pneumatic rubber suit[27,28].

The commonly adopted technique for some years was to approach the heart from the abdomen or, in experimental animals, by rhythmically squeezing the chest[29] – not to be wondered at considering that the chest was still pretty fearsome territory and the surgeon had to open a pleural cavity to get adequate access. In these cases the heart was sometimes massaged through the intact diaphragm and sometimes through an incision in the diaphragm. But whichever route was adopted, the success rate was low, though it improved as the years went by. A review of the world literature in 1952 recorded 178 cases with 69 recoveries; this is not as dismal as may at first sight appear, because the form of arrest is about equally divided between cardiac asystole and ventricular fibrillation and massage alone can never be successful in fibrillation.

For a long time it was believed that cardiac massage was a technique only occasionally applicable, and then directly to the heart, usually when the patient was already on the operating table. No one really believed that pressure on the unopened chest over the heart could maintain an adequate circulation, despite the publication in 1883, in his surgical textbook, of six successful cases by Franz Koenig, a German surgeon[30]. Another German, Maass, modified Koenig's technique (which depended mainly on artificial respiration) and was able to report a success with rapid and powerful compressions over the area of the heart at a rate of 120 per minute. His patient was nine-and-a-half-year-old Heinrich A whose heart stopped on October 26, 1891, when his cleft palate was being repaired[31]. But these were isolated cases, and even the first of more modern days attracted little or no attention at the time and was not widely published until 14 years afterwards when experimental work and other clinical successes had established the technique.

A thick-set obese, French Canadian of 60 was in St Anne's Military Hospital, Montreal, with angina pectoris due to hardening of the coronary arteries. On November 27, 1947, he developed signs of impending coronary occlusion and the next day, after lunch, became greatly distressed; his condition deteriorated rapidly. As a priest finished the last rites the patient suddenly became limp, his head fell back on the pillows, and respiration ceased. To all appearances he was dead, an impression confirmed by examination.

As the body was being stripped of rings and dentures, a slight twitch was noticed in the muscles at the front of the neck. 'For some inexplicable reason', wrote Ralph McKendry[32], 'this prompted the application of firm pressure with both hands over the lower part of the sternum, causing considerable depression of the front of the thoracic cage. This manoeuvre was carried out not less than four minutes after the heart had stopped. On release of the pressure the patient took several jerky breaths.' Lighter rhythmic pressure was continued until the patient recovered. Three months after his admission to hospital he was allowed to go home.

The movement to start the heart beating again without opening the chest began in 1957 when two papers describing rather similar techniques were published in America and England. Hugh Stout of Oklahoma[33] became unhappy after doing postmortems on three adults who had not recovered after cardiac arrest and internal massage in the operating theatre. 'Obviously massage of the heart in adults should not include massage of sclerotic [hardened] coronary arteries and essentially all adults have this.' He went on to describe a case in which a man's heart stopped while he was aspirating bone marrow from the sternum. He tried artificial respiration but suddenly remembered seeing in 1938 August Krogh, of Copenhagen University, demonstrate that almost a gallon of blood would gravitate into the legs when the feet were lowered[34]. Why not use this blood to stretch the heart internally? 'I therefore put my right arm under the patient's knees and jack-knifed the patient, thrusting the knees up into the epigastrium and on to the lower chest, actually rocking the hips off the table with the buttocks higher than the heart.' After three or so jack-knives the patient gave a convulsive movement and sat up. Stout reckoned that the pumping action could be continued at a rate of 60 times a minute.

The English paper came from Ernest Rainer, an ear, nose and throat surgeon, who described a method he had developed and used successfully in children from eight weeks to 13 years old[35]. He put one arm behind the child's neck and the other under the knees. He then flexed the legs and buttocks on the chest which was thereby compressed – the same manoeuvre as Stout's but a different explanation for its merit. Three years later he reported its use on an adult woman whose heart stopped during anaesthesia for the setting of a broken nose; after resuscitation the operation was satisfactorily concluded[36]. Although Rainer only used the technique in the operating theatre, he believed it might have a wider application. But this was not to be; a more practical technique was already on the horizon.

The paper that really convinced the medical world of the value of external cardiac massage came from Johns Hopkins University School of Medicine in 1960. William Kouwenhoven had been professor of electrical engineering at the university and since 1930 had been interested in the effect of electricity on the heart, and in particular in resuscitating people who had been accidentally electrocuted and whose hearts had gone into ventricular fibrillation[37]. When he retired, his enthusiasm did not retire with him and he was granted his wish of working in the surgical laboratories.

One day he and his colleagues, James Jude and Guy Knickerbocker, noticed quite by accident that pressure on the two heavy defibrillating electrodes on a dog's chest caused the blood pressure (which they were monitoring) in the fibrillating heart to rise slightly. This chance observation made them think, and thinking led to action. By pressing regularly on the chest they found they could easily keep an adequate circulation going for as long as 30 minutes in the fibrillating dogs.

The next step was to adapt the method for human use. 'With the patient in a supine position,' they wrote, 'preferably on a rigid support, the heel of one hand with the other on top of it is placed on the sternum just cephalad to the xiphoid. Firm pressure is applied vertically downward about 60 times per minute. At the end of each pressure stroke the hands are lifted slightly to permit full expansion of the chest. The operator should be so positioned that he can use his body weight in applying the pressure. Sufficient pressure should be used to move the sternum 3 or 4cm towards the vertebral column.... If there are two or more persons present, one should massage the heart while the other gives mouth-to-nose respiration.'[38]

A year later they reviewed their experience with patients aged from two months to 80 years. Massage had lasted between a few minutes and an hour; 96 percent of arrests occurring in the operating theatre and recovery room, and 70 percent of those in patients who had undergone cardiac surgery were successful[39].

The first unequivocal demonstration that adequate arterial blood pressures were produced by closed-chest massage was given by Peter Nixon[40], then of Leeds. The patient was a 43-year-old woman with severe disease of her mitral valve. On July 14, 1961, she was undergoing catheterization of the left side of her heart, when her heart stopped beating. Nixon thumped the front of her chest over the heart but, as this had no effect, he massaged the heart in the manner described by Kouwenhoven. 'The chest wall was so flaccid that the heart could be felt filling and emptying under the hand.' Nixon continued massaging for 18 minutes by which time the heart was beating again. As an arterial needle was already in place accurate recording of the brachial artery pressures was possible, and this showed that pulse pressures of more than 100mm of mercury were easily obtained by massage at a rate of 80-90 strokes per minute.

Kouwenhoven had drawn attention to a second person performing mouth-to-nose respiration. This method had recently been brought in from the cold, although, as we have already seen, it had been responsible for the resuscitation of some of the first patients to 'die' from chloroform syncope. But its origins go back even further, for it is sometimes known as the Biblical method, on the rather dubious grounds that this was how Elisha brought the Shunammite's son back from the dead.

The story is told in II Kings, 4, verses 18-37. The boy was out in the fields with the reapers 'and he said unto his father, My head, my head. And he said to a lad, Carry him to his mother. And when he had taken him, and brought him to his mother, he sat on her knees till noon, and then he died.'

His mother thereupon saddled an ass and set out to fetch Elisha who was at Mount Carmel, some 15 to 20 miles (24-32km) away. But Elisha at first would not go, and sent his servant Gehazi with instructions to lay his (Elisha's) staff on the face of the child. Only when Gehazi returned to report that he had done as ordered, and that there was neither voice nor hearing, did Elisha go to the boy. 'He went in therefore, and shut the door upon them twain; and prayed unto the Lord. And he went up, and lay upon the child, and put his mouth upon his mouth, and his eyes upon his eyes, and his hands upon his hands:

and he stretched himself upon the child; and the flesh of the child waxed warm. Then he returned, and walked in the house to and fro; and went up, and stretched himself upon him: and the child sneezed seven times, and the child opened his eyes.'

This tale gives a perfect example of the near-impossibility of making diagnoses of illnesses way back in history; more often than not there just is not sufficient clinical information. But from the facts we have been given, particularly those relating to the time interval between 'death' and resuscitation, the one sure thing is that, whatever else he may have done, Elisha did not perform mouth-to-mouth respiration – with 'his hands upon his hands' Elisha's breath would have come out of the child's nostrils. Nevertheless, the story does provide an early example of a long-term follow-up as chapter 8, verse 5, notes that the boy was still alive seven years later.

For a long time, probably since the days of Vesalius, anatomists had been aware that they could revive the failing hearts of animals by inflating the lungs. But the first account of this technique being used in human beings did not appear until the 18th century.

On December 3, 1732, James Blair was involved in a fire in a coal mine. When he was rescued, William Tossach, a Scottish surgeon in Alloa, found 'there was not the least pulse in either heart or arteries, and not the least breathing could be observed : So that he was in all appearance dead. I applied my mouth close to his, and blowed my breath as strong as I could: but having neglected to close his nostrils all the air came out of them: Wherefore taking hold of them with one hand, and holding my other on his breast at the left pap, I blew again my breath as strong as I could, raising his chest fully with it; and immediately I felt six or seven very quick beats of the heart.' Blair recovered consciousness in an hour, and a few hours later he walked home[41].

The method seemed to be home and dry when, in 1774, the Royal Humane Society was founded to promote effective artificial respiration; at first they recommended mouth-to-mouth respiration together with warmth, stimulants, and so forth. Perhaps because of the recent discovery of carbon dioxide, which was believed to be lethal if inhaled into the lungs, they changed their minds and in 1782 promoted the use of bellows instead[42,43]. It seems likely that this method was fairly well known (though how extensively practised is another matter) because at the end of the century the indomitable Larrey, awaiting a posting at Nice, resuscitated drowned men by blowing air into their noses with bellows. 'How is the surgeon transported,' he tells us in his *Memoirs*, 'to discover motion returning to the lips and eyelids of a man apparently dead, and when he perceives that the heart palpitates, and respiration is restored! It is the rapture of a Pygmalion, when he perceives the marble becoming animated under his fingers! In proportion as the torch of life is returned, I redouble my exertions, and the patient is at length placed in a warm bed, where he usually remains some days.'[44] What tremendous humanity there is in those words.

Yet even the idea of bellows did not last long, for within 50 years the Society had only warmth and rubbing left on their list of recommendations.

Mouth-to-mouth respiration began its comeback in the late 1930s, slowly at first because of the popularity of techniques that involved pressure on the chest in one form or another, but by the mid-1950s it was accepted as the method of choice. So with the arrival of external cardiac massage a few years later the vital functions of the heart and lungs could be kept going without the need for any apparatus. The importance of this cannot be overestimated, because it meant that, even in cases of doubt, action could be taken at once, whether the patient was in the operating theatre or on the street. The medical man no longer had to take the momentous decision of opening the chest and massaging the heart directly – the taking of which may well have lost valuable minutes. He can now act immediately and then think while doing so.

So far we have only made passing reference to the form of cardiac arrest known as ventricular fibrillation. This is responsible for roughly half the number of arrests and the only really effective treatment is electrical defibrillation, although massage will maintain an adequate circulation if the apparatus is not to hand, and may indeed be necessary to make the fibrillation more vigorous and so more susceptible to defibrillation. Claude Beck of Cleveland reported the first success in 1947; it was his sixth attempt. The patient was a boy of 14 who was having part of his breastbone removed because of a severe funnel chest. When the wound was being closed his pulse suddenly stopped. The wound was reopened and cardiac massage started at once. Beck noted that the heart was fibrillating and this was confirmed by an electrocardiogram. A series of shocks was necessary before the fibrillation stopped, but massage was continued throughout. After more than an hour Beck's persistence was rewarded and at the follow-up examination three months later the boy was in fine fettle[45].

However, the arrival of open-heart surgery with its growing variety of operations brought fresh hazards with which surgeons had to contend. One of these was damage to the conducting mechanism during closure of holes between the two ventricles; when this happened the patient almost invariably died because the heart stopped. Search for an answer to the problem led to the development of the now well-known artificial pacemakers, although initially drugs such as isoprenaline were used and did lower the mortality rate quite considerably.

The electrodes of the early pacemakers were attached to the skin, but this was a highly unsatisfactory arrangement leading to such troubles as dermal burns. So, after much experimental work on animals, it was decided to put the positive electrode directly into the heart muscle. This was first done by Henry Bahnson and his team at Johns Hopkins Hospital, on November 8, 1956. The patient was an 11-month-old girl who had had a patent ductus arteriosus ligated and an interventricular septal defect repaired. Sadly she died a few hours later[46]. However, success came shortly afterwards to Walton Lillehei and his team at the University of Minnesota. They first used a myocardial electrode and artificial pacemaker on January 30, 1957. At the time of their report later that year they had used this method 18 times with only one death, which had come about because the indifferent electrode became unstuck from the skin; thereafter they inserted it under the skin[47].

Russell Brock of Guy's Hospital was the first to use a myocardial electrode in Great Britain, and his case illustrates how the technique works. Celia Williams, aged seven, developed dissociation of the heart-beat between the atria and ventricles after closure of a ventricular septal defect. The bared ends of two electrodes (one was a spare) were sewn into the anterior surface of the right ventricle about 2cm apart. The pacemaker, set to deliver a rate of 120 beats per minute, was used intermittently as required by Celia's clinical state. From the 11th day isoprenaline was given by mouth, and on the 21st day after operation, as there was no further need for it, the pacemaker was withdrawn[48]. Since then pacemakers have developed tremendously; they can now be buried in the body as self-contained transistorized units.

Finally, there remains one point – and a most important one it is too. How do these people react who have been 'brought back from the dead'? The experience is novel, to say the least, and one for which there is no prototype. Two Americans, Richard Druss and Donald Kornfeld of New York, in 1967 reported a psychiatric study they had made of 10 survivors. Not one of these patients could face the full implications of the arrest. They developed emotional problems, irritability, insomnia, frightening and violent dreams, and restricted their activities more than was medically necessary. They also produced a variety of theories to enable them to integrate the experience of having been dead and reborn. Druss and Kornfeld concluded, 'If anything, the experience of arrest leads to a sense of isolation and uniqueness which, when bridged, adds greatly to the patients' mental health and physical well-being.'[49] The evident problem is the bridging, which indicates that there is a great deal more to the treatment of cardiac arrest than restoring the heart-beat.

6

PULMONARY EMBOLISM

Tuffier's failure at cardiac massage came about through a misdiagnosis. That he should make the mistake is more than understandable: when a patient dies suddenly from a clot of blood blocking a major pulmonary artery the diagnosis is by no means always obvious, and Tuffier had no time to be concerned with differential diagnosis. He could only assume the condition to be cardiac arrest and act on the assumption; had he known it was a pulmonary embolus there was nothing he could have done.

Ten years later another surgeon correctly diagnosed a pulmonary embolus and made a deliberate attempt to remove the clot from the pulmonary artery – the operation of pulmonary embolectomy, forever linked with the name of this man, Friedrich Trendelenburg.

Small clots of blood can travel quite a long way down the arterial system of the lung before they become stuck, but our concern is the one that lodges in the main pulmonary artery or its two major branches. These large clots, by a mixture of direct and reflex mechanisms, kill immediately or within minutes, and during these minutes the patient is very severely ill – an obvious remark perhaps, but worth emphasizing because the embolus has widespread effects which do nothing to help recovery.

The usual places where these clots originate are the deep veins of the legs and the pelvis. The reasons for the thrombosis are not fully understood, but bed rest, sluggish blood flow in the veins, injury, and surgical operations are among the precipitating causes. When a thrombus starts in one of the leg veins it is attached to the wall of the vein, but as time goes on it grows a tail which waves freely in the blood stream, and it is not hard to imagine how part of this may get broken off. In at least half the cases of pulmonary embolism there is no evidence of peripheral thrombosis and, by some sheer perversity of nature, when a leg is known to be affected by thrombosis, the killing embolus may shoot off from a vein in the other leg that was thought to be normal.

Pulmonary embolism may thus be utterly unexpected and is a dreaded complication in medical practice. Pulmonary embolectomy is in one sense an admission of defeat, as the real problem is to prevent the original thrombus from forming; but in spite of a great deal of research into the cause and prevention of thrombosis, pulmonary embolism continues to take a regular toll of life that is not significantly lower than it was in Trendelenburg's day.

Trendelenburg's fame does not rest solely on his having had the temerity to make two attempts – both of which failed – at one of the most exacting and hazardous operations in surgery. A surgeon does not achieve fame lightly. As befitted a one-time assistant to the great Langenbeck, he did memorable work on strictures of the trachea and introduced the idea of feeding patients through a hole in the stomach wall when they were unable to swallow due to a disease of the oesophagus. His name is also attached to the position, used by surgeons when operating on the bladder and pelvic organs, in which the table is tilted so that the patient's pelvis is raised and the intestines tend to fall back out of the pelvic cavity. In 1872 he was a founder of the German Surgical Society and later became its president and historian. But it is for the operation of pulmonary embolectomy – Trendelenburg's operation – that he is chiefly remembered today. The basic technique he devised stood the test of time, and of repeated failure; only when modern cardiac surgery came into its own were the limiting factors overcome.

Nine patients who had died in Leipzig Hospital from pulmonary embolism came to Trendelenburg's notice. Two had died suddenly, but the other seven had survived for intervals varying from 10 minutes to an hour. Surely, he thought, it should be possible to do something surgical to remove the clot in those few minutes – provided the surgeon was ready and knew precisely what to do.

So the first thing Trendelenburg did was to produce a pulmonary embolus experimentally in a calf by introducing long narrow strips of lung tissue, removed from another animal, into the deep jugular vein; he then successfully removed the artificial embolus. The animal was sacrificed four months later and no permanent damage found. This convinced him that the operation was a practical proposition.

Next, he took himself off to the postmortem room and worked tirelessly until he had perfected a technique suitable for use in a human patient. But remember, anaesthesia was primitive, the pleural cavities were entered at great risk, and speed was vital. Today these limitations seem almost crippling.

In 1908 Trendelenburg was ready. He did not have long to wait, but unfortunately the first patient, a man of 70, died on the table. The next patient was actually operated on by his assistant, Sievers – emphasizing the importance of teamwork and preparedness, for one man cannot possibly be ready all the time. The patient died 15 hours afterwards from heart failure. Later that same year Trendelenburg himself operated again[1,2]. He made a transverse incision over the second rib on the left and a vertical incision on the left side of the sternum. He then resected 10-12cm of the second rib and cartilage and made a vertical incision through the pleura and pericardium. Next he passed a rubber tube behind the aorta and pulmonary artery; when he pulled on this the blood flow was halted. From this moment speed was essential. He incised the pulmonary artery, pulled out the clot with special forceps – all in no more than 45 seconds. Regrettably the patient died 37 hours later from haemorrhage of the internal mammary artery which had been accidentally damaged. For some reason Trendelenburg never again attempted the operation. Probably he felt that his age (he was 64) was against him, and, having shown the way, he could leave the struggle to other, younger, men.

His enthusiasm aroused only a desultory sort of interest. In 1909, Hermann Krüger of Jena[3] reported another failure: the patient lived for five-and-a-quarter days before succumbing to infection of the left pleural cavity which had been entered at operation. In 1914, Emil Schumacher, who worked in Sauerbruch's clinic, lost a patient after 50 hours from recurrent embolism[4].

The triumph of being the first surgeon to discharge his patient from hospital fit and well belongs to Martin Kirschner of Königsberg, and a deserved success it was too – 38-year-old Johanna Kempf was his 11th case[5]. Perhaps with this record it is no surprise to learn that Kirschner had been a pupil of Trendelenburg, and like his teacher he was a surgeon of no mean merit. In 1909, he had used strips of fascia lata from the thigh in the repair of inguinal hernias[6], but the surgical world was not quite ready, and the value of fascial grafts remained unappreciated for another 12 years. Then, in 1920, Kirschner opened both chest and abdomen (the thoraco-abdominal approach) to get the necessary wide exposure for operations on the lower oesophagus and upper part of the stomach[7]. But again he was unlucky, and did not receive the credit for introducing the approach to modern surgery; this went instead to a Japanese in 1930[8,9]. (Nevertheless, see Duval's case on page 131.)

Johanna Kempf's memorable operation took place on March 18, 1924: her embolus followed a hernia operation. Kirschner used Trendelenburg's technique; all went well on the table but afterward Johanna was alternately delirious and comatose. Kirschner had to wait in an agony of suspense for four days before she recovered consciousness. Thrilled by the success, Trendelenburg presented Kirschner with a set of the instruments he had specially designed for the operation[10]. This was to be one of the last acts of the great man, for he died later that year on December 16; his obituary notices in both the *British Medical*

Journal[1] and the *Lancet*[2] contained no reference to pulmonary embolectomy. Yet even though Kirschner had shown the way, surgeons found it no easy matter to follow. Most of those who thought they were equal to the challenge retired discouraged from the fray. By the early 1930s more than 300 attempts had been made with only eight more successes to add to the list – and these eight were achieved by three men. To gain some idea of the remarkable performance of these surgeons in the face of the seemingly impossible, consider further that by 1958, the start of the modern upsurge of interest, the total of successes had been increased by only three.

Neither Arthur Meyer of Berlin, Clarence Crafoord of Stockholm, nor Erik Gunnar Nyström of Uppsala was the sort of man who gave up easily. They failed, they persisted, and they succeeded. Meyer three times (in 1927, 1928 and 1931)[13,14], Crafoord three times (1927, 1928[15], and 1933), and Nyström twice (1928 and 1929)[16].

Meyer modified Trendelenburg's original operation by not opening the pleura, although he underestimated the difficulties of this as the pleura can at times be as thin as tissue paper and it may be impossible to dissect a clear way through. Crafoord, too, emphasized the danger of opening the pleura because of the likelihood of shock and infection. To add weight to this he told how, in 1926, he had operated and had opened the left pleura widely; the patient breathed no more. Another of his patients died after seven-and-a-half days from mediastinal sepsis.

Nevertheless, an outstanding cause of death in those who left the operating table alive (and they were very few) was recurrent pulmonary embolus. In a sense this means that some of the cases that ended in this way could be accounted successful; Meyer, for instance, did actually so regard one of his patients who died from this cause after 25 days[14].

Besides his modification of the operation, Meyer set another example, that was to be followed for many years, of watching the patients before deciding to operate, first in the ward, and then, as their condition deteriorated, in the theatre. He opened their chests only if signs of cardiac standstill or of increased pressure in the neck veins developed. It was calculated that for every patient operated on, three were returned to their beds; but this policy also meant that for many patients surgery came too late to save their lives. Nyström also advised waiting until the patient was at the point of death.

Before leaving this early period, we should mention that one other surgeon made numerous unsuccessful attempts. The failure of Ferdinand Sauerbruch seems all the more surprising when we realize that he was the most famous German thoracic surgeon of his day and, as we shall see later, was largely responsible for breaking through the barrier created by the negative pressure within the chest[17]. Maybe his erratic temperament had something to do with his lack of success in such a demanding operation, although, on the other hand, he was a perfectionist. A reasonable conclusion might well be that luck just never smiled upon him.

The scene now moved away from Germany and Sweden (although Crafoord operated another seven times between 1933 and 1949[18]) and became pretty dismal and overcast with only three flashes of brilliance to lighten the growing darkness. These came from Pietro Valdoni of Rome, on November 27, 1935[19]; Ivor Lewis of Wales in 1938[20]; and Pierre Marion of Lyon in 1952[21]. Marion operated on June 4, 40 hours after the embolus had occurred. In the discussion of the paper this interval was queried and also the fact that only two small clots were removed; the inference was that the patient could already have been out of danger. Lewis's case was particularly dramatic; good fortune certainly was on his side. The patient was a 40-year-old woman, and her embolus occurred on September 12, 1938, eight days after she had had an infected bursa of the knee incised. Her postoperative course was stormy, to say the least, but she overcame the many complications which included pronounced cerebral symptoms (due to the temporary lack of blood to the brain), suppurative pericarditis (which was drained), and empyema (for which rib resection was performed).

Despite the tremendous advances in chest surgery and particularly in cardiac surgery, the decade after the Second World War saw the reputation of pulmonary embolectomy reach rock bottom. Surgeons were utterly disheartened by the seeming inevitability of failure; but more significant was the appearance of a new group of drugs, the anticoagulants. Everyone hoped that here was something to make the operation obsolete. Thrombosis could be prevented. In 1944, Alton Ochsner, an American thoracic surgeon, told the American Surgical Association[22]:

'I hope we will not have any more papers on the removal of pulmonary emboli before this organization, an operation which should be of historic interest only. Certainly the way to prevent death from pulmonary embolism is to prevent the clot from becoming detached and getting into the pulmonary artery if thrombosis does occur.' But as experience with the use of these drugs increased it became only too apparent that they were not the answer. Thrombosis and pulmonary emboli were still as much a problem as ever. Richard Steenburg and his colleagues, writing from the Peter Bent Brigham Hospital, Boston, in 1958 reckoned that they continued to see about five major massive pulmonary embolisms per year on a surgical service performing 2500 operations annually.

In their paper, which is generally considered to mark the revival of interest in Trendelenburg's operation, they recorded the first American success[23]. It was the 15th attempt at the hospital; all the others had been performed between 1933 and 1943 as a result of the stimulus provided by Elliott Cutler, one of the pioneers of modern cardiac surgery. All the patients had died, the longest survival being two hours. This lack of success discouraged other attempts although the authors did think it strange that a revival of the operation had not already taken place in view of some modern innovations – intratracheal anaesthesia, antibiotics, better availability of electrocardiography, the cardiac defibrillator, and the concept of vein ligation, all of which contributed to the successful management of their patient.

A 64-year-old woman had had an uneventful cholecystectomy and choledochostomy (removal of the gall bladder and a procedure on the bile ducts) on January 8, 1958. Six days later she developed a pulmonary embolism. The operation of embolectomy was begun 45 minutes after the initial episode and 25 minutes after the blood pressure had last been obtainable. A left parasternal incision was made and extended laterally in the submammary fold; the first five left costal cartilages were exposed, transected, and retracted. Tapes were used to control the aorta and pulmonary artery, although, in retrospect, the authors considered these to have been unnecessary. Then, through a longitudinal incision in the pulmonary artery, two large clots were removed with a sponge forceps from the right main artery. No anaesthetic was needed throughout the whole procedure, and at the end of wound closure the woman was moving spontaneously.

Five hours later she was brought back to theatre, and both femoral veins were interrupted under local anaesthesia. The reason for this was to prevent further emboli and was based on the assumption that the clots had come from the leg veins, even though she had had no signs of thrombosis before the embolism, and no clot was found in the veins at the level where they were divided and tied. (The surgeon would have preferred to have ligated the inferior vena cava, but the patient's condition precluded this.) Eight weeks after all this the patient was discharged from hospital with only minor disability.

Surgeons began to stir out of their despondency. Anticoagulants had not removed the need for surgery, and perhaps the prognosis of pulmonary embolectomy was not quite as bad as they had feared if modern advances could be exploited. Philip Allison of Oxford took the next step forward when he used general hypothermia (achieved by surface cooling of the body) to allow him to interrupt the circulation and take more time over the operation. This he did twice in patients with subacute pulmonary embolus – meaning that the embolus was not a sudden catastrophe. In fact, in his one success, on March 21, 1958, Allison operated when the 29-year-old man began to deteriorate markedly after emboli had been thrown off for a month, so it does not fall into the category of acute massive embolism that has been our primary concern. However, this does not detract from the success, as Allison removed tough thrombus and softer tailed clots from both main branches of the pulmonary artery. At the end of the operation he ligated the right external iliac vein as the clots had originated from an injury to the right thigh[24].

This operation was a pointer to what could be achieved, and surgeons began thinking of the possibility of surgery as a planned undertaking in these subacute cases when life or the function of the lungs became in danger. They considered the main indication for surgery should be increasing heart failure, although they recognized the great difficulty of deciding when to operate. But in the acute massive cases surgeons on the whole still believed Trendelenburg's operation to be extremely dangerous and felt it should only be attempted when the heart had stopped beating and the patient was virtually dead. Fortunately, events soon changed this view.

A few months after Allison had reported his cases and leader writers had assessed the situation, the first successful pulmonary embolectomy using cardiopulmonary bypass (the heart-lung machine, which takes over the work of the heart and lungs and allows the surgeon immeasurably better operating conditions) was performed by Denton Cooley and his team at Houston, Texas.

In April, 1961, a 37-year-old woman had a total abdominal hysterectomy and a right salpingo-oophorectomy (removal of the fallopian tube and ovary), at the Jefferson Davis Hospital, for a ruptured tubal pregnancy. She was discharged on April 15, but the next day was readmitted in a state of profound vascular collapse. Massive pulmonary embolus was diagnosed. Medical treatment to support the heart and circulation, and anticoagulants, were given. On the 17th her condition was deteriorating and so, at 2am on April 18, two hours after the decision was taken, emergency embolectomy was started, using a disposable bubble-diffusion oxygenator and roller pumps. (The story of the development of heart-lung machines is told in a later chapter.)

The main pulmonary artery was opened longitudinally and at first no emboli were found. Suction, however, produced many long thrombi from both main branches. The pleural spaces were therefore opened, the lungs repeatedly compressed, and the pulmonary arterial tree irrigated until no more fragments of emboli were recovered. The inferior vena cava was immediately ligated through an extraperitoneal incision in the right flank. No thrombi were seen, although the vena cava was deliberately opened in search of the source of the emboli. When the woman was examined three months after the operation she was completely free of symptoms.

In their report the authors wrote: 'Although many patients die instantly following massive pulmonary embolism, it is not unusual for patients to survive one or more hours before death occurs from pulmonary vascular obstruction or visceral reflex mechanisms. An aggressive attitude towards surgical treatment of these cases should permit the saving of many patients who otherwise are doomed. As a rule, recognition of the potentially fatal cases of pulmonary embolism is not difficult, and for these patients immediate plans should be made for operation using the pump bypass.'[25]

As must be all too evident by now, the prognosis of massive pulmonary embolism is poor; some patients die immediately from circulatory failure or a ventricular arrhythmia; some survive for hours or even days, but those who recover remain at risk of further emboli. Although medical treatment, including anticoagulants and drugs designed to dissolve the clot, is top priority there is still a place for pulmonary embolectomy in centres where the surgeon is a skilled enthusiast and has at his immediate disposal a trained team and a theatre and equipment prepared for the emergency.

7

EARLY EXPERIMENTS AND ARGUMENTS

Thus far we have considered only the fringes of cardiac surgery, but each has taught us a lesson and each either played an important role in the development of the subject or showed quite plainly how the land lay in the early days. Work on pericardial disease and then the success in suturing wounds of the heart gradually eroded the belief in the inviolability of the heart. The ability to start an arrested heart beating again was vital if sophisticated operations were to become possible, and pulmonary embolectomy showed how a technically feasible undertaking was nevertheless so hazardous as to be virtually abandoned until modern aids to surgery and diagnosis came to its rescue.

Yet none of these operations was first and foremost an attack on a diseased or deformed heart. And how understandable. It was one thing to resort to heroic measures when the patient was to all intents and purposes dead; it was quite another deliberately to operate inside the heart of a patient who was merely sick (and a 'medical case' at that). Still, there were one or two adventurous souls who, before the end of the 19th century, began to dream of what might be achieved. And the stimulus to the realization of their dreams was rheumatic fever with its frequent and tragic effects on the heart.

Rheumatic fever is a vicious disease. No one knows for certain how infection with the group A streptococcus leads to the condition, though poverty, with its associated malnutrition, overcrowding, and dampness, predisposes to the illness and to repeated attacks. Seventy and more years ago it was extremely common; today it is on the decline but is still responsible for over 90 percent of all heart disease in young people. The more dramatic and newsworthy congenital defects – blue babies and so forth – account for only some 2-3 percent.

The clinical course and manifestations of rheumatic fever are extremely variable; the disease essentially involves the whole body, but the really unpleasant consequences affect the joints, the heart or, uncommonly nowadays, lead to Sydenham's chorea (St Vitus's dance). Permanent damage to the heart is likely, especially when the first attack of fever comes at an early age or when the attacks are frequently repeated.

There are two significant points to remember about rheumatic fever and the heart: One, that after the rheumatic disease has burned itself out, the physical damage to the heart continues. And two, that the damage can affect both the heart muscle and the valves, though one or other usually predominates as the cause of disability. The second point is particularly important in the historical context because in the days before valve surgery, muscle damage was thought to be vastly the more important; and then later in the first flush of success with valve operations, the muscle damage was almost lost sight of. Once again modern techniques of diagnosis were necessary before surgeons could sort out the relative importance of each factor in tricky cases.

The valve most usually affected by rheumatic disease is the mitral, between the left atrium and ventricle. It may then hinder the flow of blood through its orifice (mitral stenosis) or be incompetent and allow blood to flow in the wrong direction (mitral incompetence or regurgitation); or both effects may be combined in varying degree. The valve next most often involved is the aortic, through which the blood leaves the left ventricle to start on its journey round the body.

So, in view of the frequency of mitral valve disease, we can well understand why some doctors – physicians as well as surgeons – dreamed of relieving the mechanical effects by surgery.

However, experimental studies on the heart valves were initially undertaken with no thought of their application to human surgery. Otto Becker, a German ophthalmologist, in 1872, was first on the scene[1]. He wanted to prove that the changes seen in the retina in aortic incompetence were due to the heart condition and not to disease of the eye. The way he did this was to produce aortic incompetence in healthy dogs by passing a glass rod down the left common carotid artery and making holes in the cusps of the aortic valve. He proved his point.

In the middle years of the same decade more animal experiments were carried out, this time to study the effects of artificially produced valve lesions. It is probably no coincidence that two of the men concerned were pupils of Rudolf Virchow, a Pomeranian and the founder of 'cellular pathology', for the greatness of a teacher can usually be measured in the quality of those he has taught. One who came under Virchow's spell was Edwin Klebs, a pioneer in the new science of bacteriology (the diphtheria bacillus was named after him). In those days scientists often had many interests, and in 1876, while professor of pathology in Prague, Klebs decided he would do some work on the heart. He used a small knife at the end of a rod-like handle to produce lesions of the aortic and tricuspid valves[2].

The other gifted pupil of Virchow to experiment on the heart was Julius Cohnheim, professor of pathology at Breslau and famous for his research on inflammation. He wanted to confirm that the work done by the healthy heart increased in the same ratio as the demands made upon it; so, using a thin metallic sound with a button at its tip he lacerated the segments of the aortic valve in rabbits and dogs. Stenosis of the pulmonary artery or aorta he produced by first paralysing a dog with curare and maintaining its respiration artificially; then, through an ample resection of the ribs on the left, he opened the pericardium, passed a strong thread around the artery in question and tied a loop knot. He found that constriction had no effect until a certain point was reached[3,4]. The implication was that natural disease would also have to produce a definite degree of narrowing of the valvular orifice before symptoms appeared – not entirely true, for in human disease the narrowing can progress slowly and the heart can adapt to the added burden up to a point which varies from person to person.

Cohnheim, in his turn, inspired his colleague, Ottomar Rosenbach, to perform other experiments to study the effects of lesions of the aortic, mitral and tricuspid valves in dogs[5]. But despite the eminence of Klebs and Cohnheim in their own particular fields, the general response seems to have been 'Yes, that's all very nice, but now let's get on with something else, shall we?' And get on with other things everyone did until Rehn's successful wound suture in 1896 led to a spurt of speculation on the further possibilities of heart surgery.

In 1897, Herbert Milton at the Kasr el Aini Hospital in Cairo wrote an article for the *Lancet* in which he described his sternum-splitting incision for access to the chest – an important clinical advance[6]. Among his conclusions, though, was a remark that, in view of prevailing opinion, might easily have damned his work: 'Heart surgery is still quite in its infancy, but it requires not a great stretch of fancy to imagine the possibility of plastic operations in some, at all events, of its valvular lesions.' But perhaps the medical powers felt his fancies could do little harm in far-off Cairo.

The next year Daniel Samways stated, in the *British Medical Journal*, that the characteristic alteration of the left auricle (atrium) in mitral stenosis was hypertrophy and not dilatation; the latter was 'an old age phenomenon in the history of mitral stenosis'[7]. He was saying that, contrary to popular belief, the atrium responded well to the extra work put on it by the narrowed valve; only in the late stages of the disease did it give up the ghost and dilate. A second article, in the *Lancet*, he concluded with the prophecy: '.... and I anticipate that with the progress of cardiac surgery some of the severest cases of mitral stenosis will be relieved by slightly notching the mitral orifice and trusting to the auricle to continue its defence'[8]. Even he was not prepared to commit himself to foreseeing anything more than a slight notching, for fear of producing a most unwelcome regurgitation. In view of the considerable interest taken by the French in thoracic surgery, it is perhaps noteworthy that Samways had a Paris as well as a British qualification and wrote his second article from Mentone [*sic*] in the South of France.

These comments produced scarcely a ripple, and all was calm until the first half of 1902 when a note in the *Lancet* by Sir Lauder Brunton ignited a correspondence that quickly put any thought of heart surgery in Britain firmly in its place and kept it there for many years to come.

Sir Thomas Lauder Brunton was a physician at St Bartholomew's Hospital, London, with a lifelong interest in cardiology and especially in the action of drugs on the heart. While still a house-physician in Edinburgh in 1867[9] he had described the beneficial effect of amyl nitrite in relieving the pain of angina pectoris, a treatment still used today. He was a kindly and respected man and a Fellow of The Royal Society – which makes the subsequent vitriolic attack on his integrity all the more surprising.

In his 'Preliminary note on the possibility of treating mitral stenosis by surgical methods'[10] he drew attention to the hopelessness of ever finding a medical treatment that would do anything for the incapacitating symptoms of the severe forms of the disease. In the postmortem room though, he had found he could separate the adherent cusps of the valve quite easily. So, he asked, why not consider the possibility of surgery? Admittedly the risks were great but, if successful, the patient would have a life worth living again.

He had in mind plunging a suitable instrument blindly through the wall of the left ventricle and, by sense of touch, separating the fused cusps. He said he would prefer going in through the ventricle rather than the atrium for practical reasons: when on one of the commissions investigating the effect of chloroform on the heart in 1889 he had noted that wounds of the ventricles bled less than those of the atria. Furthermore, he had been experimenting on the hearts of animals for 35 years and had found that they stood up to the manhandling very well indeed. Thus, as far as he could, he was speaking from experience and with a genuine desire to help the many seriously afflicted patients who filled his clinics and wards.

But, as he pointed out, he was a physician proposing an operation; he merely hoped his thoughts would encourage surgeons to take the matter up and see if anything practical could be done.

The first reaction came the following week in a leading article in the *Lancet* which viewed his idea with 'disapprobation'[11]. More strongly, it criticized him for recommending so momentous an undertaking on the basis of dead-room experiments, and said that the invitation to others to pursue the work could not absolve him from the responsibility for what he had started. But in any case the *Lancet* thought the difficulties of the operation had been underestimated and that the technique itself would 'prove fatal to its adoption'.

Sir Lauder was indignant; he replied at once saying he had no intention of abandoning his idea, and firmly reiterated the need for surgeons to find a solution[12]. He hoped also to perform animal experiments himself – but whether from disillusionment or pressure of other work, he never did.

Only two people rallied to Brunton's support: Samways[13], who drew attention to his earlier articles, and Arbuthnot Lane[14]. Lane said the idea of surgical relief had been suggested to him some years previously by Lauriston Shaw, and he had actually worked out on cadavers an approach to the valve through the ventricle. He 'was quite prepared to act as soon as Dr Shaw succeeded in finding a case likely to derive benefit.'

Shaw seemed not to like this one little bit – despite Lane's preparedness he (Shaw) had now decided quite definitely that there was no benefit to be gained by operation which he felt to be an unjustifiable form of treatment. 'It is possible to do many things that are useless and some things that are harmful.'[15] Nevertheless he did agree that the operation was technically feasible; Sir Lauder's task, he said, was to persuade his medical colleagues of the usefulness of the procedure.

But it was Theodore Fisher[16] who sounded the note that put paid to any further discussion; fibrosis of the heart muscle was, in his view, the important factor – meaning that even if a patient survived operation he would be no better off.

This belief pervaded *medical* thought until surgeons were able to prove otherwise. The physicians hitched their wagon to their own interpretation of the writings of Sir James Mackenzie, the great British cardiologist. Where Sir James led, other cardiologists were bound to follow. But was he really leading along the path of muscle damage and away from the valve lesion, or were his colleagues following their own inclinations?

Today, reading his book, *Diseases of the heart*, we can see his clear grasp of the situation, but we can also understand how contemporary cardiologists interpreted the text (which remained unaltered in the essentials we are considering between the first edition in 1908[17] and the fourth and last in 1925[18]) to fit in with the beliefs they were clinging to so desperately.

'In chronic valvular affections,' Mackenzie wrote, 'the symptoms only arise where exhaustion of the heart muscle sets in.' However, in discussing mitral stenosis specifically, he said, 'It is important to bear in mind the progressive nature of the lesion, for it accounts for the varying changes in the symptoms. It should also be borne in mind that the cicatrizing process may be going on in the muscle, causing contraction of the chordae tendineae, impairing at other places the functional activity of the heart muscle.... The manner in which heart failure is brought about in many cases is somewhat complicated.'

Sir James quite clearly recognized that either the muscle or the valves could be primarily affected: 'With the increased narrowing of the orifice ... the heart becomes much embarrassed, the symptoms become much more distressing, and finally dilatation of the heart (failure of tonicity) may set in. But even without the progressive narrowing dilatation may appear early, and then it may be inferred with certainty that the rheumatic process has permanently injured the heart muscle.'

Discussing the heart changes in rheumatic fever, he wrote: "The myocardium rarely escapes, and the changes in it are of great importance, both for the acute condition and for the subsequent integrity of the heart muscle.' And that was quite enough for those who, for whatever reason, feared the introduction of the scalpel inside the heart in rheumatic disease.

In America a proposal to operate on a common congenital defect met with a similar fate. John Cummings Munro of Boston showed remarkable foresight when, in 1907, he suggested ligation of a patent ductus arteriosus[19]. This anomaly is the persistence of a normal embryological vessel. In the fetus the ductus carries blood from the pulmonary artery straight into the aorta, bypassing the lungs, which are not functioning and so do not need a full supply of blood. After birth the ductus should close naturally, but if it fails to do so some of the blood circulating in the body is inadequately oxygenated. Additional complications may arise because congenital defects of the heart are prone to become infected – resulting in subacute bacterial endocarditis.

Munro said he had long ago demonstrated the feasibility of his technique 'on the cadaver of newborn children and felt that it was justifiable on the living.' His object was to prevent complications. When he tried to inspire his paediatric colleague he was out of luck, as this gentleman, in common with many others, was not at all reassuring about making the diagnosis during life.

The last thing we should do today is to criticize the clinicians of nearly 100 years ago for their timidity. Accurate diagnosis during life was exceedingly difficult, and in many cases impossible; heart diseases were 'medical'; modern surgery was still in its infancy, though making great strides; and operations inside the chest were few, infrequent, and hazardous. The profession was neither physically nor mentally prepared for cardiac surgery. Nevertheless the ball was rolling.

The next stage was a progression of the work of Klebs and Cohnheim, though this time the experimental lesions of the valves were made directly through the thorax, and were designed mainly for the teaching of students. Harvey Cushing of Johns Hopkins in Baltimore is rightly remembered for his immense contribution to neurosurgery, and it is little exaggeration to say that neurosurgery and neurology were advanced every time he picked up his scalpel to operate or his pen to write. His articles were a model of perfection, lucid, complete in every detail, and beautifully illustrated with his own superb drawings. In particular he laid emphasis on the need to study both at the bedside and in the laboratory.

But despite his comment that if there was to be advancement in neuro-surgery there must be 'concentration of thoughts and energies along given lines', he found time while stepping over the threshold to greatness to experi-ment with the heart. This he began in December, 1905[20]. William MacCallum, a colleague, had devised a cutting hook or valvulotome which was introduced, usually through the ventricle but sometimes through the atrium, to create valvular incompetence. Stenosis they produced by passing a stout ligature on a curved needle around the valve orifice. The animals were anaesthetized by direct inflation of the lungs through an opening in the trachea. Although Cushing speculated on the benefit of operations on the mitral valve in man, both he and MacCallum felt that the main value of the work was in teaching students, who could listen through their stethoscopes to known lesions of the valves, and could study alterations in the blood-pressure tracings[21,22].

This work was continued by Bertram Bernheim who operated to relieve experimentally-created stenoses, but in only one case was relief obtained. He also used an opening in the trachea for giving the anaesthetic, and employed bellows to keep the lungs inflated. As a result of these experiments Bernheim had a thought about the effect of the pericardium in heart disease: 'It might be of therapeutic benefit to open the pericardium of certain patients who have become bedridden from chronic myocarditis, with the object of relieving the excessive pressure and of allowing room for the overburdened and dilated heart.'[23] Echoes of Alexander Morison.

Finally we come to three men of genius whose work stands out like the Pole Star suddenly glimpsed by sailors lost in an uncharted sea. The tragedy of Théodore Tuffier, Alexis Carrel, and Ernst Jeger is, perhaps, that they lived too soon. Their work was of today, not of three generations ago. Their written accounts take one's breath away to leave an agony of wonder at what they might have achieved had they had the resources of modern science to add to their inspiration and technical ability. Instead they had to contrive that which lay in the future.

(The situation is not unlike the more familiar one in athletics where the progression of world records can be predicted. Fluctuations occur, but the graph overall follows a steady curve. From time to time a fluctuation is exceptional as was the case with Jesse Owens's long-jump record in 1935 which remained unbeaten for 25 years.)

What was so remarkable about the work of these men was their incredible grasp of the issues involved in heart surgery. It was almost as though the specialty was already acknowledged instead of being a dream – perhaps to some a nightmare. In their minds they had progressed far beyond speculation as to whether the heart could ever be operated on: it could be, and they were concerned only with developing the techniques that one feels they knew to be just around the corner. But it took many years for others even to glimpse around that bend.

Alexis Carrel was a Frenchman from Sainte-Foy-les Lyon; he was born in 1873 and graduated in 1900 from the University of Lyons. Five years later he went to America where he joined the staff of the Rockefeller Institute; but despite this geographical dislocation he was still able to work closely with his friend and colleague, Tuffier. Carrel was the experimental surgeon, Tuffier the practical surgeon. Both bubbled over with ideas, both were technically extraordinarily competent, and together they made a truly fantastic combination. They appear again in this story in guises both clinical and exper- imental, but as our concern here is with the nature of the experimental operations, we may give pride of place to Carrel. Between 1902 and 1905 he had improved the technique for sewing together the cut ends of arteries[24,25,26], and this really provided the cornerstone for much of his work in the ensuing years, as the logical progression – or so it would seem now – was to graft lengths of artery or vein to bridge a gap if the ends of the vessel could not be brought together. Then in 1907 he carried this a stage further[27]: he removed a section of carotid artery from one dog, 35 minutes after its death, preserved it in cold storage for eight days and then grafted it into another dog with complete success. The animal was still alive more than a year later. Throughout this period he was also working on the transplantation of organs – for which a satisfactory method of joining blood vessels is one essential. He transplanted a kidney from one cat to another and the donor organ functioned for a while in its new home. In 1912 he won the Nobel prize for medicine. Later his interests moved toward cytology and he developed a technique for isolating cells in tissue culture and studying their physiological properties.

By some strange quirk of fate, Carrel's name is probably most remembered in association with the Carrel-Dakin treatment of wounds. In the First World War, wound infection was a terrible problem and there was great need for a suitable antiseptic. Carrel and Henry Drysdale Dakin (an Englishman who also settled in America) studied two hundred or more substances. They found that the most effective were those containing chlorine and the best was sodium hypochlorite. As this was too alkaline and damaging to the tissues, Dakin neutralized it with boric acid and Carrel christened the result 'Dakin's solution'[28]. It killed the bacteria all right, but had the disadvantage of a short- lived action. So between them Carrel and Dakin devised a rather complicated system for irrigating the wound through rubber tubes with little holes in their walls[29]. Although the technique demanded patience and attention to detail, it served a vital function in the treatment of contaminated or potentially contaminated wounds in the conditions prevailing during that war.

In 1910 Carrel had published a paper 'On the experimental surgery of the thoracic aorta and the heart'[30]. In this he stressed the simplicity of his approach to the problem, thereby giving further evidence of his wisdom: if the approach was not simple, surgeons would be even more frightened of attempting operations on the heart than they were; and if only the occasional wizard could perform the technique, again the hope of progress would be small. Using the Meltzer-Auer method of insufflation anaesthesia (which we shall discuss in the next chapter) Carrel had successfully used a preserved graft to anastomose the left ventricle to the descending aorta, thus bypassing the aortic arch. While excising a part of the aorta he had been able to maintain the circulation through a paraffined tube. The practical use Carrel foresaw for such an operation was in the treatment of aneurysm – a bulging and weakening of the aorta (or other blood vessel) which may eventually burst. There are now known to be various objections to an aortic bypass of this precise nature and aneurysms of the aortic arch are now usually treated surgically by excision of the affected length and replacement with a prosthetic graft – provided the patient is considered suitable for the operation. Nevertheless, in other situations the principle of bypassing a diseased area that cannot be excised remains valid.

A few years later, in 1914, Carrel and Tuffier together developed a technique whereby the pulmonary orifice of the heart could be enlarged[31]. The operation consisted in suturing a patch (made from a vein) to the anterior side of the orifice. This allowed the circumference to increase after the valvular ring had been divided with scissors slipped in under the patch.

They did this on eight dogs, only two of which died; and it was their belief that operations of this type might come to be used in the treatment of pulmonary stenosis in the human patient[32]. How right they were.

The star of the third man, Ernst Jeger of Berlin, shone maybe less brightly, yet in his book on the surgery of the heart and blood vessels[33], published in 1913, he recorded a set of quite remarkable experiments including some on organ transplantation. As far as the heart was concerned, though, he began with trials in which he used valve-bearing veins as replacements for the heart valves. Then on December 11, 1912, he used a graft of jugular vein as an anastomosis between the left ventricle and the proximal end of the innominate artery. This bypassed the aortic valve. The animal lived for four days before dying of pulmonary complications, but at the postmortem the graft was found to be still patent. Jeger saw no reason why the mitral valve could not be similarly bypassed, and he described a technique in which the graft was carried from the pulmonary veins to the left ventricle.

Experimental work on animals is not always easy to translate to surgical operations on the human patient, yet the first step was taken towards the end of this particular experimental phase. That the man who took it should have been Tuffier was no accident. But before moving on in this direction it would be as well to pause and think about a formidable barrier to open chest surgery and see how it was overcome.

8

THE PROBLEM OF THE OPEN THORAX

From our rarefied height it is easy to look down at those who struggled in years gone by and point out smugly just where they went astray. Yet today's endeavours may well be a source of amusement to our grandsons, especially if the present rate of progress is maintained. The final answer to obtaining the ideal conditions for cardiac surgery may be just as simple as the endotracheal tube was in overcoming the problem of the open thorax.

Strangely enough, the endotracheal tube had been there all the time, but apart from a few instances it was not used in the early days of chest surgery, and the reason is not far to seek. Although physiologists were working hard at their subject and making steady progress, there was a tremendous amount to learn, advances tended to be linked to practical problems and were governed by the apparatus available. They knew relatively very little about the physiology of respiration, particularly about the physics and chemistry of gases in the body.

The obvious difficulty of operating inside the chest is how to keep the lungs from collapsing when the pleural cavities are opened. The effects of pneumothorax were discussed in the first chapter and these effects explain why a collapsed lung could not be tolerated in surgery. As we shall see, various and contrasting methods were tried to keep the lungs inflated; but at the root of the whole matter were ignorance and misunderstanding of the elimination of carbon dioxide. Oxygen is breathed in and passes through the lung membrane into the blood stream; when it reaches the capillaries it passes through their walls to nourish the tissues. In return, carbon dioxide, a waste product, passes from the tissues into the capillaries, and is carried in the venous blood to the lungs where it is exhaled. If the body does not get its oxygen it is in trouble; but also if it does not get rid of its carbon dioxide, it quickly builds up problems for itself.

Unfortunately, things are not as simple as that, and the behaviour of gases fooled the early workers. In 1917, Donald Van Slyke[1], a New York biochemist, introduced his method of measuring the carbon dioxide content of blood, and for years it was believed that the *content* was the important factor – it was in fact all they could measure. But work was going on in the laboratory, and in the early 1950s research workers showed that the carbon dioxide *tension* was what mattered[2]; this depends on the amount of the gas dissolved in the blood, and this in turn is governed by the Law of Partial Pressure.

We now know that it is possible for the *tension* of carbon dioxide to rise to quite alarmingly high levels, even though the *content* may be within reasonable limits. This may happen, for example, if the airways are obstructed, or if the anaesthetic technique is incorrect. In open chest surgery the tension can, however, be controlled by the anaesthetist assisting the respiration. Sudden lowering of a prolonged high carbon dioxide tension can adversely affect the heart.

If this seems complex, it is! Probably few other than respiratory physiologists and anaesthetists have more than a working knowledge of the subject, but for our purpose this does not matter so long as we realize that there were problems, unconnected with the actual manipulation of the heart, which were holding back progress. At the beginning of the 20th century the very nature of some of these problems was not even suspected, and so those whose guardian angels had led along a successful path could not explain the reasons for their success to others less fortunate. The basic mechanisms of respiration had to be unravelled, and this took time.

An endotracheal tube is nothing complicated; it is just a tube passed into the windpipe for the patient to breathe through. The idea is to give a clear airway uncluttered by the natural potential obstructions. Andreas Vesalius[3], in the 16th century, was probably the first person to use one – not on human beings but to maintain respiration with bellows during his anatomy demonstrations on animals. He introduced a cane tube through a tracheostomy (a hole cut into the trachea). Two hundred years later scattered references began to appear to the use of narrowish tubes (usually of metal) to revive newborn babies or drowned persons. These were inserted blindly through the mouth. But the adoption of the tube into anaesthesia had to wait until there was such a thing as an anaesthetic. Even so, its first use in surgery was not primarily for anaesthetic purposes.

With the discovery of anaesthesia in 1846 the number of surgical operations increased and surgeons soon noticed that those on the upper respiratory tract were followed rather too frequently by pneumonia consequent on the patient's inhaling blood and secretions. This worried our old friend Trendelenburg, who at this period (1869) was still Langenbeck's assistant in Berlin. His answer was a curved metal tube introduced through a tracheostomy and with a gauze mask attached to its outer end enabling a satisfactory anaesthetic to be given[4]. Before long he modified this by incorporating an inflatable rubber cuff on the part inside the trachea. Although this was effective for its purpose, it had the disadvantage of the tracheostomy.

The next major advance came from an extremely versatile Glasgow surgeon, Sir William Macewen, whose work in the early days of modern surgery was outstanding. He played a part in the development of operations for hernia[5]; he stood alone for a number of years in the treacherous field of neurosurgery, and in particular his results with brain abscesses were unsurpassed until antibiotics appeared on the scene[6]; he was the first to perform a bone-grafting operation[7]; and he may have been the first to remove a whole lung in stages[8], although the precise nature of this operation is in doubt. All in all, a remarkable and magnificent record for a 'general' surgeon. His contribution to anaesthesia was made in 1878 when, unhappy with the need to perform a tracheostomy in operations on the upper respiratory tract, he invented a flexible brass tube which he passed into the trachea through the mouth by sense of touch[9], a feat demanding considerable dexterity in the conscious patient, whose coughs and splutterings were, however, soon quelled by the chloroform.

In America during the last decades of the 19th century, work was proceeding on a number of seemingly unrelated problems. First Joseph O'Dwyer, a New York ear, nose and throat surgeon, in 1885, devised a tube which could be passed into the larynx in cases of diphtheritic obstruction[10]. It was of narrow bore, but O'Dwyer later gave it a bulbous end so that it would make an airtight seal in the larynx[11]. Meanwhile, in 1887, George Edward Fell, of Buffalo, had invented some bellows for giving artificial respiration in cases of opium poisoning[12]. These were combined with O'Dwyer's tube to become the Fell-O'Dwyer apparatus, which was adapted in 1899 by Rudolph Matas[13], the New Orleans surgeon, for giving an anaesthetic directly into the trachea – the positive pressure produced by the bellows kept the lungs inflated when the chest was opened.

The invention in 1895 of the laryngoscope (an instrument for examining the inside of the larynx) by Alfred Kirstein[14], of Berlin, was a godsend to patients and surgeons alike. Apart from its great value in the diagnosis of throat diseases it meant that endotracheal tubes could now be inserted under direct vision. His primitive apparatus was improved upon the next year by Gustav Killian, of Freiburg, whose instrument consisted of an illuminated split tube, rather like a rounded duck's bill, which was passed over the tongue[15]. By introducing another tube through his laryngoscope he soon found he could get beyond the larynx into the windpipe and even into the larger branches within the lungs.

In 1902, Franz Kuhn[16], of Kassel in Germany, emphasized that the tube must be wide enough to allow easy expiration as well as inspiration – many of the tubes were narrow-bore catheters, the idea being that expiration took place around the tube. He also showed how the tube could be passed through the nose, and he introduced the use of cocaine as a local anaesthetic before intubation to reduce the gagging and coughing. Kuhn was probably the first person to realize the importance of the tube in providing an adequate airway and thereby a smooth anaesthetic.

Thus by the opening years of the 20th century anaesthetists had at their disposal a very simple piece of apparatus upon which the whole of thoracic-surgery anaesthesia has been built up. But it should come as no surprise to learn that endotracheal anaesthesia enjoyed a considerable lack of popularity owing to the difficulties of intubation, despite the help given by the laryngoscope. And anyway, only a few crazy individuals operated on the chest, so there was no great urgency to master the technique. The situation improved after the First World War.

Having got our basic piece of equipment, we must now go back for a moment to see what was being done about keeping the lungs inflated during open-chest surgery. And to get a glimmering of understanding we must remember, once again, that no one knew very much about respiratory physiology.

The problem of the open thorax was tackled along two major lines. First, the lungs could be kept inflated by giving the anaesthetic through a tube in the trachea. There were two ways of doing this: (1) by inhalational endotracheal anaesthesia, in which the patient breathed the anaesthetic agent under pressure. This technique was the final answer, although it needed to undergo considerable development to reach today's standards; (2) insufflation anaesthesia, in which the anaesthetic gas was blown, or insufflated, into the trachea and by its presence in the lungs kept them inflated and oxygenated, and the patient asleep. The excess gas 'exsufflated' either around the sides of the narrow tube or through a second one. At one stage this technique ousted the inhalational method from popularity – if this word can be used in the present context.

Secondly, there were methods of differential pressure anaesthesia and these also can be divided into two: (1) the creation of a negative pressure around the chest, so that the lungs noticed no change when the pleural cavities were opened – the air breathed remained at atmospheric pressure; (2) the creation of a positive pressure around the patient's head. We shall deal with these differential methods first, as they eventually fell by the wayside, although to its proponents at the time the negative-pressure method seemed the only suitable answer in view of the supposed difficulties of other techniques.

The man who conceived the idea of putting the patient in a negative-pressure cabinet with his head outside was Ferdinand Sauerbruch. Sauerbruch had qualified at Leipzig in 1901 but found practice uncongenial until he was appointed assistant to Johannes von Mikulicz-Radecki (better known without the Radecki), the Polish professor of surgery at Breslau. As befitted a pupil of Billroth, Mikulicz had done outstanding work in abdominal surgery; he was now anxious to complete his hand by devising a satisfactory operation for cancer of the oesophagus (gullet). Although in 1886 he had removed a cancer from its upper part in the neck and restored continuity with a skin flap[17], he was still searching for a method that would prevent the lungs from collapsing when the chest was opened – a necessary manoeuvre to expose the lower part.

When Sauerbruch arrived at his clinic, Mikulicz infected him with his enthusiasm and set him to work to find a solution. In 1903, Mikulicz had taken a leaf out of the physiologists' notebook, and while operating on a dog's oesophagus had kept the lungs inflated by rhythmically pumping air into them. But the result was bad and he concluded the method had little promise. Nevertheless, Sauerbruch began on the same tack, and after much experimental work on animals, both anaesthetized and unanaesthetized, came to the same conclusion. The flaws he found were intimidating: air was forced out of the lung spaces into the surrounding lung tissue; the animals' body temperatures dropped alarmingly; the need for a tracheostomy was a great disadvantage; postoperative pneumonia was common and the pleural cavity was likely to become infected; the anaesthetic was difficult to administer; and so on[18]. Most of these he attributed to the artificial respiration; quite correctly, in fact, but without realizing that had he been a little less energetic with his pressure, the hazards could largely have been avoided. His firm conviction that positive-pressure anaesthesia was actively harmful influenced others when he became famous, and held back progress along what we now know to be the right lines.

If positive pressure on the inside would not work, perhaps, Sauerbruch reasoned, negative pressure from the outside might be effective.

'My first apparatus was very simple,' he wrote[19],'a glass cylinder closed at each end with sheets of gutta-percha. At one end were three holes (two small and one large), at the other just one larger opening. The experimental animal was pulled through the two larger openings so that it lay with its head protruding at one end and its lower abdomen and hind legs at the other. The thorax and upper abdomen were inside the cylinder. After inserting the instruments I would need, I passed my hands through the two smaller holes. All the openings were then hermetically sealed with rubber bands and adhesive material. My assistant withdrew the air from the cylinder through a tube until a negative pressure of 10mm of mercury obtained inside the cylinder. Both sides of the chest were opened; the lungs did not collapse and the animal's breathing continued undisturbed.' Then, as if to emphasize the success of the experiment, one of the gutta-percha sheets tore, the dog's lungs collapsed, and it died violently trying to breathe.

Sauerbruch next used rubber sheets for closing the ends, and showed conclusively that the chest could be widely opened with safety. Greatly encouraged, he had his technician build a little chamber in which he and his assistant could sit at either side of the table, totally enclosed, with only the dog's head outside. A suction pump was used to create and control the negative pressure in such a way that the air remaining inside was exchanged every four minutes. Even though it became very humid and the temperature rose by several degrees, he found he could work inside for more than two hours without too great discomfort. With a bigger chamber such as would be necessary for operations on human beings, he hoped these problems would be overcome.

But before moving on to this expensive idea, he decided to reverse the positions by putting the animal's head in the chamber and *raising* the pressure inside – in other words, back to a positive pressure but without the bellows. Although he and his assistant worked in normal atmospheric conditions, the anaesthetist had to be inside with the animal's head. At the end of the first experiment, with things this way round, the unfortunate anaesthetist staggered out completely overcome by the chloroform vapour. This decided Sauerbruch: the method was just not practical, and he was now firmly convinced that positive pressure was unphysiological. There was a negative pressure inside the chest and, in his view, this demanded a negative pressure cabinet to maintain the normal physiological workings.

By now Mikulicz was satisfied with the merits of the negative pressure chamber and had ordered a large one to be built for human operations. However, before this was ready, the two surgeons went to a Congress of the German Society for Surgery early in April, 1904. Both read papers. Sauerbruch's was a straightforward account of his work[20]; Mikulicz speculated on the revolution the chamber would cause in thoracic surgery; perhaps, he said, it would even allow operations to be performed on the heart[21]. In his paper Mikulicz also mentioned their experiments with high pressure but only to condemn them as unphysiological.

The next two speakers were Ludolph Brauer and Walther Petersen from Heidelberg – they, it will be remembered, had been concerned with the operation of cardiolysis in pericardial disease. Sauerbruch knew what they were going to discuss, for Brauer had a short while earlier published work on the high-pressure method which he had described as an improvement on Sauerbruch's technique[22,23]. As may well be imagined. Sauerbruch did not like this at all, and was prepared to defend his views to the last ditch. He was also incensed because Petersen had visited Breslau and seen the negative-pressure chamber in action, although he had been told nothing about the high-pressure experiments. The stage was set for a battle over priorities.

Brauer acknowledged his debt to Sauerbruch for starting his train of thought but emphasized that he and Petersen had worked out their high-pressure technique completely on their own[24]. He had foreseen the problems a chamber would create for the anaesthetist, and also the difficulties of having the patient's head and anaesthetist's hands only in the chamber. His solution, therefore, was to do away both with the chamber and with a pump for inflating the lungs: he created a tracheostomy through which he passed a tube connected to an oxygen cylinder in such a way that the oxygen flowed over a flask of ether before entering the lungs. The pressure of oxygen flow kept the lungs inflated and the flow could also be regulated so as to prevent overinflation.

Petersen, the surgeon of the pair, had used this method successfully in animals, and he and Brauer felt sure it was a better answer to the problem of the open thorax than the expensive and complicated negative-pressure chamber[25]. They were nearly correct in this, although much water had to flow under the bridge before positive-pressure anaesthesia was generally adopted; but, as it turned out, their work was a tributary rather than part of the mainstream of future events.

Sauerbruch, naturally, did not agree with them; he could hardly be expected to, as it would mean all his hard work had been brought to naught before it was fairly off the ground. He reacted strongly to the Heidelberg men's papers and the subsequent discussion was acrimonious[26]. In the end he came away with the credit for the basic idea, but with both sides saying that history would show who was right.

This whole episode probably explains Sauerbruch's subsequent blind determination to prove his cabinet and to see no good, only danger, in positive-pressure techniques.

In June, 1904, a glass chamber, large enough to walk around in and equipped with a telephone, was ready. Animal experiments had gone off without a hitch, but the suction apparatus failed during the first operation on a human patient. However, during the next few weeks Mikulicz and Sauerbruch carried out more than a dozen technically successful operations on lungs and oesophaguses. Despite the size, however, the temperature inside the cabinet still became unpleasantly high and there was the disadvantage that the patient could not be moved because of the airtight join around his neck[27]. Nevertheless, intrathoracic operations could now be undertaken in conditions which gave the surgeon a degree of confidence he might not otherwise have felt.

Then disaster struck. Almost exactly a year later Mikulicz died of stomach cancer – a disease he had done so much to alleviate – and Sauerbruch was deprived of his sponsor. He had hoped he might be promoted to Mikulicz's job, but this was not to be. Even worse, though, the new professor had little interest in chest surgery and had brought with him his two assistants. Sauerbruch was out in the cold. For five more years he held a variety of posts in none of which could he raise the money or enthusiasm for building a cabinet. Then in 1910 he was appointed to the chair of surgery in Zurich. Here, patients with chest troubles gathered to enjoy the clear Swiss mountain air, and a thoracic surgeon was welcomed with open arms. Sauerbruch at last was his own master; with a new cabinet he went from strength to strength and his fame spread throughout the world. After the First World War he moved to Munich and there constructed a perfect negative-pressure chamber. But it was destined to lie idle: even Sauerbruch's stubbornness could no longer hold out against positive-pressure methods.

So back we must go to the 1890s in France. In 1891, Tuffier had successfully removed the apex of a lung for tuberculosis[28]; he described his anaesthetic technique five years later as artificial respiration by insufflation, and to this end he had designed an improved endotracheal tube with an inflatable cuff[29]. At the same period two other Frenchmen, Quénu and Longuet[30], were working at the problem of lung surgery using dogs as their experimental animal. They realized there were two ways of equalizing the pressures and preventing the lungs from collapsing. One was to reduce the pressure outside the thorax (thus they had the idea before Sauerbruch) and the other was to increase the pressure inside the airways. They decided on the second, and achieved it by putting the animal's head in an airtight bag under pressure. Although there were difficulties, the technique did give them good conditions for operating on the lungs.

The next step was Brauer's positive-pressure method, but this, as we have seen, necessitated a tracheostomy. An alternative was an airtight face mask for administering the anaesthetic under pressure; this had the disadvantage of inflating the stomach and also meant that secretions could not be removed from the respiratory tract.

In 1907, two more Frenchmen, Barthélemy and Dufour[31] of Nancy, began the movement that brought the insufflation method to general notice. They passed a thin rubber catheter down to the bifurcation of the trachea (the point where the windpipe divides into the two main bronchi to the lungs); in the course of the tube was a hand bulb. A mixture of chloroform and air was delivered through the tube, and each time the patient breathed in the anaesthetist squeezed the bulb. Expiration took place up the trachea around the outside of the catheter.

The following year Franz Volhard[32] of Munich drew attention to the problem of carbon dioxide elimination. He found he could keep animals alive for only a short time by continuous insufflation of oxygen down the trachea. What was needed, he said, was a rhythmic inflation of the lungs with oxygen to give the carbon dioxide an opportunity to be expelled. And he devised a machine for doing this. Although Volhard's work inspired others to continue experimenting, the essence of his technique tended to be lost to sight. For instance, in 1909, a notable paper was published by Samuel James Meltzer and

John Auer[33], of the Rockefeller Institute, New York, in which they reported their finding that respiration could, in animals paralysed by the intravenous injection of curare, be carried on by keeping the lungs continuously inflated with air 'by the Brauer method of over pressure'. Once again, a tracheostomy was needed, as they found an O'Dwyer tube did not give consistent results. They also noted that, to ensure the exchange of gases, two tubes had to be put in the trachea, one for air to enter and the other for it to leave.

This paper aroused widespread interest and in 1910 the underlying principle was adapted to human anaesthesia by Charles Elsberg[34], who, among other things, used an endotracheal tube introduced under direct vision with a laryngoscope. An apparent advantage of this endotracheal insufflation anaesthesia was the absence of undue movements of the lungs which had previously hampered operations. Yet it did mean that the lungs were distended, unfortunately not an ideal feature for the surgeon. But worst of all was the problem of carbon dioxide, and this went largely unappreciated.

For a few years this method of anaesthesia was far more favoured than the endotracheal inhalational technique for such few lung operations as were performed. Tuffier's views on the matter in 1913[35] were that the operator should use whichever he was most familiar with or preferred, thus emphasizing the lack of understanding in those days of gaseous exchange in the lungs. Nevertheless the flag of inhalational positive-pressure anaesthesia was being kept flying, notably by Kuhn. Yet he and other enthusiasts had to contend with some pretty devastating criticism. There was Sauerbruch for instance, whose opinions found much support around this period. Positive pressure, it was said, reversed the normal respiratory rhythm; it forced air into the lung tissues; it caused the right side of the heart to dilate; and it lowered the body temperature by excessive evaporation. Only after the First World War did the situation begin to clarify.

Two anaesthetists, Ivan Magill and Edgar Stanley Rowbotham, were working at Sir Harold Gillies's plastic surgery hospital at Sidcup, in Kent. Here great work was being done for the casualties of the war whose faces were badly burned or wounded. Reconstruction operations were likely to take a long time, and anaesthetic face masks obviously could not be used; endotracheal anaesthesia was essential to leave the face free for the surgeon. At first Magill and Rowbotham employed the insufflation method, but soon they found this left a lot to be desired, despite the claims made for it: carbon dioxide elimination was poor (as Volhard had shown 10 or more years previously); secretions could be inhaled, and if the return flow became obstructed the lungs could blow up quite alarmingly. Their first move was to do what Meltzer and Auer had done and pass a second tube down the trachea to allow the gases to escape. But why two tubes? Why not a single wide-bore one? And so a single endotracheal tube was what they used; and with this they reverted to the positive-pressure inhalational technique with bellows, which proved far more physiological and gave rise to fewer postoperative complications in the lungs[36]. At last the battle was over and all that remained were modifications and improvements, of which an important one was Magill's invention in 1936 of a method of intermittent suction to remove secretions in the air passages[37]. He simply passed a catheter down the inside of the endotracheal tube.

Carbon dioxide was still a problem. Because of its presence, all the expired air had to be breathed into the atmosphere – that is, it was an open system. If it could be disposed of, the anaesthetic system could become closed with a saving of the agent used and a greater control of respiration, which meant the patient could rebreathe, and oxygen and anaesthetic agent could be introduced into the system as required. Help was not far off. In 1915 an American, Dennis Jackson, had performed successful rebreathing experiments on animals using sodium hydrate and calcium hydrate to absorb the carbon dioxide[38]. Ralph Milton Waters[39] of Minnesota, in 1924, provided some finishing touches and the carbon dioxide absorption technique was added to clinical anaesthetic practice.

These advances still did not solve the problem of the actual administration of the anaesthetic, and it was not until 1938 that the answer was seen to lie in some apparatus that would give good control of the respiration. To meet this need, Clarence Crafoord invented a machine[40], but in 1941 Michael Dennis Nosworthy, a British anaesthetist, achieved the same effect by intermittently squeezing the anaesthetic bag with his hand[41]. With these techniques respiration could be assisted or controlled with great accuracy, and the needs of the surgeon met relatively easily.

Finally, by paralysing the patient's muscles, the anaesthetist can obtain complete control of his breathing. This was a bonus, for the primary purpose of the paralysing drugs was to relax the muscles of the body for the surgeon's benefit. In days gone by, the surgeon doing a major operation on the abdomen was constantly crying for more relaxation of the abdominal muscles; the anaesthetist would do his best with the anaesthetic agents at his disposal but his difficulty was often that adequate surgical relaxation meant too deep an anaesthesia. Then, in 1942, Harold Griffith and Enid Johnson of Montreal introduced muscular paralysis as an anaesthetic technique by the injection of a purified preparation of curare[42]. For many centuries this drug has been used by South American Indians to tip their arrowheads; the victim dies from paralysis of the muscles of respiration. In 1595, Sir Walter Raleigh brought the drug to Europe, but it was not until the 19th century that its properties were studied by the great French physiologist, Claude Bernard[43,44]. Subsequently it was used in physiological experiments, such as those of Meltzer and Auer on insufflation anaesthesia. Since 1942 a number of preparations, with two main different modes of action, have been introduced to provide muscular relaxation during surgery.

This digression into the realm of anaesthesia shows how important the subject is to chest and heart surgery. Although surgeons could, and did, operate inside the chest from the 1890s onward, they did so in most difficult circumstances and with only the most confused and hazy notions of what was going on. In the 1920s, light began to dawn and techniques to improve. But it was the 1940s, with the urgency provided by the Second World War, that saw conditions really take on a favourable shape. By this time, too, blood transfusion, another essential to modern cardiac surgery, had come into its own, and the antibiotic era had started. Real progress in cardiac surgery had to wait until the scientific stage was set. Yet this did not stop men of the calibre of Tuffier from lifting the edge of the curtain to show what the future held.

9

THE CURTAIN RISES

July 13, 1912. Tuffier had at last decided to put his experimental work to the test in a human patient. The decision had not been reached lightly; for some while the physician in charge of a young man had been begging the surgeon to operate – a measure of the confidence his colleagues placed in Tuffier's ability and judgment. But Tuffier held off; he had to be sure of what he was attempting, and he could only be so on the evidence brought to him through his stethoscope and by his observation and examination of the patient. He had no special tests he could rely on to give a clear picture of what was going on inside the heart. He could only guess intelligently as to the effect of operation.

The 26-year-old patient had a severe and progressive stenosis of the aortic valve[1,2]. Whether Tuffier was aware of just what he was undertaking is uncertain. But we now know that the aortic valve is the most difficult and problematic of the heart's valves to operate on. Maybe, though, he thought it would be easier than tackling a mitral valve because he could reach it through the aorta without delving into the inside of the heart.

Whatever his thoughts, he was no fool. He knew full well the responsibility he was accepting. With his experience it needed great courage to operate, and this quality he certainly did not lack. And so on that summer's day in 1912 his operating theatre was prepared. Immaculately clean and every detail attended to. His friend, Alexis Carrel, was there to give advice, encouragement and moral support.

The patient was brought to the theatre and anaesthetized; Tuffier set to work. He opened the chest and exposed the heart and the great vessels that enter and leave it. Then he stopped. He laid down his scalpel and looked over his mask at Carrel. The same thought was going through both their minds. This was the point of no return. Should he take the tremendous step of incising the aorta and reaching the valve directly? Might there not be another and safer approach? The murmur of their voices was the only sound in that theatre for the next few minutes.

Then Tuffier returned to his task. But the scalpel still lay on the draped tray. Instead, he grasped the heart to steady it and with his index finger invaginated the wall of the aorta a short distance above the valve. By pushing his finger downwards, with the intact wall in front of it, he reached the diseased valve and, although unable to penetrate far into the orifice, he slowly dilated the narrow ring of the valve. As he remarked afterwards he was 'most impressed with the extremely lively vibrations' he felt.

He removed his finger, again looked at Carrel and nodded. This was all he would do. Without doubt he had improved the flow of blood through the stenotic valve and that was what he had set out to do. Twelve days later the patient returned to his home in Belgium[1], but he was not lost sight of, for in July, 1920, Tuffier reported to the fifth congress of the International Surgical Society that he and Carrel had seen the man three months previously and that he had been in fair spirits, having been temporarily improved by the operation[3].

The interest taken by the general public in heart operations has undergone a quite remarkable change since those days. Had Tuffier made this advance today he would have been feted internationally and appeared on the television screens of the world. As it was, his achievement aroused very little enthusiasm even among the medical profession. They simply were not ready, and there were no mass communications media eager to whip up excitement, despite the fact that the next and perhaps more dramatic operation followed within a few months. It also took place in France.

Eugène Louis Doyen, the surgeon on this occasion, was a flamboyant character whose operating technique was quite dazzling. In the last decade of the 19th century he had been instrumental in popularizing the bypass operation of gastroenterostomy for peptic ulcer[4]; but he was really a hangover from the early days of modern surgery when surgeons, although resourceful and often brilliant, were spectacular in a way that would not be tolerated today. Perhaps it was a characteristic forced on them to cover up the deficiencies of their adolescent art. They were not unlike the Italian opera singers of the same period who revelled in showing off their vocal skill and who had to be brought to heel to prevent that art-form from deteriorating. However, by the first decade of the 20th century, surgeons as a rule no longer played to the gallery; they had learnt the merits of painstaking, conscientious operation. But not Doyen. He delighted in the spectacular and when the opportunity to operate on the heart presented itself, he seized it with both hands. Nevertheless, he was not unprepared, although the amount of experimental work he had done could in no way compare with that of Tuffier.

A 20-year-old girl had what Doyen had diagnosed as a stricture of the infundibulum of the pulmonary artery. This is a narrowing of the outflow tract of the right ventricle before the flow of blood from the ventricle reaches the pulmonary valve and the pulmonary artery proper. It is a congenital defect. The girl was severely ill, and Doyen thought that in view of the satisfactory results of heart suture it should be possible to try to section the orifice of the valve, and for this purpose he devised a special tenotome (strictly speaking, an instrument for dividing tendons).

He introduced the tenotome through the right ventricle and blindly cut the obstruction. However, he was not rewarded by an increased flow of blood to the lungs, the cyanosis remained and the girl died later that morning. The postmortem produced some interesting findings: the stenosis was 'quite other than had been expected'. From the description given it appears that there was no infundibular stenosis, but the valve itself was reduced to a 'septum' in the middle of which was a small orifice of 4mm with inflamed edges. In addition, there was an interventricular septal defect. This shows how important it is to have a complete picture of the defects in the heart before operating – something that Doyen was denied. But even had he been correct in his diagnosis we know now that what he planned was a risky adventure, since blind relief of infundibular stenosis is quite likely to damage the papillary muscles of the tricuspid valve and lead to tricuspid incompetence.

In his report[5,6], Doyen stated that he had studied the problems of mitral stenosis and had worked out a precise technique for its surgical treatment. What he had in mind, and whether it would have succeeded we shall never know, for he died three years later, in 1916, at the age of 57.

The First World War then intervened and gave surgeons other problems to think about. It also brought a geographical shift, for it drove the heart out of the adventurous French, and the United States came to the fore. The first indication of their interest was a paper from St Louis, Missouri, in 1922. Evarts Graham and Duff Allen had decided that if they were to operate satisfactorily they must be able to see what they were doing. So they invented a cardioscope. Because blood is opaque, the essential feature of the instrument was a lens at the very tip that would come in direct contact with the desired structure. Admittedly the view was somewhat fuzzy, but it did allow them to see where they were. The knife with which they proposed to cut the stenosed valve was carried alongside the tube of the cardioscope and had a sharp blade set at right angles to the lens[7].

At first, in their experiments on dogs, they introduced the instrument through the left ventricle, but later changed to an approach through the left atrial appendage. The mortality rate among their animals was very low, yet when they came to try the operation clinically in August, 1923, the 31-year-old woman died on the table before the cardioscope was even used[8]. Such was the feeling among their colleagues that they were unable to get another patient.

Elliott Cutler and his two assistants, Claude Beck and Samuel Levine, were more fortunate, doubtless because their first case was a success, but it was the only one to be so out of their seven attempts. Cutler also had the good fortune to inherit a fairly long tradition of experimental heart surgery since he was working in Harvey Cushing's laboratory at Harvard, where, it will be remembered, work had started in 1905, and had continued on and off ever since. For instance, in 1913, Lawrence Rhea and Isaac Walker had devised a fairly sophisticated instrument on the lines of a cystoscope (a thin tube with lenses for examining the interior of the urinary bladder). It had an electric bulb at the tip and, just behind the bulb, a knife which could be operated by the surgeon. These two research workers had not published their results because no animals survived the experiments[9]. When Cutler fell heir to their instrument and tried to use it, he realized why they had failed – he could not see what he was doing through the blood, and so he abandoned the idea for the time being.

Cutler was, nevertheless, determined to find a surgical solution to the problem of mitral stenosis. He reasoned that mitral incompetence was a far less serious condition than mitral stenosis. Patients with incompetence, he said, often lived to an advanced age, whereas those with stenosis uncommonly reached full maturity and, when their disease was fully established, their activities were severely and permanently curtailed. His experiments on animals bore out these views. Accordingly, he planned to cut part of the stenosed valve to allow the blood to flow through more freely, even though this meant deliberately producing a moderate degree of insufficiency. (Here we must remember that the patients he was considering were late cases with thickened, hardened, and often calcified valves. The procedures used at a later date whereby the competence of the valves could be retained would have been inapplicable.)

So Cutler began to experiment on dogs, cats and goats, using a tenotome type of knife, similar to those used by Klebs and Cushing in the past. Then on May 20, 1923, feeling sufficiently prepared, he operated on an 11-year-old girl who was bedridden, extremely short of breath and coughing up such alarming quantities of blood that she was expected to die at any moment. The little girl's parents had had the risks explained to them and they knew that no similar operation had ever been performed. But they gladly gave their permission.

The operation, at the Peter Bent Brigham Hospital, Boston, lasted one-and-a-quarter hours. The incision was an elaboration of Milton's sternotomy, known as the Duval-Barasty (after two Frenchmen) in which the breastbone was split down the middle and the cut continued to two inches (5cm) above the umbilicus. This gave a full exposure of the heart and enabled the pleura to be dissected out of harm's way without opening its cavities. The tenotome was inserted through the left ventricle[10].

The girl lived for another four-and-a half-years, 'apparently improved'. The signs of mitral stenosis did not disappear and her activities were still restricted, but she coughed up no more blood and gained weight. Her final illness was short and she died suddenly in November, 1927. The postmortem examination showed that without doubt the mitral orifice had been enlarged by the incision[11].

Moderately pleased with his success, Cutler operated twice more during the next few months, using the tenotome, but the patients died 10 and 20 hours afterwards. Examination of their hearts showed him that the instrument was insufficient for the task it had to perform, as it had to be manipulated at a great mechanical disadvantage. He therefore set about designing a strong instrument which he called a cardiovalvulotome. This was a circular tube, with a blunted point that was separated from the rest of the tube by the cutting mechanism. The instrument was introduced through the left ventricle and the point passed through the valve into the atrium. By operating the spring-loaded handle, the point closed onto the body of the tube, cutting off a segment of the valve.

Two more patients were operated on with this new cardiovalvulotome, but they only survived for seven and three days. In the latter case Cutler had been unable to reach the stenotic valve and this made him feel it would be unwise to attempt any more operations on human beings until he could be sure of placing the instrument accurately against the valve[11]. By this time he had read Graham and Allen's paper[7], which gave him the clue to the design of a new cardioscopic valvulotome – a 'see-and-cut' instrument that he used successfully on animals but one that was never applied to human surgery[12].

In retrospect[13], Cutler said that all the four fatal cases had features that made them unsuitable for surgery: advanced disease of the heart muscle; adherent pericardium; unexplained attacks of fever before operation that probably led to the fatal pneumonia; and another unexplained fever which had been thought due to pulmonary tuberculosis. 'These experiences, however,' said Cutler, 'had to be learned for the first time; there were no previous ideas to guide us.'

Although we shall return to America for Cutler's last two operations, the spotlight now falls once again on Europe. For some years Strickland Goodall, a cardiologist and physiologist at The Middlesex Hospital, London, had been working on the problem of the surgical relief of mitral stenosis and with the help of Lambert Rogers had done many operations on cadavers, using a specially designed double-edged knife to slit the fused cusps of the valve. They thrashed out the relative merits and demerits of entering through the ventricle or the atrium and concluded in favour of the atrial approach[14]. They saw quite clearly that the mitral stenosis could be relieved surgically, but emphasized the great importance of practice in perfecting the technique. (An alternative method which they mentioned was to bypass the valve by a tubed sleeve of pericardium carried outside the heart from the left atrium to ventricle. This, however, they did not pursue.) It is, perhaps, an indication of the authors' assessment of the climate of opinion in Britain that their report was published in 1924 in an American journal and in the *New Zealand Medical Journal*[15] – this latter may seem a strange choice but maybe the fact that both were born and raised in Australia had something to do with it. When Goodall died in 1934 at the age of 59 his obituary notice in the *British Medical Journal* contained no mention of this work nor, more surprisingly, did an accompanying note written by Lambert Rogers[16].

The next episode was a momentous one in the history of heart surgery, although not appreciated as such for many a year afterwards. On May 6, 1925, an operation a generation ahead of its time was performed at The London Hospital by Henry Souttar, a general surgeon, whose name until after the Second World War was far more familiarly associated with a tube passed through growths of the oesophagus to keep the gullet open. Lilian Hine, born and bred in Bethnal Green, in the East End of London, was the patient. She was one of six children of a tuberculous labourer and in early childhood had suffered from asthma and bronchitis. She had also had three attacks of acute rheumatism. At the age of 10 she was admitted to The London Hospital under Lord Dawson of Penn with Sydenham's chorea and rheumatic carditis affecting the mitral valve. In 1925, when she was 15, she was admitted again with mitral stenosis, shortness of breath, coughing up blood, and all the signs of heart failure. By some miracle the physicians decided to give her the chance, remote though it was, of benefiting from surgery, and her case was discussed at length with Souttar.

The anaesthetic was ether vapour given by intratracheal insufflation, the pressure of insufflation being increased as necessary to keep the left lung expanded when the pleural cavity was opened. Throughout the operation Lily's breathing caused no problems. Souttar entered the chest by incising along the fourth space between the ribs on the left, up beside the sternum and then along the first space. After dividing the appropriate ribs, he turned the whole rectangular flap (including pleura) outward, and opened the pericardium. After a moment's pause while the heart-beat settled, he clamped off the atrial appendage (a small ear-like pouch of the atrium which nature might almost have included in the anatomy of the heart for the benefit of surgeons). He then incised the appendage between two stay sutures and, removing the clamp, inserted a finger right down to the ventricle. The finger passed easily through the valve – more easily than Souttar had expected because it indicated a degree of regurgitation he later described as 'terrific'. He had been intending to divide the valve cusps with a hernia bistoury, but in view of the regurgitation he decided against it. So apart from this digital exploration and the division of a few adhesions in the process, nothing was done to the valve. Nevertheless, this proved sufficient to ease the stenosis.

Then came '10 secs touch and go'. As he was withdrawing his finger, the lower stay suture tore out and he was faced with a 'voluminous gush of blood'. Keeping his head, Souttar gripped the appendage and squeezed it against the atrium; a clamp was put on and crisis averted. The operation was then completed without further incident. It had taken just one minute over the hour[17].

Although Lily was improved subjectively and could do more, circumstances were against her, for the next year she had another attack of rheumatic fever and thereafter spent a lot of time in bed with heart failure and bronchitis. In 1932 she was admitted for the last time in severe heart failure and atrial fibrillation. In July of that year she developed a hemiplegia and lost her power of speech. She died three weeks later from multiple cerebral emboli which had probably come from clots in the atrium[18].

Even though the operation had been a success, the physicians got cold feet and would not let Souttar have another patient to operate on. It seems they reverted to type, and after their one lapse continued in their unshakable belief that the state of the heart muscle, not of the valves, was the salient factor in rheumatic disease of the heart. The performance was not to be repeated for 20 years.

Cutler's work had earned him editorial notice in the *British Medical Journal*[19]; admittedly it was a pretty noncommittal note, but Souttar's paper resulted only in four letters[20], [21], [22], [23]. These were all congratulatory in tone and included one from Goodall and Rogers referring to their previous articles, and one from Samways who could not resist the temptation of drawing attention to his correspondence in the *Lancet* a quarter of a century before; progress, he said, had been slower than he thought it would have been.

Meanwhile news of Cutler's doings had reached Germany, and on November 14, 1925, Bruno Oskar Pribram, of Berlin, operated for what appeared to be a clear-cut case of mitral stenosis in a woman of 38 who was steadily losing ground under medical treatment. He followed Cutler's technique, and with a cardiovalvulotome succeeded in excising a portion of the stenotic valve. The immediate results were good, but on the third day fever developed and the patient died on the fifth from pneumonia. Postmortem examination revealed the cause of the failure: there was a considerable degree of aortic stenosis, but the signs and symptoms of the mitral lesion had obscured this. In addition there was a fresh vegetative endocarditis (an infection) of the aortic valve. The mitral valve was, however, clear of infection and the heart wound had healed perfectly. As Pribram observed, this showed how vitally important was precise diagnosis, and how difficult it was to achieve it in those days[24].

And now back to Cutler for the last two operations of this era on the mitral valve – and, not to put too fine a point on it, what a shambles they turned out to be. The first of these (his sixth) was on a man of 34 and took place on December 8, 1926. Cutler inserted his cardiovalvulotome through the left ventricle, as in his earlier operations, but this time had great difficulty in finding the valve orifice. Eventually he managed to get the instrument in place and excised a segment of the valve. The man died 15 hours later. Despite his previous concern about placing the instrument accurately, so obviously justified by this operation, Cutler did not use the cardioscope because the vision it gave was 'so slight'[11].

For his last mitral valvectomy, on April 15, 1928, Cutler changed his tactics. This time he went in through the atrium, as he believed it would give an easier approach to the valve, but again he had difficulty placing the cardiovalvulotome. The 47-year-old man survived for only three hours[11].

In their paper, written in 1929 from the department of surgery of the Western Reserve University School of Medicine, Cleveland, he and Claude Beck analysed their own experience and reviewed all the operations to that year. A sense of puzzled despondency is apparent right from the beginning: the subtitle was 'Final report of all surgical cases.' Cutler admitted that his approach to the ventricle through the long mid-line sternum-splitting incision might put an unnecessarily heavy strain on an already weak patient, but in its favour were the facts that the ventricle presented itself immediately in the incision and that the pleural cavities were not opened. Other experimenters had reported that introducing the instrument through the ventricle was liable to induce irregularities in the heart-beat, but apparently these were not so serious in Cutler's experience.

His dislike of opening the pleura influenced his views on the atrial approach. He agreed that the opening in the chest was smaller; the trouble came from the left atrium lying too deeply. To get at it, the surgeon needed either to enter a pleural cavity, or to use a curved instrument. However, entering through the atrium had the advantage that the instrument tended to be funnelled towards the valve, whereas just the opposite applied with a ventricular approach. The surgeon came to the valve from the wrong side of the 'funnel' – towards its narrow end – and had to contend with the beating ventricle and all the structural irregularities on the inside of that chamber.

The authors' despair became yet more evident when they considered the total situation. The useful information derived from the 12 cases was meagre, but the fact remained that the only patients surviving at that time were those two (Tuffier's and Souttar's) who had merely had a finger dilatation of a valve. Could this be, they asked, because only a small change had been made in the state of the valve? Was the human heart unable to endure the sudden change from long-standing severe stenosis to marked incompetence? Experiments had been unable to help them because it had so far proved impossible to produce surgically-treatable mitral stenosis in animals[11].

But guidance was on its way had Cutler stayed the course a little longer. In the department of experimental surgery at the University of Edinburgh, William C Wilson was working on this very problem, and after a number of false starts managed to give dogs mitral stenosis by fixing strips of rolled pericardium across the orifice. Then after a suitable interval, he operated to relieve the obstruction. For this purpose he designed an operating cardioscope. The light was reflected from a bulb in the handle; a ring trapped the valve against the distal window of the tube and a circular shear cut off the trapped part of the valve. With this instrument inserted through the atrium he could take a number of bites without fear of losing the excised tissue. (Cutler's instrument allowed one bite only.) In his paper, published in 1930, Wilson noted that the experiments were too few to draw conclusions, but they indicated that the heart could not easily withstand a sudden change from stenosis to incompetence[25].

We now know the truth of this, for severe incompetence created at operation for mitral stenosis will lead either to death from congestive heart failure or to a poor result. But, as we have seen, it was not the only explanation for the failures up to the 1930s. Most were due to associated conditions and in Cutler's last two cases the trauma of the operations played a major role.

Although the story we have been following as it developed through heart wounds and the early experiments and operations represents the main stream of cardiac surgery, there were other facets developing alongside, all serving to keep the subject alive through difficult times. These, too, often ran into troubled waters, as happened with pulmonary embolus and cardiac arrest. Yet an interesting aspect of the main stream during the 1920s and 1930s was the isolated nature of much of the work. Apart from Cutler's sustained effort lasting for most of a decade and the tail end of Tuffier's remarkable career, the few participants made only a single appearance in the limelight and the whole period lacked continuity.

But by the end of the 1930s the rumblings of a great revolution were heard. Experimental work that was to prove the foundation of modern cardiac surgery was beginning, and young men, destined to perform operations then undreamed of, were starting out on their careers; some were not yet qualified. The first indication of what the future held in store came in 1937. On March 16, John W Strieder of Boston attempted to close a patent ductus arteriosus in a young woman with subacute bacterial endocarditis[26]. The infecting organism was *Streptococcus viridans*, and in those pre-penicillin days recovery was uncommon. 'Because there was nothing to offer in the way of medical treatment, the idea of attempting to obliterate the patent ductus by surgical means had some appeal.' The reason underlying the proposition was the fact that a heart with a congenital anomaly is more liable to subacute bacterial endocarditis than a normal one. Therefore if the ductus could be closed, the infection might resolve. It was indeed an heroic measure, but C McK was only 22 and seriously ill.

At operation, Strieder could only partially close the ductus with a series of plicating sutures, as its posterior end was bound to the right pulmonary artery by fibrous tissue – a result of extensive vegetations in the artery. All went well postoperatively until the evening of the fifth day, when the patient died from acute dilatation of the stomach.

Then, 18 months later, Robert Edward Gross, also of Boston, carried out the operation that announced the arrival of a new era. On August 26, 1938, he successfully closed a patent ductus in a seven-and-a-half-year-old girl. There was no infection on this occasion; the closure was done as an end in itself[27]. Why this operation should stand out as a landmark is difficult to say; there is just something about the 'feel' of it that separates it from all that had gone before and stamps it as undeniably modern. The surgical world was at last ready, and before long other surgeons followed Gross's lead. Soon ligation or division of a patent ductus was found to prevent bacterial infection of the heart as well as prolonging life. The mortality was low and within three decades had fallen to less than one percent in children who had not developed complications.

But before surgeons grasped the full implications of what was happening, another war broke out, and before we return to see how the main stream flowed onwards there are one or two tributaries to be explored, not the least important of which were the discoveries that led to improved diagnosis.

10

CARDIAC CATHETERIZATION

Without techniques for accurate diagnosis and assessment before operation, cardiac surgery could not have progressed much beyond the state at which we left it in the last chapter. Operations frequently came unstuck because the unexpected was found, and it was all too apparent that existing diagnostic methods were inadequate. Information given by the patient's history, by physical examination, by the electrocardiogram, and by plain x-rays was insufficiently detailed, although it met the requirements of the fairly limited medical treatment then available. But medical cardiologists themselves were beginning to feel restricted, and slowly their opposition to cardiac surgery faded as they realized that the demands of the surgeons would bring rich rewards to them also.

For centuries physicians had felt the pulse and built up its study into a complex pseudo-science. Although in the Edwin Smith papyrus[1] of ancient Egypt a feeble pulse was described as a 'heart too weak to speak', it would be wrong to imagine that the pulse told doctors anything about the state of the heart until Harvey discovered that the blood circulated. Before his time the pulse was in some way thought to be due to the bounding liveliness of the pneuma contained in the arteries; a minute study of its real and imagined characteristics had therefore great significance in the diagnosis of practically any disease.

In the 18th century Morgagni's work[2] relating the postmortem findings to the symptoms during life altered the whole approach to diagnosis; physicians became concerned with detecting the evidence of pathology in their patients and slowly they evolved methods of achieving this. Leopold Auenbrugger, an Austrian, discovered the value of percussion and published his treatise in 1761[3] although it was not brought to popular notice until 1808 when the Frenchman, Jean-Nicholas Corvisart, published a translation and commentary[4]. Then, in 1819, René-Théophile-Hyacinthe Laënnec[5] invented the stethoscope which completely transformed the diagnosis of chest diseases. At first these advances were applied to diseases of the lungs, but as time went on their importance in diagnosing heart conditions was realized; the size and outline of the heart was studied by percussion and the heart sounds and murmurs, heard through the stethoscope, were identified and correlated with the underlying pathology.

The second half of the 19th century saw a tremendous amount of work on the heart and circulation culminating, from the practical, diagnostic, point of view, in the invention of the electrocardiograph. In the 1880s the electrical impulses produced by the heart had been discovered and in 1889 Augustus Waller[6], a general practitioner in Kensington, London, decided to measure them, but unfortunately the recording apparatus was not sufficiently sensitive to give a true result. The necessary accuracy was achieved a few years later, in 1902, by Willem Einthoven[7], of Leyden, who connected the electrodes to a string galvanometer. It was he who gave the initials P,Q,R,S and T to the waves that are still used today. Initially the apparatus was extremely cumbersome and the subject had to sit with his feet in a tub of salt solution. The electrocardiograph is now thoroughly sophisticated and, besides there being light portable models, the positions of the numerous skin electrodes are variable so that the maximum information can be obtained.

Nevertheless, what the electrocardiograph can reveal still does not tell the surgeon all he needs to know. One crucial piece of apparatus is the cardiac catheter, for this enables contrast medium to be injected into the heart so that its chambers and vessels can be visualized on the x-ray screen and photographed; it allows the pressures to be measured and samples of blood to be withdrawn from inside the heart for analysis of the gaseous content and tension. It is also the means by which therapeutic interventions can take place within the heart and coronary vessels.

Once again it was the French who showed the way, for as long ago as 1855 they were experimenting with cardiac catheterization. Auguste Chauveau and Etienne Marey[8], two physiologists, were experimenting on the horse (they reckoned the bigger the animal the easier would be their task). Their purpose was to study the intracardiac pressures and find out whether or not all the chambers contracted simultaneously.

For the right side of the heart they used an almost modern appearing catheter inserted through an incision in the jugular vein. The device had two separate tiny sausage-shaped recording balloons (one to lie in the ventricle, the other in the atrium), the tubes from which ran up inside the catheter to pens that recorded the pressure changes on a revolving drum. For the left side of the heart, they used a rigid metal tube which was passed down the carotid artery. The tube had to be rigid as it was being passed against the blood flow.

Next on the scene was Claude Bernard, the great French physiologist and founder of the modern experimental method in medicine. He catheterized the heart and great vessels for biochemical and temperature research on the blood as it entered or left the organs under study. Dogs were his experimental animals, and he had no difficulty passing the catheter through the jugular vein directly into the heart. He also reached the right atrium from below by inserting the catheter through the left femoral vein. The left side of the heart caused him more trouble but, by choosing the correct moment when the aortic valve was open, he succeeded in entering the left ventricle down the left carotid artery[9].

This work was published in 1879, the year after his death at the age of 65. His genius had been recognized during his lifetime for Napoleon III had two laboratories specially built for him and appointed him a senator in 1869. But although his physiological researches set the pace for the years to come, cardiac catheterization did not move outside the laboratory – if it was considered at all, it was believed too dangerous and of no practical application to medicine.

The scene now moves to Germany where this view was shared by Fritz Bleichroder after some experiments in 1905 in which he passed a ureteric catheter through a femoral vein into his own inferior vena cava. As he saw no future for the technique, he did not publish his work at the time and forgot about it until 1912. By then, however, a fundamental change was taking place in medical treatment due to Paul Ehrlich's discovery in 1909 of salvarsan – his so-called 'magic bullet' – as a remedy for syphilis[10]. For the first time chemical substances were seen to have a specific effect on the course of infective diseases; the science of chemotherapy was born.

Bleichroder started thinking[11]. How about getting the appropriate chemical straight to the organ that needed it? He knew it was possible to pass catheters into human blood vessels; now here was a chance to give an experimental exercise a practical purpose. His colleagues, Ernst Unger[12] and Walter Löb[13], agreed with the idea, and after a trial run in which Unger passed a catheter up one of Bleichroder's arm veins to the level of the axilla, they injected a chemical (Collargol) into four women suffering from puerperal sepsis – not into a vein but directly into the aorta through a catheter inserted in the femoral artery. And that was that as far as that particular piece of research went.

Nevertheless, the idea of getting drugs into the body as directly as possible did not die completely; it was thought up again by another German, Werner Forssmann of Eberswalde, in 1929. Forssmann was unaware of Bleichroder's work, but anyway his plan was rather different, as he intended to use cardiac catheterization as a method for giving drugs rapidly in an emergency on the operating table. Amazed at the ease with which he could slip a ureteric catheter up an arm vein and into the right atrium in a cadaver, he asked his assistant to try it on himself, Forssmann. The man reluctantly agreed, but as he was inserting the catheter his nerve failed and his hand started to shake. This was enough for Forssmann. Without further ado he took over and, under local anaesthesia, cut down on a vein in the front of his left elbow and threaded a ureteric catheter through a wide-bore needle already in place in the vein. Then with a mirror rigged up so that he could see the x-ray screen, he manipulated the catheter into the right side of his heart. Still not satisfied, since he wanted an x-ray picture as incontrovertible proof, he walked out of the door and up the stairs to the radiography department, with no discomfort whatsoever. The picture came out excellently and was reproduced in his article[14].

Two years later Forssmann reported on his experiments to obtain contrast x-rays of the heart. In dogs he was successful and got good pictures outlining the cavities by injecting a contrast medium through the catheter, but when he injected the medium through a catheter inserted into his own heart via his femoral vein, the contrast failed to show[15].

Surprisingly quickly after x-rays were discovered by Wilhelm Röntgen in 1895[16], research workers set about finding substances opaque to x-rays and suitable for outlining body cavities. Soon barium was chosen for the stomach and intestines and air for the ventricles of the brain. Certain iodine-containing compounds were found suitable for the air-passages, gallbladder, spinal canal and urinary bladder. All these organs had been visualized in this way by 1922, but the problem of injecting contrast media into blood vessels took longer to overcome. Egas Moniz of Lisbon provided the answer when, in 1927, he obtained pictures of the arteries of the brain[17]. Vessels in other parts of the body were visualized not long afterwards, but the heart itself, the aorta and, in particular, the coronary arteries were a far more difficult proposition. Despite Forssmann's having shown that the heart could safely be catheterized, to others it seemed a major and hazardous undertaking. Contrast media were toxic and in an early stage of development; added to which the site of the studies meant that the medium was rapidly diluted and dispersed.

The essentials of contrast investigations are accuracy, dependability, and reproducibility. If the surgeon cannot have faith in what the x-ray picture shows him, it is no good, no matter how clear and beautiful some of it may appear. For instance, if he is contemplating a coronary artery procedure he must be sure in his mind that a small, absent or blocked coronary artery is what it seems to be and not a technical failure to fill the artery with contrast. Reproducibility means that other people besides the originator must be able to undertake the investigation and get the same satisfactory results.

These essentials took a long time to be fulfilled and it was not until 1938 that George Robb and Israel Steinberg of New York City developed 'A practical method of visualization of the chambers of the heart, the pulmonary circulation, and the great blood vessels in man' as they entitled the first of their articles[18]. They were influenced in their choice of technique by the difficult nature of cardiac catheterization which, they said, had precluded its general use. The right side of the heart had admittedly been outlined by other workers when doing pulmonary arteriography, but only occasionally. Their experiments, which led to consistent results, had begun in January, 1936, on rabbits. By January 30, 1937, they achieved their first successful visualization of the right side of the heart and pulmonary circulation, and by May 23, 1937, of the left chambers and aorta.

Their technique depended on speed and timing. Between 20 and 45ml of Diodrast was injected in less than two seconds into a vein in the patient's raised arm and the film taken 3-5 seconds later[18,19]. The side-effects included a fall in blood pressure, increase in heart rate, and a transient feeling of great heat spreading over the body; but although unpleasant, they did not prevent the technique's being an important landmark in cardiac investigation and one, moreover, that appeared at the right time to encourage surgical progress.

Hard on its heels came another advance which ended the objections to cardiac catheterization and really opened the human heart to physiological examination. In 1941, André Cournand and Hilmert Ranges[20], in New York, passed a radio-opaque catheter into the right atrium under x-ray control without the risks of clotting or psychic effects that had bothered previous experimenters. Their object was to gain information on the blood gasses and thereby gather a great deal of information about the functioning of the heart and lungs. For his work in cardiac physiology, Cournand, who was born in France and educated at Paris University, won, jointly, the Nobel prize for medicine in 1956; his co-laureate was Werner Forssmann.

So, it would seem, the troubles were over. Both sides of the heart could be visualized and the progress of the medium as it passed through the chambers could be monitored on the x-ray screen. Pictures and, later, cine films could be taken. But, unfortunately, it was not good enough for the left side of the heart, as the opacification in the right side and the pulmonary circulation obscured the details when the contrast medium reached the left side.

The story of left ventricular visualization had actually started as far back as March, 1932, with the experiments of two Frenchmen, Henri Reboul and Maurice Racine, on dogs. Realizing that catheterization of the left ventricle (with the apparatus available) could be dangerous to the integrity of the aortic valve, they went straight to the heart of the problem and injected between the ribs directly into both the right and left ventricles. The procedure, carried out under general anaesthesia, did not upset the animals and gave good, consistent results, showing up the first parts of the great vessels as well[21].

But the idea failed to attract attention because the risks of heart puncture were still considered to outweigh the benefits of the information provided, which anyway had no practical application in surgery at that time. Thus there was a hiatus until after the Second World War, when Elmo Ponsdomenech and Virgilio Núñez of Havana reported their work in 1951[22]. They punctured the left ventricle by inserting a trocar under the xiphoid process at the lower end of the sternum. They were aware that they might accidentally hit a coronary vessel, but their experiments on dogs showed their fears to be unfounded. In 30 patients who underwent the procedure 45 times, there were no untoward results and they obtained good pictures. They called the examination cardioangiography from the order in which first the heart and then the aorta were visualized, although it is now more usually referred to as angiocardiography.

Angiocardiography by ventricular puncture was, however, soon ousted from popularity by a new technique of catheterization. In the 1940s the brachial artery had been catheterized on a very few occasions, but the work was abandoned on account of severe arterial spasm. But in 1946 Pedro Fariñas[23], also of Havana, had successfully catheterized the abdominal aorta and obtained good contrast pictures of that part of the aorta and of the iliac arteries. He had dissected out the femoral artery in the thigh and inserted the catheter through a small incision. Fortunately, he had not been troubled by spasm.

Although the technique of retrograde arterial catheterization came into use, no one was really enamoured of it until Sven Seldinger of Stockholm published his method of percutaneous catheterization in 1953[24]. Like so many great advances the idea was simple: the artery is punctured through the skin by a hollow needle; a thin flexible leader or guide-wire is passed down inside the needle and into the artery; the needle is withdrawn; the catheter is threaded over the guide-wire and on into the artery; the guide-wire (which must be long enough to protrude from one end of the catheter as the other passes into the vessel) is withdrawn; the catheter is manipulated on to its destination. The tremendous advantages of the technique are that tiny catheters of the size of the needle's bore can be used, and the artery is not dissected out. Complications remained, however, including the risk of arterial spasm and ventricular fibrillation, but the procedure was practical and became routine.

If the left side of the heart had its problems, they were as nothing compared with the difficulties of visualizing the coronary arteries. The mouths of these are situated in the aortic bulb just above the aortic valve and until 1962 it seemed as if it would be impossible to find a reliable way of getting contrast medium into them. Before then most pictures of the coronary arteries were a bonus on contrast films of the heart and aorta, or if intentionally obtained were inconsistent.

Peter Rousthöi[25] of Stockholm made the earliest deliberate attempts to x-ray the coronary arteries of animals in 1933, and very successful they were too. At first he injected contrast medium directly into the aorta but later he catheterized the aortic bulb through the carotid artery. Then, in the strange way these things seem to happen, interest flagged until 1945 when Stig Radner[26] of Lund in Sweden injected the contrast medium into the ascending aorta but, unlike Rousthöi, he went in through a puncture hole in the sternum. The opacification of the coronary arteries was 'moderate'; unfortunately, complications in two of his five patients made him give up further attempts. Nevertheless in 1948, Jorge Meneses Hoyos and Carlos Gomez del Campo of Mexico City reported that they achieved good pictures of the thoracic aorta, its main branches, and the coronary arteries by injecting 30ml of medium into the aorta through a needle inserted in the space between the second and third ribs just to the left of the sternum[27].

Retrograde arterial catheterization then began to make its presence felt, and in 1952 an encouraging paper was published by two Italians, Lucio di Guglielmo and Mariano Guttadauro[28], working in Stockholm. They passed a catheter through the radial artery (apparently not unduly troubled by spasm) into the ascending aorta and then injected contrast medium. With correct technique and provided there were no adverse pathological conditions such as aortic incompetence, they said it should be possible to obtain 100 percent contrast filling of the coronary arteries.

However, as experience was gathered, it became apparent that different investigators were getting results of different value, and the x-ray pictures by no means always agreed with subsequent findings at operation or postmortem. By the end of the 1950s the possibility of surgical reconstruction of blocked thrombosed coronary arteries stimulated the search for a reliable technique and a variety of modifications were introduced. The simple ones included putting side holes at the end of the catheter and other special design features. The complex ones were aimed at slowing or even stopping the blood flow of the region while the medium was injected[29,30,31]. Methods such as temporarily arresting the heart by injection of acetylcholine and blocking the aorta above the level of the mouths of the coronary arteries by means of an inflatable balloon on the catheter, all had their day which lasted until 1962, when Mason Sones and Earl Shirey[32] of Cleveland showed how to get the contrast medium into the mouths of the coronary arteries.

Between 1956 and 1958 they had studied dogs and human beings and had found it impossible to obtain dependable opacification of the coronary tree with existing methods. So in October, 1958, they made their first deliberate attempts at 'selective' coronary arteriography. With considerable ingenuity they developed a technique whereby they could manoeuvre the tip of the catheter from the brachial artery, under x-ray control, into the immediate area of each coronary orifice – and occasionally they catheterized the orifice itself without harm. Once the catheter was in place they injected a small amount of contrast medium (2-5ml) and watched the filling take place on a screen intensifier; a permanent record was taken on a cine film at 60 frames a second.

The technique is time-consuming and calls for an experienced team but it gives invaluable information and is an essential investigation before coronary bypass or angioplasty. It has also given insight into the results of operations to improve the circulation to the heart muscle in angina pectoris – operations that had their beginning long before any of these special investigations on the heart were of any practical use.

11

ANGINA PECTORIS

When, during his last illness, Samuel Johnson was asked who attended him, he replied: 'Dr. Heberden, ultimus Romanorum, the last of our learned physicians.' And he was not far off the mark. William Heberden was indeed an outstanding Latin and Hebrew scholar and a man of great culture; he was also an astute physician, loved by his patients and respected for his wisdom by his contemporaries. In 1768 he gave the first medical description of the behaviour and progress of angina pectoris, introducing the term to the literature[1]. Having mentioned other pains in the chest he went on, 'But there is a disorder of the breast marked with strong and peculiar symptoms....The seat of it, and the sense of strangling, and anxiety with which it is attended, may make it not improperly be called angina pectoris.' Yet the cause eluded him: 'On opening the body of one who died suddenly of the disease, a very skillful anatomist could discover no fault in the heart, in the valves, in the arteries, or neighboring veins, excepting some small rudiments of ossification in the aorta.'

A few years later, John Fothergill[2,3] described a case of angina in which the patient eventually dropped dead in a fit of anger. The postmortem, carried out by John Hunter, revealed 'The two coronary arteries, from their origin to many of their ramifications upon the heart, were become one piece of bone.' Hunter himself suffered from angina and after his death in 1793 the coronary arteries were found to be calcified. There was other pathology in the heart and aorta, but Edward Jenner, of vaccination fame, correctly attributed the anginal attacks of his friend and teacher to the state of the coronary arteries.

After this excellent start, the situation deteriorated and angina pectoris became a most confused subject. There were many reasons for this, and amongst them was an inability to distinguish anginal pain from the many other pains in the chest, some associated with the heart and some not. National preferences were very much in evidence too. The Germans thought angina had a rheumatic or gouty origin; the Italians believed that it was due to enlargement of the liver disturbing or paralysing the function of the heart; and the French that it was due to a neuralgia of the cardiac plexus, or of the vagus or phrenic nerve[4]. Each country stuck obstinately to its opinions.

Even in the British Isles there was scepticism. Angina pectoris was evidently not as common as it is today (for one reason, life was shorter then), and although an association between the symptom and coronary disease was occasionally mentioned, no one was prepared to admit a cause-and-effect relationship. The postmortem findings help to explain this, for coronary artery disease, with or without narrowing, was and is quite commonly seen in patients who had no angina during life. Again, patients who had had angina were sometimes found to have relatively healthy coronary arteries; their pain came from disease of the aortic valve or of the aorta. And finally no cause of death could be found in some patients who died suddenly from a 'heart attack'.

The first person to make a diagnosis of coronary thrombosis while the patient was still alive was the German-born Adam Hammer, of St Louis, on May 4, 1876. He reasoned correctly that the sudden appearance and rapid progression of the symptoms could only be due to a cutting off of the supply of nourishment to the heart, and that such an obstruction could only be due to a thrombotic occlusion of at least one of the coronary arteries.

'I mentioned my conviction to my colleague at the bedside. He however had a non-plussed expression and burst out, "I have never heard of such a diagnosis in my life," and I answered, "Nor I also."' But the postmortem examination proved Hammer correct[5].

The opening of the 20th century brought some clarification, and acceptance of the fact that angina pectoris and coronary thrombosis are due to disease of the coronary arteries began with the work of James Bryan Herrick[6], of Chicago, in 1912. With his lucid explanations he showed why the clinical picture could vary greatly from patient to patient, thus clearing away much of the confusion of the past. Yet even he was obviously perplexed by some aspects as he could not differentiate between angina pectoris (due to ischaemia of the heart muscle – insufficient blood supply) and mild degrees of occlusion (causing necrosis or death of a small area of heart muscle because no blood was getting through to it).

This distinction had to wait until electrocardiography came into general use in the 1920s and 1930s, when recognition of the electrical changes of ischaemia and necrosis enabled the two states to be separated.

To understand what the various surgical operations were designed to achieve, it is important to have a clear mental picture of the meaning of the different terms and of what goes on when the coronary arteries that carry the blood to the heart muscle are affected by disease.

When the demand of the heart muscle for oxygen cannot be met by its blood supply the heart reacts by producing the pain of angina pectoris. This term simply means 'pain in the breast', but over the years it has come to refer to this one particular sort of pain. Angina pectoris is not a disease, it is a *symptom* of disease, usually (in more than 90 percent of cases) of the coronary arteries, but also of the aortic valve and aorta; sometimes atypical attacks occur in severe anaemia when the oxygen-carrying capacity of the blood is reduced.

Since we will be concentrating on disease of the coronary arteries, we must differentiate between angina pectoris and the pain of a 'heart attack'. In angina the pain comes on when the heart muscle becomes ischaemic; the coronary arteries are narrowed and sufficient oxygen-carrying blood does not reach the muscle. In the early stages the pain appears when increased demands are made on the heart by exercise. As the disease progresses, strong emotion, such as perhaps the excitement of watching a boxing fight, or anger, or a large meal may precipitate an attack. Later still the heart may have difficulty in getting enough oxygen to do its ordinary work and so anginal attacks may occur at rest. The pain is not always confined to the chest, for it may radiate up into the neck and jaws, or down an arm. But with angina, no matter how narrowed the arteries become, some blood manages to reach the heart muscle and it does not die. If the work the heart has to do can be reduced to a level at which the blood supply is adequate, there will be no pain. Angina is thus an indicator to the patient that his heart needs more oxygen. It is a temporary phenomenon that passes off when the heart gets sufficient oxygen again. In the so-called angina of effort, the obvious answer is to stop making the particular effort; patients often learn precisely how much they can do without bringing on an attack.

A 'heart attack' is another matter. Here a main coronary artery or one of its branches becomes blocked, and depending on the area supplied by that artery, a large or a small area of heart muscle is completely deprived of oxygen and dies – it becomes infarcted and causes pain, sometimes agonizing; this must not be confused with the pain of angina pectoris, though when the area infarct-ed is very small the pain may seem like a prolonged anginal attack. The effects of an obstruction vary greatly and depend on the artery affected, whether the hardening process has been going on for some time and other vessels have been able to open up and help it in its work, how badly the other arteries are affected, and so on. Generally speaking, though, if the area is large or affects the tissue conducting the nervous impulses of the heart-beat, the patient dies, often suddenly. If it is small he lives – though the 'shock' may stop the heart, in which case immediate cardiac massage may revive him. As the patient convalesces, the area of dead heart muscle becomes converted into whitish scar tissue. A heart attack may occur without previous angina, though angina due to coronary disease leads eventually to a heart attack.

The main disease that affects the coronary arteries is atherosclerosis – hardening and narrowing of the arteries. (The other conditions that may affect the coronary arteries, directly or indirectly, are of lesser importance and need not concern us here.) Blood may clot at the site of disease and suddenly block the artery – coronary thrombosis.

So much, then, for what happens. Why it happens, no one knows. There are many theories, all of which play a part in the cause of atherosclerosis: dietary factors, cigarette smoking, and lack of exercise are the chief ones, but they do not tell the whole story. Other diseases, such as diabetes mellitus, hypertension and obesity, predispose to coronary atherosclerosis. Thus the first lines of treatment are becoming apparent, and they are medical not surgical.

Now we return to a consideration of the main symptom of coronary artery disease – angina pectoris. This is treated by drugs, a mainstay still being glyceryl trinitrate, one of the nitrites first introduced for this purpose by Sir Lauder Brunton some four generations ago[7]. The benefit of this drug is greatest when taken to prevent the pain, as before exercise. It acts by an effect on the peripheral circulation which eases the work of the heart, and not by a direct improvement of the flow of blood through the coronary arteries. In recent decades other drugs have been discovered which slow the heart rate and indirectly improve the blood flow to the heart muscle. If all these medical measures are unavailing and angina still seriously troubles the patient, the possibility of relief by surgery will probably be discussed.

When the idea of relief by surgical means first dawned at the beginning of the 20th century, a tremendous amount of energy and ingenuity was expended in the search for a suitable answer to the problem. Although there were reports of undoubted clinical improvement, it had to be admitted that the surgeon was still groping in uncertain territory. The assessment of results in terms of what a particular procedure achieved was excessively difficult, for pain is a subjective phenomenon. The mere fact of having had an operation may have had a beneficial psychological effect; the stress reaction to any operative procedure probably entered the picture. Indeed, patients were improved when only a skin incision was made. Opening the pericardium was an essential part of many of the operations and this in itself may have been beneficial, though possibly the reason here may have been the cutting of some of the nerves to the heart. Also the rapidity with which some patients were relieved of their symptoms after operation would seem to point rather to an interference with the nerve supply than to an improvement in the blood supply when that was the intention. Factors of this nature are extremely complex and defy analysis. However, the arrival of coronary arteriography has made objective studies a reality.

Historically, the surgical procedures designed to relieve the pain of angina pectoris can be divided broadly into three groups: (1) interference with the nerve supply to the heart; (2) lowering the metabolic needs of the heart muscle; and (3) improving the blood supply to the muscle.

Charles Émile François-Franck, professor of physiology in Paris, made the first move when, in 1899, he tentatively suggested thoraco-cervical sympathectomy as a treatment[8]. His reasoning was exquisitely involved and based on ideas that have no substance today, and all tied in with the French obsession with neuralgias. In his day they were treating thyrotoxicosis (overactivity of the thyroid gland, known as Graves's disease to us and as Basedow's disease on the Continent) by excising part of the sympathetic nervous system in the neck. Some of François-Franck's thyrotoxic patients also had aortitis and angina which, he thought, might have contributed to the thyroid disease. So, if the sympathetic nerves to the heart were also cut, he reasoned it should be possible to get a yet more complete cure of the thyrotoxicosis. Hence the suggestion of excising the appropriate part of the sympathetic system as a treatment for angina itself.

Sympathectomy had many other strange applications on the Continent in those days – epilepsy, idiocy, glaucoma and migraine, for instance – and Thomas Jonnesco, a Bucharest surgeon, devoted most of his career between 1896 and his death in 1925, to the sympathetic system and operations for its removal. But not until April 2, 1916, did he put François-Franck's suggestion into practice. The patient was a 28-year-old man whose angina was due to syphilitic aortitis; Jonnesco removed the last two cervical ganglia and the first thoracic ganglion on the left side. Before discharging him from hospital, Jonnesco wanted to operate on the right side as well, but the man was well content with the result and declined the offer. When he was seen again four years later he said he was completely relieved of his angina and able to do heavy work; his heart action and respiration were completely normal[9].

In fact, Jonnesco was not the first surgeon to perform a sympathectomy for angina, but this was not generally realized until 1925 when, in a discussion of a paper on the subject Charles H Mayo, one of the famous Mayo brothers, who with their father had founded the Mayo Clinic in Rochester, Minnesota, reported that 12 years previously he had done a cervical sympathectomy on a major in the United States army. The major was still able to get about and no longer suffered from angina[10].

The sympathetic nervous system is part of the autonomic nervous system that is concerned with the involuntary functioning of the body. As far as the heart is concerned, one of its jobs is to convey sensory impulses from nerve plexuses around the heart to the brain. Although normally these sensations do not reach consciousness, it seemed reasonable to interrupt the nerve pathway in cases of angina when somehow or other pain did get through to the conscious mind. However, some of the early workers believed that interruption of the sensory fibres would improve the blood flow to the heart muscle, and indeed in the late 1930s experimental evidence showed that sympathectomy could have a slight protective effect on subsequent coronary occlusion. Nevertheless, this effect was only short-lived and it was not considered worthwhile introducing the idea to clinical practice.

Another way in which the vaguely understood nervous pathways could be interrupted was suggested by Gastineau Earle and Strickland Goodall before, in fact, sympathectomy had been tried. Their plan was to cut the sensory roots as they entered the spinal cord, an operation known as posterior rhizotomy. In 1913 they persuaded their surgical colleague at The Middlesex Hospital, London, William Sampson Handley, to see if the operation was feasible and, on a cadaver, he cut the second, third, and fourth thoracic roots. However, they all concluded that injection of alcohol or novocaine into these roots would be simpler and just as effective[11].

The idea of posterior root section, nevertheless, cropped up again 10 years later when Daniel Daniélopolu, director of the Second Medical Clinic at the University of Bucharest, objected to Jonnesco's type of sympathectomy on the grounds that it produced irremediable disturbances of cardiac function and damage to the heart muscle owing to the fact that the motor sympathetic fibres as well as the sensory fibres were also interrupted. So he persuaded his surgical colleague, Hristide, to cut the posterior roots of the upper thoracic spinal nerves, by which means only sensory fibres were divided[12].

By the next year, 1924, Daniélopolu seems to have forgotten all about posterior rhizotomy and returned to sympathectomy – but with a difference. (Here, some more anatomy is necessary: the part of the sympathetic system concerned is composed of a chain of ganglia (nerve stations) running down the neck and into the chest beside the backbone and under cover of the muscles. In about 65 percent of cases the lower cervical and first thoracic ganglia are amalgamated and known as the stellate ganglion. From the ganglia the sympathetic nerves pass out to the viscera and back eventually to the brain – if only it was as simple as that; their ramifications are vastly complex.)

'Cervico-thoracic sympathectomy has been disastrous from the therapeutic point of view,' wrote Daniélopolu[13], 'but it has at any rate made it clear that removal of the stellate ganglion in angina is incompatible with life. The operation must, then, be definitely abandoned, but the idea of surgical treatment of angina need not be given up.'

For the next two years he made extensive anatomical studies, so that the operation he developed caught more and more of the sensory fibres, leaving the motor ones intact. It was still a cervical sympathectomy but did not touch the stellate ganglion[14]. The inescapable conclusion from reading his papers is that Daniélopolu was jealous of Jonnesco, for removal of the lower cervical and first thoracic ganglia (the composite stellate ganglion) was Jonnesco's operation. Somehow or other Daniélopolu had got his experiments to prove that stellate ganglionectomy did damage the heart and he reiterated his belief that the operation for angina in the human patient was lethal. Obviously he was blaming the postmortem appearance of the heart disease on to the results of the operation in those patients who died fairly soon after Jonnesco's sympathectomies. His explanation of the survivors was crafty: excision had been incomplete as the operation was very difficult and not everyone possessed Jonnesco's skill.

Others, such as Elliot Cutler[15], who were able to view the situation dispassionately did not agree with him and brought forward the fact that Jonnesco had done at least 200 of his sympathectomies for a variety of conditions with no signs of ill-effect on the heart.

Despite posterior rhizotomy requiring removal of part of the vertebrae (laminectomy) to get at the nerve roots it was still occasionally performed and in 1957 James C White, a Harvard neurosurgeon, said that it was undoubtedly the surest method of securing permanent relief from angina; nervous function was capable of regeneration after sympathectomy or alcohol injection of the roots. The postoperative complications were bearable, he said, and 'giving the patient a reprieve from suffering is often an effective method for promoting the spontaneous recovery of a more adequate coronary circulation.'[16]

Since the 1920s many forms of sympathectomy have been proposed and carried out: alcohol injection into the upper thoracic sympathetic ganglia or into the nerve roots as well as posterior rhizotomy. But even though a sympathectomy might relieve the anginal pain, it could lead to other annoyances and pains which, in severe cases might make the cure worse than the disease. Sometimes, too, if only one side was operated on anginal pain might continue, but on the opposite side only. Probably about a third to three-quarters of the patients were relieved of their anginal pain, but the variety of the procedures and the inconsistent results reflected the ignorance of the true nature of the pain and of the nerve pathways to the heart. And, in any case, the operations were only palliative and did nothing to treat the disease responsible for the pain.

Methods for lowering the metabolic needs of the body are again palliative since they only make life easier for the heart and do not strike at the cause of the angina. In overactivity of the thyroid gland the body's metabolic rate is increased; in underactivity it is decreased. The idea of deliberately creating thyroid underactivity as a treatment for angina came in stages. Since thyroidectomies became commonplace at the beginning of the 20th century, there had been the occasional observation of a patient whose congestive heart failure had improved after subtotal removal of the thyroid for hyperthyroidism.

But no one thought of this sort of operation for heart disease, in the absence of thyroid overactivity, until 1927, and even then it was the possibility of thyroid disease that was the governing factor. Elliot Cutler and his colleagues at Harvard had a woman patient of 61 with severe congestive heart failure; because they thought she might be suffering from latent hyperthyroidism they decided to perform a subtotal removal of the thyroid. At the operation on June 27, the gland appeared normal but as the surgeon had been warned of this and told to press on regardless, he completed his task. Subsequent histological examination of the removed tissue confirmed its normality. However, the patient was greatly improved for four years and this made Cutler wonder whether removal of part of the normal thyroid might not lower the metabolism sufficiently to ease the burden on an exhausted heart. So, on June 15, 1932, he carried out the first subtotal thyroidectomy which had for its objective the relief of angina. The patient, a 53-year-old man, was improved[17].

The Harvard workers then joined up with Herrman Blumgart and David Berlin at the Beth Israel Hospital where Berlin performed another similar operation on October 17 of that year. In the December, Cutler acted on a suggestion of Blumgart, and removed all the thyroid gland in a man of 43 with angina and heart failure[17,18].

Thus was the idea of surgery for angina born, but the disease process, obviously, was not arrested and eventually even the lowered metabolic demands became too great for the heart. Surgery, and alcohol injection of the thyroid which was also tried, conceivably owed part of their action to interference with a nerve pathway, for relief from the angina often occurred before the metabolic rate had time to fall. These techniques fell by the wayside after about a decade since the operation carried a significant mortality rate in these patients and the complications of thyroid ablation, such as tetany (due to accidental removal of the parathyroid glands), damage to the recurrent laryngeal nerve with subsequent voice changes, and severe myxoedema, showed themselves in full measure. The passing of this phase of surgery for angina pectoris has not been regretted.

In the mid-1940s the thiouracil drugs were introduced for the treatment of hyperthroidism; they were a given a trial in heart failure with angina but without a great deal of success owing to their toxic effects, and to the facts that they had to be taken for the remainder of the patient's life and were not effective in every case.

But all this time Herrman Blumgart had been tenaciously pursuing his beliefs in the value of treating heart disease by the creation of thyroid insufficiency. So when radioactive iodine made its appearance in medicine, he used it for this purpose. It works because iodine is selectively taken up by thyroid tissue where it gives off its radiation which then destroys the function of the gland. Blumgart began this form of treatment in March, 1947[19], and in

1952 reported on 26 patients with angina; 13 were improved[20]. Neverthless, a thought should be given to the role of lipid metabolism in the pathogenesis of coronary heart disease and to the raised blood cholesterol that occurs in hypofunction of the thyroid. For these reasons, the treatment never proved popular.

12

MYOCARDIAL REVASCULARIZATION

The surgical battle against angina pectoris reached the heart itself with the start of attempts to improve the blood supply of the cardiac muscle. Once more the variety of procedures contemplated and in many instances put into practice is quite staggering. The literature is littered with enthusiastic descriptions of operations that have been tried, possibly only once or twice, and then forgotten about. Some were persevered with in their original form or in a multitude of minor variations at a number of surgical centres, but none of those we shall discuss has survived.

In this chapter we are dealing with operations designed to bring blood to the heart muscle either from outside sources or from sources already existing in the heart but not fully utilized. They have no effect on the diseased coronary arteries; instead, they are intended to circumvent the problems created by their narrowing or occlusion.

The reason why so much effort has been put into finding an answer to coronary artery disease is its great frequency. Precise figures are difficult to arrive at, not least because of the problem of obtaining, from death certificates, exact information on diseases within broader groups. As if the mortality was not bad enough, there is the morbidity to be considered. Probably something like a quarter of those who have an acute coronary occlusion die in the first attack. Many of the remaining three-quarters are able to return to work thanks to modern medical management. Still speaking very generally, and bearing in mind that the presence of co-existing disease such as hypertension influences the outcome, the average length of life after a coronary attack has increased over the past few decades; however, the risk of another attack remains, though the chances of its happening lessen with the passage of time. Thus it is not hard to see why surgeons regard coronary artery disease as well worth their attention.

The heart muscle is supplied with blood through the two coronary arteries (left and right) – in some people there is a third, or accessory artery. These branch and branch again and again, but there is very little communication between the branches of the two arteries in the normal heart. However, when the arteries become narrowed or obstructed, the degree of communication increases markedly and can do so quite rapidly. In addition, the heart gets a small quantity of blood through branches from other arteries such as the internal mammary; when more blood is needed these branches can increase their supply and join up with the intercoronary communications. In other words, when the heart is distressed by a poor blood supply it has many normally closed channels that it can open up, and is grateful for any extra blood it can get.

The first experiments designed to give the heart some extra blood vessels began in February, 1932. Claude Beck[1], of the Western Reserve School of Medicine, Cleveland, who worked indefatigably at the problem for the rest of his professional career, had had his attention drawn by his colleague, Alan Moritz, to a case reported by Christen Thorel in 1903[2]. At the postmortem, both major coronary arteries were found to be obliterated, and the patient had obviously been living with them in that state for some time. But there were adhesions around the heart and Thorel suggested that the heart had managed to get sufficient blood through the vessels in these adhesions. So, thought Beck, why not deliberately bring a source of blood from elsewhere and make it adhere to the surface of the heart. After a great deal of experimentation he operated on his first patient, 48-year-old Joseph Krchmar, on February 13, 1935. He used a burr to roughen the inside of the pericardial sac and to remove the epicardium (the thin fibrous layer covering the heart muscle) in shreds. Between these two raw surfaces he then grafted part of a pectoral muscle with its blood supply intact. Seven months later Krchmar claimed he was cured[1].

During his experiments Beck had used the pericardium itself, pericardial fat, and omentum as well as the pectoral muscle for the extra source of blood, and he showed how, after these procedures, his animals would survive almost total occlusion of both coronary arteries. For human surgery, though, he doubted whether the omentum (the fatty apron hanging down in front of the intestines) would prove practical owing to the problems involved in bringing it up through the diaphragm.

Such doubts did not assail Laurence O'Shaughnessy. In 1930, he had been attracted to the thoracic oesophagus and had worked out methods for excising part of it and restoring continuity. However, the only way he found he could satisfactorily ensure the safety of the suture line at the join was by bringing up a large portion of the greater omentum as a pedicle graft, complete with its blood supply, and wrapping it around the oesophagus in the chest. At this time he was also experimenting with coronary occlusion in animals and in April, 1933, at the Buckston Browne Farm in Downe, Kent, he brought his two interests together and showed that when omentum was grafted to the heart, vascular connections developed in great numbers and very rapidly[3,4].

Then, one day, he happened to read that greyhounds were prone to a type of heart failure that he thought could be relieved by his grafting operation and, indeed, those animals he tried it on were able to run again. The next step was to tie off a greyhound's left coronary artery and in due course graft omentum to its heart: when the animal had recovered, it was able to put up a respectable performance on the track. The first human patient to be treated with an omental graft was a 64-year-old man on whom O'Shaughnessy operated at Lewisham Hospital (south-east London, close to the Catford Greyhound Stadium!) on January 4, 1936[5]. In subsequent operations, worried at inserting sutures into a degenerated heart, he stitched the omentum to the pericardium and applied a special adhesion-producing paste (aleuronat) between the graft and the heart.

In 1938 he reported that all his patients who had survived for six months or more were improved; those who had been bed-ridden could walk, and those unable to work could do so[6]. All in all he reckoned the results justified the procedure. But alas! O'Shaughnessy was to be denied the place in the forefront of British cardiac surgery that would undoubtedly have been his. The Second World War broke out and he was killed at Dunkirk while still only 40.

A fair variety of other tissues – skin, jejunum and stomach – were tried experimentally as the graft during the 1950s, but the only one to have had any sort of a run for its money was lung. This had in fact first been used by Albert Lezius, a German surgeon, in 1937; he considered it to be the ideal source of extra blood. He removed a window of pericardium, painted acriflavine (an antiseptic) on the heart muscle and then sutured the adjacent lung to this area. He was able to produce radiographic evidence of anastomoses developing between coronary and pulmonary vessels in his experimental material[7]. This simple approach was elaborated by several enthusiasts in the 1950s, but as with so many operations for angina only a few patients were submitted to the procedures even though the results were reported as good or satisfactory.

In an attempt to increase the added blood supply still further and possibly open up more intercoronary connections, an adhesive pericarditis was created either at the time of grafting or in its own right. The idea was to set up a sterile inflammation by introducing various substances into the pericardial cavity. The cavity was thereby obliterated by adhesions which contained blood vessels. O'Shaughnessy had already used aleuronat as part of his grafting operation but on November 25, 1938, sterile talc (powdered magnesium silicate) was used as the sole agent in a 39-year-old man by Samuel Thompson and Milton Raisbeck of New York[8]. After Thompson had opened the pericardium he applied 5ml of 2 percent novocaine (a local anaesthetic) to the epicardium to prevent the irritant talc from producing ventricular fibrillation. This was left on for four or five minutes before he removed it by suction and introduced the powder. The patient's symptoms were markedly improved.

Thompson used the technique extensively and 15 years later reported that most of his patients had benefited clinically[9]. He was able to complete the operation in about 20 minutes – a favourable feature as his early patients were all 'cardiac derelicts'; of the first 16, only four died in the immediate post-operative period.

A wide array of other substances were used as the inflammatory agent, both experimentally and clinically: for instance, carborundum sand and Beck's choice of powdered beef bone or asbestos (he also experimented with kaolin, iron filings, iodine, ether, alcohol, formaldehyde, cotton, human skin, and water glass and other unlikely-seeming irritants). Yet, despite the encouraging reports, doubt remained as to how the operation achieved its effect since Beck's technique was the only one in which the epicardium (a probable barrier to blood vessels entering the myocardium) was removed. The importance of this was appreciated by Dwight Harken of Boston who, in 1955, introduced 95 percent carbolic acid for the purpose, following it up with a powdering of sterile talc[10].

Grafting operations were abandoned in the general belief that they were not very effective and that such effect as they could produce was more easily achieved by simply creating adhesions after removal of the epicardium. Experimental work gave little or no objective evidence of improved circulation in the heart muscle from the adhesions, and thus conflicted with the subjective improvement. And, as with the thyroid operations, improvement was often dramatically rapid; much too fast to be attributable to the development of new vessels in the adhesions, but (apart from the possibility of nervous impulses having been cut off) it might have been due to the opening up of existing intercoronary connections. Unsurprisingly, the creation of pericardial adhesions (cardiopericardiopexy) never achieved widespread acceptance.

The attempt to force the thoroughly confusing operations for angina pectoris into a straightforward story is further confounded by the next phase which shows how impossible it is even to keep the procedures in watertight compartments. By 1941 Beck had stopped using muscle grafts and the same year began studying the effect of obstruction to the venous return from the heart muscle (about which more will be said later). This development led to what is known as the Beck I operation, first put into practice in 1954[11]. In suitable cases this comprised abrasion of the epicardium and inner surface of the pericardial sac; the application of an inflammatory agent to these surfaces; the grafting of pericardium and mediastinal fat to the surface of the heart – all of which he had been doing for many years – and partial occlusion of the coronary sinus where it entered the right atrium. (The coronary sinus is a short, wide vein into which flow nearly all the veins from the heart muscle; if it is occluded by a ligature tied round it, the blood is dammed back and the heart muscle becomes congested.)

The rationale behind operating on the coronary sinus is that normally all the oxygen is not removed from the blood, and in circumstances of congestion uptake is increased. Also the small vessels dilate. Admittedly, after a while, the congestion disappears because other minor channels of venous drainage dilate to cope with the increased load, but by this time intercoronary connections have opened up. Work on the coronary sinus had, in fact, begun in 1935 when Louis Gross and his colleagues in New York had noticed that anginal pain not infrequently disappeared if the patient had an attack of right-sided heart failure (during which the myocardium is congested). They followed this up with experiments on dogs in which they showed that complete or partial ligation of the coronary sinus would save the animal from death when they subsequently ligated a major coronary artery[12]. Later, they modified the technique to a partial ligation with similar satisfactory results.

Also in 1935, Mercier Fauteux of Montreal, working in Boston, began his experiments aimed at attacking the problem from two directions simultaneously. His original plan had been to remove the sympathetic nerves from around the coronary vessels (pericoronary neurectomy) and ligate the great cardiac vein (which drains into the coronary sinus). He carried out his first operation along these lines on a human patient in 1940 and by 1946 had operated on 16 patients all of whom had a history of coronary thrombosis, confirmed by electrocardiography, and were practically disabled by angina. In his report he stated that 11 patients were still living and that one, six years after operation, was working at the age of 65 years[13].

Having mentioned a Beck I operation, it is reasonable to expect there to be a Beck II – though with this subject one cannot be sure of anything, but there was a Beck II. Its main feature was arteriolization of the reversed coronary circulation, meaning that a functioning artery was grafted on to the coronary sinus so as to force the flow of blood in the veins backwards into the heart muscle. The idea can be traced back to 1898 when Frederick Pratt of the Harvard Medical School set out to challenge the belief that without the blood brought by the coronary arteries the heart could not continue beating. He succeeded in demonstrating experimentally two other ways in which it could be nourished. First, backwards through the Thebesian veins – small vessels normally draining blood from their minute branches in the heart wall directly into the ventricular and atrial cavities – and second through the coronary veins which may carry a backward flow of blood from the atrium into the tissues of the heart. He said this 'affords a reasonable explanation of many cases in which the cardiac tissues have survived for months or even years the closure of terminal arteries long believed to be their sole supply.'[14] (We know now, however, that the coronary arteries are not really terminal or end-arteries, but have connections that open up under the stress of ischaemia.)

Pratt's work was taken up again in 1943 by Joseph Roberts of the University of Texas Medical School, Galveston, who produced experimental results that put Claude Beck on the trail of the Beck II operation. Roberts first showed by dye studies on dog hearts that it was possible for the Thebesian veins to carry blood from the left ventricular chamber into the myocardium when the pressure in the chamber was greater than that in the coronary vessels[15]. But of greater significance were his experiments indicating that an ischaemic myocardium might be revascularized by the anastomosis of a large artery with the coronary sinus and coronary veins[16]. He did this by connecting the coronary sinus through a glass cannula with the brachiocephalic, subclavian or innominate artery. The coronary veins became distended, pulsatile and arterial in colour, and the hearts continued to beat after the coronary arteries were ligated in different combinations[17].

Beck's new series of experiments began in February, 1946, and on January 27, 1948, the first Beck II was done on a human patient. The difficulty, though, was to find an artery that could be spared from its normal duties; Beck eventually decided on the brachial artery in the patient's arm, since it was the correct size and he believed the loss would not seriously cripple the hand. A length was cut from the distal end of this artery and used for the anastomosis between the aorta and the coronary sinus; the coronary sinus itself was ligated where it entered the right atrium, otherwise the new supply of arterial blood would have taken the line of least resistance and have flowed directly into the atrium[18].

In those days vascular surgery was still in its developing phase and Beck's suggestion of using a piece of vein instead of artery for the graft had to wait a little while before it could be adopted. The operation itself was soon changed to a two-stage procedure to prevent rapid clotting within the graft and to try to make it better tolerated by the patient. The first stage was the insertion of the graft, and the second, some two to six weeks later, the partial ligation of the coronary sinus.

The Beck II produced excellent and enduring opening up of intercoronary connections, even though the graft became thrombosed after a few weeks or months and the smaller myocardial veins closed in self-defence as they were unable to withstand the pressure. However, it had a short life owing to the need for two stages and its unacceptably high operative mortality rate of 15-20 percent. As a consolation, the partial ligation of the coronary sinus became incorporated into the Beck I operation.

The 1950s were a time of great activity in the field of myocardial revascularization and many were the techniques that crossed the surgical horizon. For instance, in 1954, the Italians, M Battezzati, A Tagliaferro and G De Marchi[19], resuscitated the operation of ligating the internal mammary artery that had previously been done by their fellow countrymen Zoja and Cesa-Bianchi[20]. The idea for this had originated with a physician, D Fieschi, who in 1939 had been able to show that bilateral ligation of the artery below the origin of the pericardiacophrenic branch increased the flow of blood to the myocardium[21]. (This branch normally gives off twiglets to the pericardium which join up with other twiglets from the aorta.) Later in 1939 Fieschi persuaded Zoja and Cesa-Bianchi to carry out the operation on a man who had had a myocardial infarction; it was done under local anaesthesia and two years later the patient was well and had not had another heart attack.

Battezzati's first operation of this nature was on a 61-year-old man on December 12, 1954, and the report of 11 cases in 1955[22] brought the procedure to the notice of cardiac surgeons. It had the merits of being simple, not needing a general anaesthetic, and having virtually no mortality rate; it could safely be undertaken soon after a heart attack, though the Italians did say that it was preferable to wait for a few weeks; and it produced worthwhile results. But when we come to work out how the operation achieved its effects we are once again at a loss.

Tying off the internal mammary artery through an incision in the second space between the ribs is intended to divert the blood, that would normally flow onwards, into the branch to the heart and so increase the pressure in this branch and lead to the opening of connections with the coronary circulation and an improvement of blood supply to the heart muscle. Experimentally, such a local increase in pressure has been observed, but, haemodynamics being what they are, this cannot be the answer for two reasons. First, if there is an increase in pressure it would seem more logical for the blood to be pushed backwards up the internal mammary artery and equalize the pressures, rather than flow on into the area of higher pressure. And secondly, ligation of this artery can only increase the total peripheral resistance very slightly, if at all, and since arterial pressures balance out and are governed by the total peripheral resistance, the operation cannot achieve its effect in this way. In fact, many investigators have been unable to show that ligation produces any significant increase in the flow of blood to the heart.

Clinical experiments would seem to indicate a psychological mechanism. Patients with angina have been divided into two groups: in one the ligation was carried out; in the other the skin was incised and the motions of ligation gone through without actually tying off the artery. In all other respects the treatment of the two groups was identical – and so were the beneficial effects experienced by the patients. Another interesting observation was that when the ligation was performed on one side, the anginal pain was abolished on that side only (as we saw happened with sympathectomy); this suggests an interference with the nerve supply. So, in the absence of any objective explanation, the reason why some patients were improved remains a mystery.

Now we come to one revascularizing procedure for which there was objective support; it again involved the internal mammary artery but in a quite startling fashion: Arthur Vineberg of McGill University implanted the cut, bleeding end of the artery directly into the heart muscle. However, before we tell the story of Vineberg's struggles, two other operations are worthy of brief mention.

The underlying principle of the first was the same as that of Vineberg's operation but the technique was only used experimentally. There were two main variations. In one, Alfred Goldman and his colleagues from Duarte, California, in 1955 used either straight or U-shaped grafts of either a carotid artery (taken from the same animal) or perforated plastic tubing, so placed in the wall of the left ventricle that blood from the cavity of the chamber was channelled directly into the muscle[23]. The following year C Massino and L Boffi of Florence, influenced by Vineberg's work, carried out experiments on dogs using a T-shaped plastic tube[24]. Their tube was implanted in the wall of the left ventricle with the vertical limb opening directly into the chamber and the cross limb lying in a 'lacuna' created in the myocardium. The immediate mortality was 10 percent. Despite opinions to the contrary, the Italians stated that blood was forced into the lacuna with each contraction of the ventricle. Even so the blood ebbs and flows into the muscle and this is unlikely to supply the needs of the myocardium as efficiently as a method which keeps up a continuous arterial pressure.

The other operation was devised by Walton Lillehei at the University of Minnesota and had as its objective the opening up of intercoronary connections by deliberately lowering the oxygen content of the blood in the left side of the heart. Working with S B Day, he showed experimentally that these anastomoses would develop within a month of the creation of an arterio-venous fistula between the main pulmonary artery (which carries venous blood to the lungs) and the left atrium. Their first patient, operated on on December 26, 1958, was a 47-year-old man, and the side-to-side anastomosis was 2cm long. Before operation the patient had had severe and progressing anginal pain; coronary arteriography had shown widespread coronary atherosclerosis with complete occlusion of the right coronary artery and left anterior descending branch. After surgery, the clinical response was dramatic and sustained, and the man was free of anginal pain[25].

We can now return to Vineberg's implantation of the internal mammary artery, the only one of the many surgical procedures for angina pectoris so far discussed for which there was objective proof that it did improve the intercoronary circulation, and for which, at the time, a future was fairly confidently predicted. How was it supposed to work? If a bleeding artery were to be implanted in any other muscle, it would simply form a huge haematoma or bruise. Fortunately, the heart muscle is unlike other muscle; in this context it can best be thought of as sponge. In early embryonic life the sponge is soft and loose and derives its oxygen from the blood that is squeezed in and out of it (this, in fact, is how the hearts of many of the lower vertebrate animals, such as fishes, obtain their nutrition). As the human embryo develops the sponge tightens up and the smallest of the coronary vessels and capillaries condense out of the spongy tissue. So when the intercoronary connections are opened up under the stress of ischaemia or by an effective surgical procedure, there is, in a manner of speaking, a return towards the soft sponge state which can mop up the blood more readily. In addition, there is better distribution of blood: this point was made in 1957 by Claude Beck, who emphasized that the surgical problem was the redistribution of available blood rather than the provision of extra blood[26]. Oxygen differentials between neighbouring areas of heart muscle, he said, affected the electrical stability of the heart and caused ventricular fibrillation; this he believed to be a common cause of death, and one that could be reversible. So on theoretical grounds Vineberg's operation had much to recommend it: not only did it allow the distribution of blood to be improved, it also increased the supply. But it did not reach its eventual standing without a fight.

Vineberg began his experimental work in 1946[27]. He freed the left internal mammary artery, tied off the lower end, and implanted the upper, bleeding end into a tunnel he had made in the ventricular muscle close to a coronary artery. No haematoma formed, and he demonstrated that the artery eventually joined up with branches of the neighbouring coronary artery. In 1950, he put the experimental work to the test in a human patient. Three years later he wrote, 'from a condition of complete disability' this man 'can walk 10 miles [16km] through the bush.'[28]

Subsequently Vineberg used pads of pericardial fat grafted to the surface of the left ventricle to provide a supplementary source of blood[29], and in 1962 he developed the use of a free omental graft[30]. For this, he detached the greater omentum completely from its abdominal home and wrapped the entire heart in the fatty apron after removing the epicardium and the inner layer of the pericardial sac. But apart from these modifications, his technique of internal mammary artery implantation remained unaltered through the years. (Other research workers had implanted, experimentally, the subclavian or the splenic artery, and Sidney Smith of Bradenton, Florida, used grafts led off from the aorta and pulled through the substance of the heart muscle from base to apex. After a series of animal experiments, Smith operated on a 43-year-old man on October 4, 1955, taking the saphenous vein from the leg as the graft; 18 months later the patient was leading a normal life. For his second successful operation, on June 27, 1956, Smith used a perforated nylon prosthesis which he found made the whole operation much quicker – 1 hour 50 minutes from skin to skin[31].)

In a follow-up of 140 patients from the beginning to 1964, Vineberg[32] recorded a *total* operative mortality of 33 percent; this was high, but for the decade 1954-63 it was only 1·8 percent, showing how experience had greatly improved the results. Of the 109 patients still alive in 1964, 91 had no pain or only slight pain on effort; eight were worse. Clinical improvement was marked and a high percentage of patients had been able to return to work.

However, right from the start Vineberg and his operation were at the centre of controversy. Doctors found it hard to believe that the effects would be other than haematoma formation with occlusion of the implanted artery. Experimental work on animals produced conflicting and inconsistent results; some workers obtained good intercoronary anastomoses, others did not; most found that the implanted artery soon became obliterated. It now seems that the reason for all this lay in the experimental conditions. When the animals had normal hearts, the results were poor; when a coronary artery was previously occluded, or partially so, the results were better; but when a coronary artery was gradually occluded by special techniques, they were greatly improved. The real difficulty was to create an experimental model that resembled the state of affairs in a diseased human heart, and also – as may well be imagined in a subject such as this – to control the experiments adequately. Nevertheless, there was unequivocal experimental evidence that Vineberg's operation did what he said it did, even though questions remained unanswered regarding the functional value of the observations.

On the clinical front, too, Vineberg encountered scepticism and doubt, but he steadfastly stuck to his guns, maintaining that operative technique had been at fault in the case of those surgeons who failed to equal his results. Then we have to remember the strange behaviour of angina pectoris and the subjective improvement so often produced by a variety of likely and unlikely undertakings. The symptomatic benefit reported by patients after the Vineberg operation can indeed be matched by that experienced after other operations. But the crux of the matter lay in objective evaluation of the procedures and, regrettably, useful information, such as details about the electrocardiographic response to the stress of exercise and the coronary flow, was sparse. Nevertheless, selective coronary arteriography, both at Vineberg's own hospital and elsewhere, did show that between 70 and 80 percent of internal mammary implants gave rise to worthwhile anastomoses with the coronary circulation. Shirey and Sones[33], for instance, were able to show that implanted mammary arteries were effectively perfusing the left ventricular muscle from five to seven years after operation. But in more than 20 patients who had had a cardiopericardiopexy with partial ligation of the coronary sinus or internal mammary artery ligation, they had been unable to demonstrate any myocardial perfusion through the normal internal mammary branches that go to the heart.

13

CORONARY OCCLUSION

Since the most usual cause of angina pectoris (which, remember, is only a symptom) is clogging of one or more coronary artery, it was only a matter of time before someone came forward with the idea of operating directly on them so that a normal flow could be restored. And incredibly someone had, as long ago as the beginning of the 20th century. During his experiments on the heart and aorta in 1910, the amazing Alexis Carrel had anastomosed a blood-vessel graft between the descending aorta and the left coronary artery at a point before it branches. An operation of this nature, he said[1], might find a place in the treatment of angina pectoris when the mouths of the coronary arteries were calcified. He was almost right.

From what we know of the history of cardiac surgery in the first half of the last century, it will come as no surprise to learn that Carrel's speculation was not taken seriously for many a long year. Indeed the starting-point of modern research came not from surgeons but from investigations by pathologists into the relationship between angina pectoris during life with the pathology and distribution of the lesions postmortem. Monroe Schlesinger at the Beth Israel Hospital, Boston, in 1940 developed a technique whereby he injected radio-opaque lead-agar masses of different colours into the coronary arteries, unrolled the heart, x-rayed it, and then dissected the arteries using the radiographs as a guide. He found most of the zones of occlusion to be less than 5mm long and to be within 3mm of the mouths of the vessels. These zones were as numerous in the right coronary artery as in the left descending coronary artery (often referred to as 'the artery of coronary occlusion') and they also occurred in the left circumflex coronary artery[2,3].

This was good news, for it meant that the coronary system was not riddled with disease. If the short, affected areas could be dealt with or bypassed, the blood would find normal channels to flow through. Immediate use of the knowledge could not be made as arterial surgery was still in rather a primitive stage and only in 1945 was the modern era heralded when Robert Gross[4] of Boston and the Swede, Clarence Crafoord[5], independently announced their treatment of a coarctation of the aorta by excising the constriction and stitching the cut ends together. Subsequently, when Gross found the gap too wide, he bridged it with an arterial graft taken from a cadaver[6]. From this has developed a whole range of operations on the arteries which make use of stored artery and vein grafts and a great variety of plastic prostheses, and enabled clots to be removed and diseased segments to be replaced or bypassed.

Gordon Murray of Toronto, who played a great role in the progress of cardiac surgery, often being a long way ahead of the field, reported to the Congress of the International Society of Angiology in Lisbon in 1953[7] that in five patients he had resected the narrowest part of the anterior descending coronary artery and had replaced it with a vascular graft. He had also done experimental work on dogs in which he anastomosed either the internal mammary, the axillary, or the carotid artery to the left coronary artery. There were various objections to all these and the only technique of this nature that he considered at all feasible for use in human beings was the insertion of a free graft of carotid artery between the aorta and the left coronary artery. This, he said, would require full information on the state of the coronary lumen obtained by radiography, which in those days presented yet another challenge[8].

However, at about the same time in Russia, Vladimir Demikhov (about whom we shall have a lot more to say when we talk about transplantation of the heart) was working along similar lines, and in dogs he joined the left internal mammary artery to the left descending coronary artery a few millimetres beyond its origin. His first attempt took place on April 29, 1952, but it failed because of irreversible ventricular fibrillation. On July 29, 1953, he had the first of a number of long-term successes with the animals living normal lives.

In 1955 Demikhov developed the operation further in experiments on human cadavers and on live baboons. By now he was becoming even more adventurous and his plan was to use a three-way plastic tube to connect the internal mammary artery to two branches of the coronary arteries beyond the obstructions. In principle he felt an operation of this nature to be possible, but when writing in 1960 he considered that technical improvements and more animal experiments would be needed before attempting it on patients.

Since the Western world did not learn of Demikhov's work until 1962[9], it was Murray's successes (all his patients survived the operation) that put other surgeons on the same track. In 1956 Walton Lillehei and his Minnesota colleagues gave an account of two procedures he had been using experimentally[10]. One, performed on human cadavers, was endarterectomy – virtually a rebore of the diseased segment – and this proved to have practical possibilities. The other was a repeat of Murray's anastomosis on dogs, which Lillehei approached in two ways. First, he used a special plastic prosthetic tube to form an anastomosis between the subclavian artery and the circumflex branch of the left coronary artery, but at postmortem examination the tube was found to be occluded by thrombus. Secondly, he made a direct anastomosis between the left internal carotid or the internal mammary artery and the same coronary branch; the anastomosis was patent at postmortem in about half these dogs. Even so the rate of occlusion was felt to be too high to justify a trial on human patients.

Quite independently Angelo May, a colleague of Charles Bailey in Philadelphia, had also been experimenting with endarterectomy, this time on dogs as well as human cadaver hearts. He designed a special curette that was passed beyond the blockage and as it was pulled back again the cutting edge of its cup-shaped head scooped up the atheroma and so prevented the material from getting lost in the coronary artery. In the dogs, which had normal arteries, he simply stripped off parts of the vessel lining; all the animals developed thrombosis at these sites after operation. This work began in October, 1954, and at first he made an incision in the aorta in the region of the openings of the coronary arteries passing the curette in through their mouths. A year later he tackled the problem by a retrograde approach – the incision was made into the coronary artery itself at a point beyond the blockage and the curette passed up the vessel[11].

Charles Bailey carried out the first coronary endarterectomy on a human patient on October 29, 1956, using the retrograde approach. The 51-year-old man, who was given heparin to prevent the blood from clotting in the artery after operation, made a satisfactory recovery[12]. Encouraged by this, Bailey performed seven more similar operations; all the patients recovered and seemed to be improved[13]. But the technical limitations of the method made Bailey try the approach through the aorta, which he did successfully on November 13, 1957, with the aid of a heart-lung machine so that the heart was temporarily excluded from the circulation. Yet he was still not satisfied; curettage, he believed, could be improved upon and before long he devised a method by which he could introduce a special thin knife to cut out the diseased inner lining of the artery as a tube which was then withdrawn with forceps[14].

As Bailey pointed out, these operations had to be restricted to patients whose disease was in fact localized to a fairly short segment of coronary artery; and these patients, according to Schlesinger's postmortem studies, were in the majority. However, techniques for x-raying the coronary arteries during life were improving and in 1958 Alan Thal of the University of Minnesota Medical

School challenged the view that occlusive disease was usually localized to the first part of the arteries. His coronary arteriograms showed that patients with angina of effort appeared to have diffuse disease of the whole coronary arterial system, while those with angina at rest had poor intercoronary connections as well. In 50 patients examined, he found only two instances of segmental arterial block[15]. Although this swung the pendulum vigorously in the opposite direction, it did not affect surgical enthusiasm adversely; rather, it underlined the very great importance of accurate pre-operative assessment of the coronary arteries, which came to fruition with the work of Sones and Shirey published in 1962[16]. Probably at its height fewer than 20 percent of patients with coronary atherosclerosis had lesions suitable for treatment by endarterectomy, though in some series of cases the percentage was higher, reflecting individual opinions of what constituted operability.

One troublesome feature of coronary endarterectomy, however, arose when the dissection passed across the mouth of a branch artery. The inner lining of the branch, being no longer attached to that of the main channel rolled back on itself, clot formed, and the branch became sealed off. This problem struck Åke Senning, an associate of Clarence Crafoord in Stockholm, during his dog experiments, and more forcibly when a patient died from this cause a short while after operation. So he decided to open the artery, carefully dissect out the diseased areas under direct vision, avoiding the mouths of branch arteries, and then enlarge the artery by putting a patch along the length of the incision. Experiments showed that the plan would work, so towards the end of 1959, he operated on a 55-year-old man who was disabled by angina. Blockages were peeled out from the circumflex and descending branches of the left coronary artery, avoiding side branches, and the incisions closed with patches of the patient's saphenous vein taken from the ankle. While this was being done the heart was bypassed and the blood cooled to 23°C by passage through a heat-exchanger. The operation took about three hours and for most of the time the heart was fibrillating, but its normal beat was restored by one electric shock. Three months afterwards both grafts were seen to be patent on arteriography and two months later the patient was still free of symptoms and working part time[17].

The next development took place in 1967 when Philip Sawyer, Martin Kaplitt and Sol Sobel of the State University of New York Downstate Medical Center introduced the technique known as gas endarterectomy or carbodissection[18]. In this, jets of carbon dioxide gas were sprayed down the affected vessel separating the obstructing core, which was then removed through a small incision. Carbon dioxide was used because it did not balloon the artery and was harmlessly absorbed. During 1966 these surgeons had been using the method successfully on patients with obstructed arteries in other parts of the body such as the neck, abdomen and legs. When they decided to attack the coronaries they mastered the operation in the postmortem room, yet their first attempt on the table, in August, 1966, was doomed to failure – the patient's heart could not be started after a serious mitral-valve operation and the gas endarterectomy was a last resort; but it did show the technique to be feasible on a living patient.

Their first planned endeavour took place on January 5, 1967. A 44-year-old housewife had had two serious myocardial infarctions within a month and arteriography revealed her right coronary artery to be totally blocked for about two inches (5cm) – making her unsuitable for ordinary endarterectomy. She could take only a few steps before being crippled with angina and her future prospects were bad. The surgeons made a sternum-splitting incision, connected her to a heart-lung machine, clamped off the aorta and exposed the affected artery through its overlying layer of fat. Then they inserted an ordinary hypodermic needle, attached to the carbon-dioxide cylinder by plastic tubing, into the arterial wall beneath the diseased inner lining. The jets of gas went in at a pressure about three times that of the normal blood pressure. The core was next freed completely with a special instrument and drawn out with forceps through a short incision in the artery. Three days after operation the woman was able to walk short distances, and the early tests indicated that the blood flow to her heart muscle was significantly improved[18].

The advantages of the operation, said Sawyer, were its quickness – it took about half the time of a standard endarterectomy – and the fact that it could clear quite long stretches of artery together with its branches. A subsequent modification was to insert a type of probe used for freezing (a cryoprobe) along the length of the blockage after it had been separated by the jets of gas. The temperature was reduced to $-20°C$, freezing the core to the probe so that when the probe was withdrawn all the diseased tissue came away with it.

Thus far we have considered coronary artery surgery as it applied to the patient who was chronically ill with evidence of occlusive coronary disease localized to a relatively short segment of artery as proved by selective coronary arteriography. But what of the acute situation when a thrombosis blocked a major coronary artery?

In 1958 Bailey[14] thought that emergency thromboendarterectomy might be a possibility, in the same way that clots could be removed from, for instance, the femoral artery thus saving the leg from amputation. Animal experiments gave him reason to hope that the idea might be practical, particularly as heart-lung machines and trained personnel were then becoming commonplace. Pre-operative radiological localization would obviously be unnecessary, he said; the affected artery could be found after the chest had been opened either by its appearance, its feel, or by passing a probe down the arteries.

George Nardi and Robert Shaw of the Harvard Medical School in 1963 reported on four patients on whom they had tried the operation[19]. They failed to rescue any of them although one lived for 52 hours with a normal heart-beat. After this patient, a 42-year-old man, had failed to respond to open cardiac massage, Nardi and Shaw removed an area of blockage through an incision in the left descending coronary artery. For 24 hours after operation the man made good progress, but then he developed pneumonia and died the next day. At postmortem another area of atheroma with fresh blood clot was found about 1cm beyond the area operated on.

Yet even as all this ingenuity was being expended on endarterectomy in its variety of forms, the operation that was to supercede it was taking shape at the Cleveland Clinic, Ohio, and on May 9, 1967, the Argentine, René Favaloro who was working there, performed the first coronary artery bypass on a 51-year-old woman[20]. A length of saphenous vein from the upper thigh was used for the bypass from the aorta to beyond a total blockage of the right coronary artery in its proximal third. The patient made an uneventful recovery and cineradiographic studies 20 days after operation showed 'total reconstruction of the right coronary artery.' Since then multiple grafts have been inserted when more than one artery has been affected and, in selected cases, a length of internal mammary artery has been used as the graft.

Alexis Carrel's dream had been realized.

Ten years later, a technique that complements coronary artery bypass appeared on the scene: percutaneous transluminal coronary angioplasty. This procedure, which is almost invariably performed by a physician, was introduced by A Grüntzig of Zürich who, in 1977, reported on five patients with severe stenotic lesions associated with refractory angina[21]. He used a catheter with a sausage-shaped balloon at its tip which he inserted through the femoral artery; when the balloon was seen, radiologically, to be in position he filled it with saline solution and contrast medium under pressure and thus compressed the obstructing atheromatous lesion, leaving a smooth inner surface to the artery.

Between them these two techniques have transformed the outlook for patients with coronary artery disease and, what is important for the surgeon, their effects can be assessed objectively by a wealth of modern techniques. No longer does the value of an operation have to be judged solely on whether or not the angina is relieved.

14

CARDIAC ANEURYSM

Hardening of the coronary arteries, like atherosclerosis of all other arteries, is fundamentally a 'medical' disease. The ultimate objective is prevention, but since this is still a long way from realization (if it will ever come to pass, as the disease is probably part and parcel of the human condition) and since little or nothing can yet be done to arrest the inexorable advance of the atheroma once it has started, surgeons step in to do what they can. Nevertheless, for as long as heart attacks continue to afflict the human race there is one complication in the treatment of which the surgeon reigns supreme: cardiac aneurysm.

After a coronary thrombosis the area of heart muscle cut off from its blood supply dies and becomes softened At this stage there is a danger that the area may give way and burst, but if all goes well the infarct slowly changes into whitish scar tissue which cannot contract along with the rest of the heart muscle. This may be of no significance but in an uncertain number of cases, varying in different series from 5-38 percent, the scar is unable to withstand the pressure inside the ventricle and begins to bulge outward and form what is known as an aneurysm. The outlook is then grim. Most patients die within a short time from congestive heart failure; with each heart-beat blood fills the aneurysm, reducing the amount that gets pumped around the body; the heart fails while trying vainly to do its job. A less common cause of death comes from clots of blood breaking off from the larger clot that invariably forms in the aneurysm and shooting into the circulation to block an important artery, for example in the brain. Strangely enough, death is rarely caused by the aneurysm bursting. Cardiac aneurysms mostly follow a coronary thrombosis; other less common causes are a congenital defect, and the result of injury to the heart, or of syphilitic infection.

The first time a surgeon had operated on a cardiac aneurysm, it was quite by mistake. In 1931 a 28-year-old woman was diagnosed as having a cystic tumour of the mediastinum in the tissues near the heart. Ferdinand Sauerbruch, of negative pressure obstinacy, decided to operate and when he opened the woman's chest he was faced with a swelling the size of a child's head[1]. Still not suspecting the true diagnosis he thought it best to aspirate the contents and so make the tumour easier to remove. As he put the needle in, blood spurted out' around it; he tried to retrieve the situation by stitching the needle hole but this only made matters worse.

'Suddenly a strong column of blood spurted from the mistaken "cyst sac". I rapidly introduced my index and middle fingers into the wound and stopped the blood flow….Quickly I had an assistant pass two strong silk ligatures….The bleeding ceased! The position was now clear. The great cystic sac was an aneurysm of the right ventricle.' This called for a reorientation of surgical thought. Sauerbruch first succeeded in clamping off the swelling so that he could open it widely and remove the contained clot. After this there was really only one course he could adopt: he excised the surplus tissue constituting the walls of the aneurysm and brought the edges together with several layers of sutures. The cause of the aneurysm was not discovered.

The patient of this incredible operation was lucky to survive, but she did and seven years later Sauerbruch, in a talk to the West London Medico-Chirurgical Society, reported her to be alive and well[2]. Despite this, however, he said he had no intention of repeating the procedure as a planned undertaking.

All aspects of coronary disease intrigued Claude Beck, and in 1934 he tried to produce aneurysms experimentally so that he could work out a form of treatment, but the dogs' hearts would not co-operate. However, in 1942 he had the opportunity to put his ideas into practice[3]. The patient, a man of 42, was seriously ill and debilitated with constant anginal pain referred to the upper part of his abdomen in the epigastrium. Eighteen months previously he had had a severe bout of this epigastric pain which had been diagnosed as a perforated gastric ulcer and an exploratory operation was carried out. Two months afterwards the pain recurred but this time its cardiac origin was correctly identified. Since the man continued to go downhill Beck was asked to operate and on June 12 went in through an incision over the heart removing the fifth and sixth rib cartilages and part of the corresponding ribs. As soon as Beck incised the pericardium the aneurysm increased in size, giving him added confidence, for what he had in mind was the strengthening of the pericardium over the aneurysm to prevent its rupture (the natural behaviour of these swellings was imperfectly understood in those days), and, secondarily, to reduce its size. First, though, he wetted the surface of the aneurysm with Dakin's solution to promote an adhesive pericarditis[4]. The strengthening material Beck took from the broad band of fibrous tissue (fascia lata) on the outside of the patient's thigh; this he cut large enough to cover the whole of the aneurysm and stitched it to the inside of the pericardial sac. A few days after operation the man developed an empyema, and a litre of pus was removed from the left pleural cavity; but the infection proved too much for him and he died five weeks later. The postmortem examination showed that the fascial graft was in place and free from infection.

Beck felt the operation would have had a greater chance of success had the patient not been so ill. Nevertheless, no one attempted it again for more than 10 years, when in the mid-to-late 1950s strengthening operations enjoyed a mild vogue, particularly in Germany and Russia, and successes were achieved with grafts of skin[5], pectoralis major muscle[6], intercostal muscle, diaphragm, and omentum. But techniques of this nature were never really satisfactory, based as they were on an incorrect assessment of the dangers of cardiac aneurysm. The useless sac itself had to be removed and with progress in heart surgery this became possible.

Gordon Murray began speculating on the excision of infarcted heart muscle in an article published in 1947[7]. Although not dealing with the actual treatment of aneurysms, this marked the starting-point of subsequent work. Murray was, in fact, thinking about removing the dead area before an aneurysm had even had time to develop. His experiments on dogs were an attempt to discover why death occurred from coronary thrombosis. When a coronary artery was ligated. the area of heart muscle supplied by the artery dilated and then ceased to contract. As soon as its contraction stopped, it operated against the interests of the remainder of the ventricular muscle. So Murray excised this area to overcome its deleterious effects. This he did by bringing the boundaries of the area together so that it bulged outwards, cutting off the bulge and stitching the edges together. Most of the 25 dogs operated on made good recoveries and some were alive and well, with no limitation of function, as long as two years afterwards. His control experiments showed that the tying off of the particular coronary artery would otherwise have been fatal.

Murray reckoned that this form of treatment soon after a heart attack would not only remove the 'expansion chamber' (created by the dilatation of the infarcted area) and save the patient from collapse, but would also remove the danger of rupture of the area or its development into an aneurysm. 'While it is obviously facetious at this stage to make the following remarks,' he wrote[7], 'still I have a conviction that, as medical treatment is so ineffective, and is entirely helpless, except from a palliative point of view, the day may come, when the best plan of dealing with a coronary thrombosis, would be emergency operation.'

That day took 19 years to dawn: on July 14, 1966, Raymond O Heimbecker, working closely with Murray, carried out a successful emergency infarctectomy on a man of 56[8]. Since his previous paper of 1947, Murray had performed further experiments on calves which were extremely encouraging: with cardiac massage and heart-lung bypass he had had initial salvage rates of 12 percent and survival rates of 8 percent; but with infarctectomy he improved the figures to 100 percent and 47 percent, respectively. Murray based his belief in the value of the emergency operation on the fact that most of the patients who die from acute infarction do so within the first 48-72 hours. The 56-year-old patient fulfilled the criteria for the ideal subject as he was admitted in shock, with pulmonary oedema and failure to respond to medical treatment. At operation large infarcts were resected from both ventricles, and the necrotic, perforated ventricular septum (a result of the heart attack) was repaired.

The first person to excise a postinfarctional aneurysm was Charles Bailey on April 15, 1954[9]. His patient was a 56-year-old man whose heart attack had occurred some 15 months previously. When surgery was decided upon this man was in pain, extremely short of breath and compelled to sit upright in bed to get any rest. Bailey's incision was in the sixth space between the ribs on the left and extended from the bodies of the vertebrae behind to the internal mammary vessels in front. When he dissected away the dense, very vascular pericardium, he was greeted by a 'smooth ovoid bulge' involving the entire anterior wall of the left ventricle. This he clamped off and immediately there was an improvement in the functioning of the heart. The next step was to insert a continuous heavy silk suture on the heart side of the clamp followed by a series of interrupted mattress sutures. Bailey then removed the clamp slowly cutting away the aneurysm and sewing the raw edges together with another continuous suture as he went along. The patient stood the operation well and was in good health three years later.

In 1957 Bailey presented his report on the nine patients he had operated on[10]. All but one were alive and much improved; the failure had been due to clots dislodged from the aneurysm getting into the circulation, a recognized hazard of the technique. Another hazard was damage to the structures inside the ventricle, but Bailey had overcome this by inserting an ungloved finger through the atrium into the ventricle from time to time to keep a check on how the excision was going. He also laid considerable stress on 'tailoring' the ventricle, emphasizing that he did not necessarily attempt to remove all the scar tissue, but sufficient to restore the chamber to as near normal a size and shape as possible.

During the discussion of Bailey's paper, Beck said that not all aneurysms were of a sac-like shape; those that were merely a bulge did not need to be excised; they could be grafted. But he was flogging a dead horse, and indeed Bailey's 'closed' technique was also on the way out, as by the time his paper was published, the first 'open' excision using a heart-lung machine had already been performed.

On January 17, 1958, Denton Cooley of Baylor University, Houston, Texas, temporarily bypassed the heart so that he could more satisfactorily clear all the clot out of the aneurysm (which was 10cm in diameter), excise it and stitch the edges together with a clear view of the internal structures[11]. The patient, a man of 50, had had his heart attack only three months before operation – a short interval, as in a later paper Cooley stated the average time between infarct and surgery to be 15 months – and suffering badly from shortness of breath on exertion. After his operation the man had a fever and was mentally disorientated, but fortunately the anxiety for him only lasted a short while and 18 days later he was sent home, where he continued to improve and increase his activities.

Other surgeons were soon tackling aneurysms under these improved conditions; for instance Walton Lillehei, on June 5, that same year, excised a huge one measuring 12 by 15cm with complete success[12]. Three years later the patient was well and working full time; something that would have been only a dream a few years previously.

And so we can come to a halt in the long and complex story of surgery and coronary artery disease at a point at which a physical deformation of the heart wall made the surgeon undisputed master of the situation, and one in which he was using his skill and the resources of a rapidly developing science with increasing success.

15

FIELDS OF BATTLE

The story of cardiac surgery in both the major wars of the last century is largely that of foreign bodies in the heart. The neat stab wounds favoured by murderers, would-be suicides and the accidents of civil life were virtually non-existent. Instead surgeons had to contend with bullets and fragments of shrapnel that lodged within the pericardial cavity, the heart muscle or the chambers themselves. Missiles reached the heart directly through the chest wall or, more occasionally, migrated there from a wound elsewhere in the body usually by penetrating a blood vessel and being carried in the blood stream as an embolus[1]. When the missile entered through the chest it often produced bruising and ugly lacerations; cardiac tamponade was rare because the hole in the pericardium was too big to allow blood to accumulate in the pericardial cavity and build up a strangling pressure; it leaked out into the surrounding tissues or pleural cavities. Nevertheless, the surprising thing was really the small amount of disturbance experienced by the wounded soldiers who survived long enough to get into the right surgical hands and then be recorded in the literature. The official history of the British medical services in the Great War stated, for example: 'Further, a perusal of published cases cannot fail to emphasize the insignificant nature of the primary symptoms [of a foreign body in the heart or pericardium] in a large number of instances.'[2] However, when the wounded man later returned to service life or a civilian job, the foreign body might sometimes make its presence felt by alterations in the rate and rhythm of the heart-beat and by shortness of breath; pain was less constant, but was at times felt when lying on the injured side. Whether or not the missile was then removed depended on the individual circumstances.

At the start of the First World War very little open chest surgery was carried out. There were two reasons for this. First, surgeons were afraid of creating a pneumothorax, and second the experiences of the Boer War, where chest wounds tended to be relatively clean, had led to an official policy of conservatism. But as the war progressed, the mud of Flanders changed all this; infection was the big problem and operation was needed to allow adequate drainage of pus. So, because their hand was forced, surgeons came to lose their fear of the open chest.

The over-all picture of heart wounds in the First World War is best summed up by three quotations, two from the British and the third from the United States official histories.

'While, therefore, no records are available upon which to form a reliable opinion as to the proportionate frequency with which death follows as a consequence of uncomplicated wounds of the heart, the natural inference is to the effect that the traditional view is correct, and that the immense majority of men who receive these injuries find their end upon the field of battle.'[2]

'No doubt a considerable number of operations have been performed in which rents in the pericardium were repaired, or retained foreign bodies removed, but unfortunately few records of these are available.'[2]

'Early operations upon the heart and pericardium have been few because wounds affecting them are either promptly fatal or treated expectantly. Such injuries as are disclosed by operation are easily remedied as they require little more than simple suturing.'[3]

Before the First World War at least 380 operations had been carried out for heart wounds with a mortality rate of about 45 percent. During the war more than 60 were added to the list; Sir Charles Ballance, the British surgeon, collected the records of 58 of these and found that only 14 patients had died; this, as he said, was 'a wonderful record!'[4] The French performed all but a handful of these operations and in some cases the interval between the injury and surgery was impressive as in the case of a soldier wounded at Bapaume on August 27, 1914, and taken prisoner by the Germans. At first he had very slight symptoms but after six months he began to get worse with frequent heart attacks and a sensation of impending death. Since an x-ray showed a bullet in his heart, he was sent to Switzerland where he remained until he eventually managed to reach Paris in April 1917. Here he came into the care of Henri Hartmann who successfully excised the bullet from the wall of the right ventricle – more than two-and-a-half years after the wounding[5].

In a number of instances a bullet that had entered a ventricular cavity was later pumped out with the blood stream; for instance in 1916 another Frenchman, Deneke, removed such a bullet which had become impacted in the right axillary artery[6].

Another memorable operation was carried out by Paul Duval with the assistance of Henry Barnsby[7]. A bullet had entered through a soldier's left lung, passed through his left ventricle and interventricular septum and eventually lodged in his inferior vena cava, although only one of those who studied the x-rays was prepared to say that that was where it was, as it was extremely mobile. At Beauvais, six days after the injury, Duval operated; he decided on a long mid-line thoraco-abdominal incision (from the level of the fourth ribs to the umbilicus) which would give him a good chance of being able to cope with any eventuality. There was blood in the left chest (causing some difficulty with the anaesthetic) but only a little sero-sanguineous fluid in the pericardial cavity. Duval opened the inferior vena cava at its junction with the left atrium, and here he found the bullet 'like an egg dancing on a jet of water'. He removed it and closed the incision. The operation took 35 minutes. Nine days later the patient was doing well, and went on to complete recovery.

Of the six recorded operations on the heart by British surgeons, three were successful. John Fraser of Edinburgh and a Captain in the RAMC had seen soldiers die in six to eight hours from accumulation of blood in the pericardial cavity. Therefore he made up his mind to operate immediately should he have another case in which the symptoms raised suspicions of the heart's wall having been perforated. That case, reported in 1917[8], was a soldier with multiple wounds of the face, both eyes, arms and chest who, in spite of it all, was in fair condition. When he opened the chest, Fraser found a small flap-like perforation in the right atrium which he repaired. Four months later the soldier was in excellent health, having made an uninterrupted recovery; one eye had had to be removed, but vision in the other was adequate.

The success of Herbert Henry Sampson was with a furrow of the heart. At operation the wound was gaping with a clot already forming in its depths. Sampson left the clot undisturbed and simply sewed up the wound over it[9].

The third of the three British successes was achieved by Sir Berkeley Moynihan (later Lord Moynihan). JB, aged 34, was hit in the chest on April 11, 1917, in France. The wound became infected and an empyema (pus in the pleural cavity) developed. Nine days after the wounding, the empyema was drained surgically; for more than six months it continued to discharge and when Moynihan saw him a year later JB was short of breath on exertion, but had no pain or cough. A bullet was found embedded in the heart and on May 3, 1918, Moynihan operated. He put two stitches in the left ventricle to steady the heart and then cut down on the missile which was lifted out with a scoop. Recovery was rapid and without incident but in response to a letter from Moynihan at the end of 1919, JB wrote: 'I am not yet capable of doing my usual work.' This remaining disability was attributed to the damage to his lung. Moynihan also removed missiles from the pericardium on three occasions with success in all. He drew attention to the variable presence of symptoms with retained foreign bodies, but felt that generally they were a source of discomfort and anxiety, although there seemed to be no distinction in this respect between smooth and jagged missiles[10].

The three British cases that ended fatally were of a quite different character to those that were successful. In one, the operation was undertaken because of established infection and the patient died from severe pericarditis. In the other two, the right ventricle was actually opened and the patients died, respectively, from multiple pulmonary emboli (arising from clots in the ventricle) and from infection. This last case came under the care of Ballance himself. A 21-year-old trooper had been wounded in Salonika on November 14, 1917, and an x-ray showed the bullet in the wall of the left ventricle. He was evacuated to Malta suffering greatly from seasickness on the voyage. When Ballance saw him at St Elmo Hospital his pulse was rapid and irregular on the slightest exertion. Before operating, Ballance tested the bullets of various nations to see whether a magnet might be useful in the removal as it was virtually certain that the offending missile had come from a Bulgarian rifle. The 'modern' Bulgarian bullet was not magnetic although a 'modern' Serbian bullet was strongly so. At operation on February 16, 1918, the bullet was found firmly embedded in the inner surface of the left ventricle and had to be freed by cutting with a knife. Towards the end of the operation the patient became very anaemic and was given a blood transfusion directly from a donor. This was continued until the donor's systolic blood pressure fell to 90mmHg which was reached in five-and-a-half minutes. Some saline solution was left in the pericardial cavity and the wound closed. The bullet, true enough, was Bulgarian, but it proved to be of ancient pattern and strongly magnetic!

For a few days all went well, but then infection set in and progressed in spite of all that could be done until it killed the trooper four weeks after the operation. Ballance at first thought the symptoms and signs were due to clot forming on the surface of the wound inside the heart; he was mesmerized by what he believed to be the heart's difference from other organs, and only afterwards did he realize that he should have treated the infection like infection elsewhere and opened up the wound widely to allow good drainage[4].

'It is a common experience that bullets frequently lodge in the tissue and induce neither local nor general infection until attempts at removal are made,' said Ballance, and indeed many missiles were left undisturbed in the area of the heart, sometimes because their presence was not diagnosed, sometimes because the surgeon in charge did not feel competent to remove them, and sometimes deliberately because this was felt to be the best course. During a discussion on war wounds of the heart in 1947, Jerome R Head of Chicago said he had been dealing with the chest problems of the First World War veterans between 1926 and 1946 and although many had foreign bodies left in the chest, he had seen only two in whom these were causing trouble[11].

In the years between the two world wars a change in the approach to heart wounds slowly became apparent. The swing away from operating whenever possible towards operating in selected cases began with Albert Singleton, professor of surgery at the University of Texas, Galveston, who wrote in 1933: 'Aspiration of the pericardium is criticized as an unsafe procedure by many. We do not believe that aspiration of the pericardium is always unwise; on the contrary with definite signs and symptoms of effusion, and with reasonable care, one need not hesitate to puncture the pericardium.'[12] He was talking about aspirating the blood in cases of cardiac tamponade, one of the common causes of death in stab wounds; admittedly he believed the procedure was most useful to relieve the pressure round the heart while the patient was awaiting surgical repair of the wound, but he did say that occasionally aspiration alone might save life. Singleton also reviewed the literature on foreign bodies in the heart and concluded that their presence was not always lethal. Removal might invite trouble, he said, and should only be attempted after very careful consideration. The figures he gave showed that of 33 patients who had been operated on four died, and of 49 not submitted to surgery five died – these really only bear out the argument in favour of assessing each case individually.

In 1938, Alexander Bigger of Richmond, Virginia, reported on 17 patients and said, 'we now believe that patients with heart wounds should be operated on promptly if the indications are clear and urgent, but if the indications are not urgent some form of conservative treatment should be considered.'[13] And included in the conservative treatment was aspiration of blood in the pericardium, although this suggestion was not received with unreserved enthusiasm by all the participants in the discussion of his paper, owing to the possible risks of the undertaking, such as puncturing a coronary artery.

A short while afterwards John Strieder of Boston, who so narrowly missed success with the first operation to close a patent ductus arteriosus, was confronted with a 12-year-old Armenian boy who had been stabbed accidentally. While waiting for the theatre to be prepared he remembered Bigger's talk and decide to aspirate the pericardium. The improvement was immediate and dramatic – incidentally the 100ml of withdrawn blood was returned to the circulation by intravenous injection. Yet despite his success in averting operation, Strieder concluded, 'However, it would seem that not operating upon a patient with a stab wound is a very hazardous course to follow.'[14]

But the message was beginning to get home, helped not a little by the arrival of an adequate blood transfusion service and of the sulphonamides and penicillin to combat infection, the bugbear of heart wounds. In March, 1942, an American military manual *Guides to therapy for medical officers* included the following directions for dealing with heart wounds: '(*a*) Aspirate the blood from the pericardium by the costoxiphoid route, if possible. (*b*) Repeat if there is a recurrence. (*c*) If it again recurs, perform a cardiorrhaphy through an extrapleural exposure.'[15] (i.e. repair the heart wound through an incision that does not open the pleural cavities).

These instructions soon received the support of a study of the non-operative treatment of cardiac tamponade carried out by Alfred Blalock and Mark Ravitch at Johns Hopkins[16]. They found that the mortality rate in reported cases of patients who reached hospital and were operated on for heart wounds was almost 50 percent; in other words there had been no improvement since the years before the First World War. This made them wonder whether better results might not be achieved by delaying operation when there was no bleeding through the chest wound or into the pleural cavity. If there were symptoms of cardiac tamponade, aspiration was the order of the day, although should the fluid reaccumulate rapidly operation was essential. However, while this method of management was in progress the operating theatre should be instantly available. Their own patients who were treated in this way had blood and fluid transfusions, and the results were excellent – if the heart wound had already begun to heal and seal itself off, there was no point in operating to insert stitches.

This work marked the start of the modern treatment of heart wounds, even though some surgeons took a lot of convincing that these injuries did not always require suturing, and the only refinement came after 1953 when the heart-lung machine enabled surgeons, at a time of their own choosing to repair structures within the heart that had been damaged by the original insult.

But to return to the Second World War. Most thoracic surgeons, said the official British history[17], operated on a few casualties for removal of retained missiles from the walls of the ventricles or from the pericardium. There was no British case in which a foreign body was removed from the chambers of the heart. These laconic remarks were in striking contrast to the 44 pages devoted to heart and pericardial injuries in the Great War history and such statistics as were given tended to be lost among those for chest wounds as a whole.

After being given first aid, the soldier wounded in the chest was evacuated, having whatever was possible done for him at the various stages along the route until he arrived at a forward hospital. Here he might receive definitive treatment or be sent back to the base hospital. In 1948 Paul Samson of Oakland, California, reviewed the experiences of the Second Auxiliary Surgical Group at forward hospitals[18]. Soldiers with foreign bodies in their hearts were, in general, sent back to base, unless the haemorrhage was persistent or there were signs of cardiac dysfunction; but in spite of this, the surgeons in the group dealt with 57 patients with heart wounds and 18 with pericardial wounds.

Even at the forward hospitals diagnosis was difficult and in rather more than half of all cases the fact that the heart was wounded was not discovered until the operation had been started. Samson confirmed the unusualness, due to the size of the lacerations, of cardiac tamponade and in 10 of the 16 lacerated wounds of the myocardium found at operation no repair was attempted – and with no awkward consequences. Pericardium was frequently sutured over the heart wound, especially when apposition of the edges had been difficult, to give added strength to the repair, and in two instances free grafts of muscle were used to help stop the bleeding. Out of their 75 patients Samson's group had 30 deaths; 27 of these were among the 57 patients with injuries to the heart muscle, and three among the 18 with pericardial wounds. But, as Samson remarked, it should not be forgotten that these patients often had other wounds which might have contributed to the mortality rate.

At a base hospital in the south of England an American surgeon, Dwight Harken of Boston, truly made use of the injuries of war finally to cross the frontier between ancient and modern and show convincingly what the future could hold for cardiac surgery. Working in the thoracic centre of the 160th General Hospital in the United States Army in the European Theatre of Operations he removed 134 missiles from the mediastinum without losing a single patient. Of these missiles, 55 were pericardial and 13 were in the heart chambers – Ballance's comment on the results during the First World War, 'a wonderful record!', would be a totally inadequate footnote to this achievement.

Harken did not operate on all soldiers who came to his hospital with foreign bodies in their hearts; in fact more foreign bodies, 'presumably within the heart', were allowed to remain than were removed. He had four main reasons for deciding to operate: to forestall embolus of the missile or of blood clot associated with it; to reduce the danger of bacterial infection; to avoid recurrent pericardial effusions; and to reduce damage to the heart muscle. Admittedly, as he said, he was influenced in favour of surgery in some cases by pain or cardiac neurosis[19].

One of the difficulties to which Harken drew especial attention was that of localization of the missile by x-ray or even by fluoroscopy (in which movements can be watched on the x-ray screen). Only if the patient came to operation or postmortem could one be certain whether the foreign body was in the heart or not. This had not always been appreciated in the past to judge from the confident tone in which x-ray localization had been reported[20], although the official British history of the Great War medical services had been aware of the possibility of confusion and had noted that a bullet in the lung, completely outside the pericardium, could sometimes move in time with the heart-beat[21].

In no sense of the words did Harken have his eyes shut while operating; he used the opportunities given him to study the behaviour of the heart during the necessary manipulations and found that it did not take kindly to dislocation from its normal position – thus confirming the observations of Cutler and other surgeons in the 1920s. But his most significant contribution to the future was when, in one case, he isolated part of the right ventricle with pressure from his fingers and thumb and worked for more than three minutes to free a metallic foreign body in what was virtually an 'open' heart.

Throughout, the patient's heart continued to maintain an effective blood pressure[21].

During the discussion of the paper recording these events, which was read by Harken in 1947, another American surgeon, Laurence Miscall of New York, said that at his centre in northern England they had removed 39 foreign bodies from the heart, again with no deaths[22].

Unlike other medical and surgical spheres of endeavour, during both world conflicts the experiences of surgeons added little to the actual technique of heart surgery. In the First World War surgeons lost their fear of the open chest; the second had an intense stimulating effect on the associated activities that were to make the technical advances possible. Diagnostic facilities were improved; anaesthesia made great strides; penicillin, the first of the antibiotics, was in commercial production; the blood transfusion service as we know it today came into being; and, a point stressed by Miscall, the importance of team-work was appreciated. And Harken gave confidence for the work ahead.

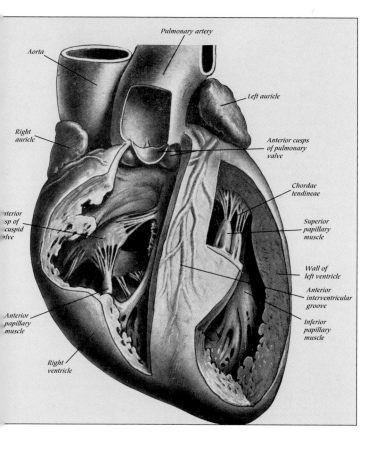

The heart. (a) The interior of the ventricles, exposed by removal of the anterior walls. (b) The interior of the right atrium and of the ventricles, showing also the interventricular septum. (Hamilton WJ. (1956). Editor, *Textbook of human anatomy*. London; Macmillan.)

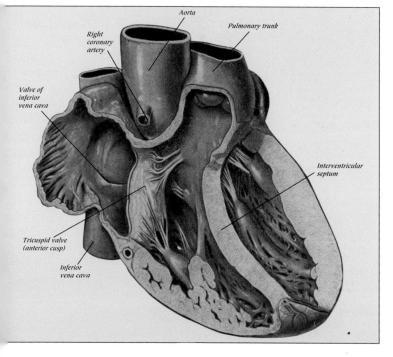

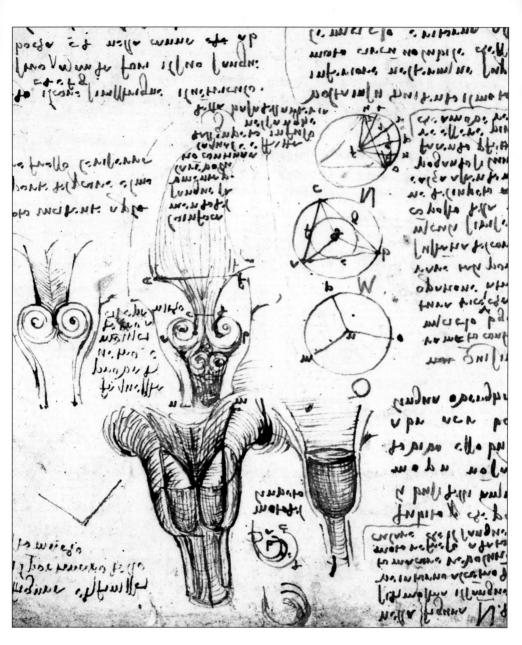

Leonardo da Vinci's diagrams of the left ventricular outflow tract, the aortic valve and the haemodynamic turbulences in the area. (Reproduced by gracious permission of Her Majesty the Queen.)

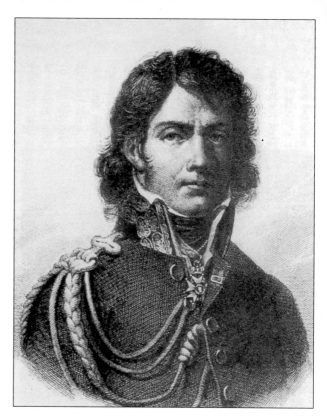

Dominique Jean Larrey, 1804. From an engraving by Pollet. (By courtesy of the Wellcome Trustees.)

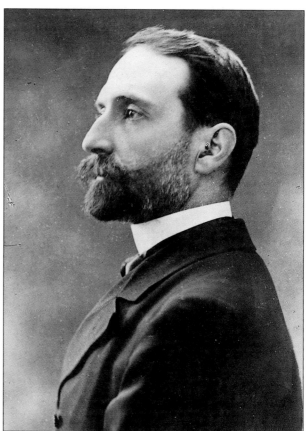

Théodore Tuffier. (From an original photograph lent by Dr EA Underwood.)

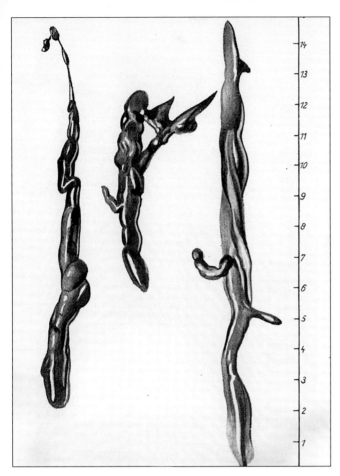

Pulmonary emboli removed from Johanna Kempf by Martin Kirschner on March 18, 1924. (Kirschner M. (1924). By courtesy of Springer Verlag.) [Chapter 6; ref. 5.]

Ferdinand Sauerbruch's experimental negative-pressure chamber. (Sauerbruch F. (1904).) [Chapter 8; ref. 18.]

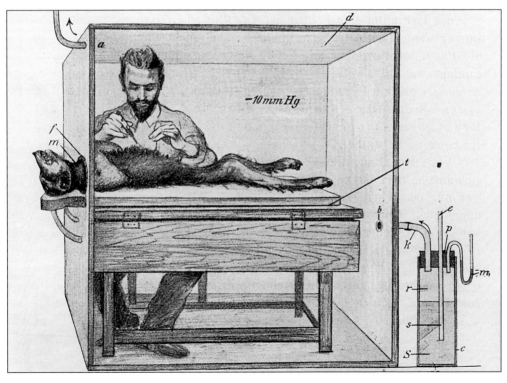

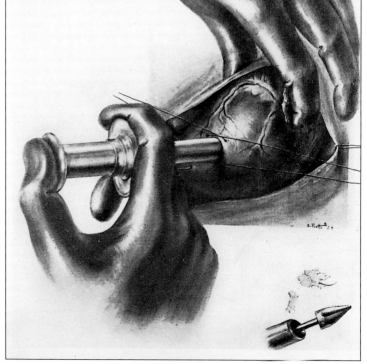

Cutler's and Beck's cardio-valvulotome. (a) The model used in their fourth patient; it carries the distal blade centrally situated. (b) The way the cardiovalvulotome was used. (Beck CS, Cutler EC. (1924). By courtesy of Dr Beck and the Editor, *Journal of Experimental Medicine*.) [Chapter 9; ref. 12.]

(a)

(b)

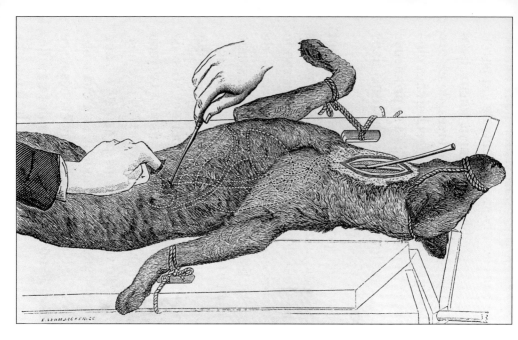

ABOVE: Claude Bernard's experiment of catheterizing the heart and both venae cavae of a dog through its jugular vein. The abdominal manipulations were part of a more extended procedure for obtaining blood flowing into the inferior vena cava from the liver. (Bernard C. (1879). [Chapter 10; ref. 9.]

BELOW: The x-ray taken by Werner Forssmann after he had passed a ureteric catheter up a vein in his arm into the right side of his heart. (Forssmann W. (1929). [Chapter 10; ref. 14.]

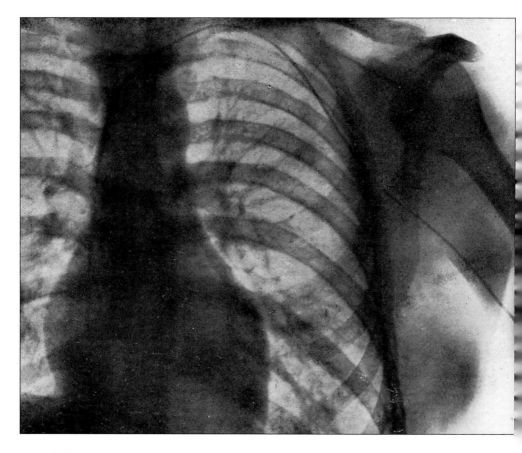

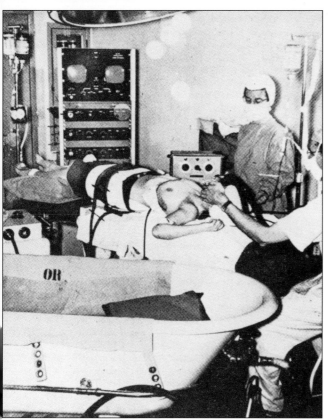

Henry Swan's operating room equipment for hypothermia. This included the tub, a rectal thermometer, a diathermy unit, a multi-channel electronic recording device, the defibrillator, a direct writing electroencephalogram, and a standard anaesthetic machine. The patient is still in the operating position immediately after wound closure. (From Swan H, *et al.* (1955). *Annals of Surgery*, **142**, 382, by courtesy of Dr Swan and the Editor, *Annals of Surgery*.) The tub and other equipment which served more than 500 open heart operations at Colorado General Hospital were displayed in the medical division at the Smithsonian Institute in Washington.

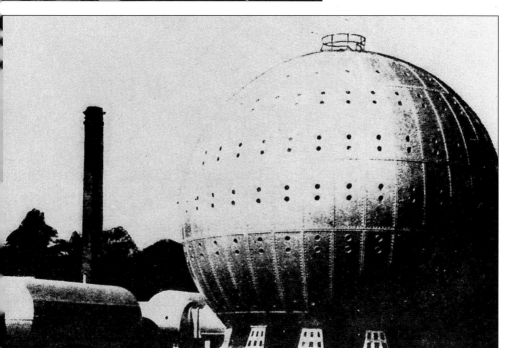

The six-storey, 72-room hyperbaric chamber built for Orval Cunningham in Cleveland, Ohio, in 1928. Jacobson JH II, Morsch JHC, Rendell-Baker L. 1964). 'Historic perspective of hyperbaric therapy.' Boerema I, Brummelkamp WH, Meijne NG, eds. *Clinical application of hyperbaric oxygen*. Amsterdam, London, New York; Elsevier. By courtesy of Dr Jacobson and the publishers.)

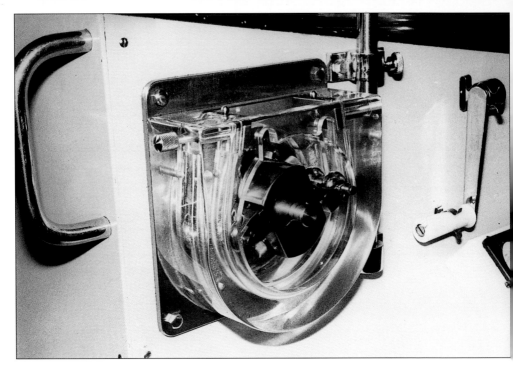

A roller pump, showing how the rollers work without coming into contact with the blood inside the polythene tubing. (By courtesy of the Department of Medical Illustration, Royal Postgraduate Medical School.)

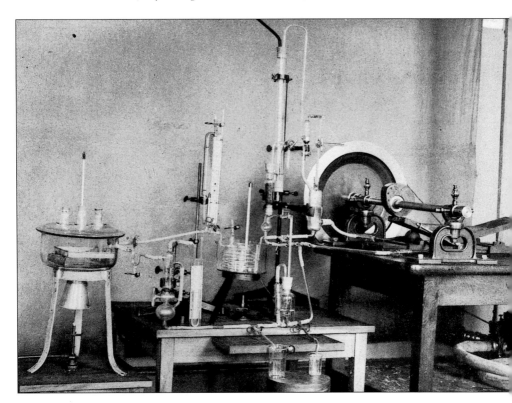

Carl Jacobj's pump-oxygenator showing the pump on the right and the oxygenating device in the centre and left. (Jacobj C. (1890).) [Chapter 24; ref. 1.]

16

BLUE BABIES AND SOME OTHERS

After the Second World War ended, surgeons were able to revert to the problems of heart disease. Some of the advances were the logical progression of research started before 1939, but the war itself had rapidly matured the outlook of the chest surgeon. More than that, it was as though the whole profession had emerged from a long dark tunnel to see an exciting new prospect. The foreground was clear and ready for exploitation; the middle distance was misty, and the beyond was impenetrable. No one at that stage could have foreseen just how quickly the apparently impenetrable was to be reached and illuminated. No other realm of surgery ever moved so fast, so surely and confidently it now seems, as did cardiac surgery after the war.

In the immediate post-war years there was tremendous activity; at first most attention was paid to congenital defects, especially those that could be treated by extracardiac or anastomotic operations. The direct attack on the heart valves was attended by a high mortality rate – not unexpected owing to the selection of seriously ill patients. But as surgeons gained in experience they were able to operate earlier and the results began to improve. In some instances palliative operations were introduced as interim measures until a definitive technique could be devised. In others, adequate treatment demanded an 'open' heart, with a bypass circulation, and until this was obtainable surgeons had to make do with 'closed' operations and adapt their procedures to the limitations currently imposed.

Since a strictly chronological account would be utterly confusing, we shall trace the story along a number of paths, all of which were running side by side. These paths were transformed from muddy tracks to metalled highways in 1953 with the arrival of hypothermia and the heart-lung machine; so, as far as is practicable, we shall use this date as a convenient staging post.

The first of our paths will be that of congenital abnormality. Here, owing to an error in embryological development, the heart is physically deformed. The outlook varies tremendously depending on the abnormality and its severity; the baby may be born dead or die soon after birth; he may die in early or middle adult life or he may live a normal existence and the defect perhaps only be discovered postmortem. About eight babies in every 1000 born in Great Britain have a cardiac malformation, and four of these, if untreated, will die before they are two years old. Medical treatment is confined to managing the symptoms, for instance of heart failure, when they occur and to getting the patients into as good shape as possible for surgery – for surgery is the only real treatment.

In some mild defects, though, there is little difficulty in deciding whether or not to operate. The first essential of all treatment is that the patient should benefit, either immediately or in the long run as a protection against complications. But before cardiac surgery came along little attention was paid to congenital heart defects, and almost nothing was known about their natural course. Knowledge of the defects was acquired in response to the increasing capability of surgery and for this very reason the natural, untreated course of some defects remained uncertain and there was no yardstick against which the results of surgery could be measured. For example, there is no doubt that patients with large interventricular septal defects (holes in the wall between the two ventricles) should be considered serious candidates for surgery, but those with small symptomless holes pose a problem. On the one hand the condition may not progress, the hole may even close spontaneously or become smaller as the child grows; on the other the lungs may be affected or various complications develop. The surgeon has to weigh up these natural possibilities and balance them against the risks inherent in any surgical operation.

There is, however, general agreement that patients with coarctation of the aorta should be operated on. Although this abnormality is not of the heart it is usually considered to come within the province of cardiac surgery. It is a limited narrowing most commonly of the arch of the aorta though it may sometimes be quite lengthy and occasionally affect the abdominal aorta. Trouble arises from the high blood pressure in the arteries of the upper part of the body that come off the aorta before the constriction. If the condition is untreated about 50 percent of affected babies die in their first year of life – often they have associated abnormalities – and most of those who survive are dead before they reach 50, usually from the effects of the high blood pressure. Thus we know sufficient of the natural course of coarctation to show that operation is beneficial, particularly if it can be done at the optimum age of seven to nine years, when the aorta is a reasonable size; and there is good evidence that its growth after treatment will keep pace with the growth of the child.

Clarence Crafoord's wealth of experience in chest surgery stood him in good stead when on October 19, 1944, he and Gustav Nylin excised a coarctation and joined the two cut ends of the aorta together. Their first patient was a 12-year-old boy; 12 days later they repeated the performance on a 27-year-old farmer[1].

Meanwhile, in America, Robert Gross of Boston was bringing to fulfilment the experiments he had started in March 1938[2]. He had subsequently been joined by Charles Hufnagel and on June 28, 1945, they operated on a five-year-old boy; regrettably the clamps used to seal off the blood flow were released too quickly and the lad died of cardiac dilatation. But, profiting from this error, they achieved complete success with their next patient, a girl of 12. Her operation took place on July 6, and 10 minutes of the three-and-a-half hour operation were spent in the slow removal of the clamps[3].

It is much to the credit of Crafoord and Gross that their technique, arrived at quite independently, is essentially that still used in uncomplicated cases. Modifications have, of course, been necessary to meet the demands imposed by coarctations in different parts of the aorta and especially to overcome the problems of a long stricture or a relatively inelastic aorta when the two ends cannot be brought together. In the days before arterial grafting became commonplace recourse was had to a method devised by Alfred Blalock and Edwards Park at Johns Hopkins. They produced an experimental coarctation in dogs with elastic bands and then bypassed it by freeing the left subclavian artery (which comes off the aorta before the coarctation in most human cases), ligating and dividing it at a suitable level, and anastomosing it end-to-side to the aorta below the stricture. The aorta itself was divided between ligatures at the level of narrowing[4]. The first time this was done clinically was quite unintentional and not because the coarctation was lengthy:

On August 6, 1946, Theron Clagett was operating on a 34-year-old man (the oldest patient reported up to that time) at the Mayo Clinic. He had every intention of resecting the coarctation in the usual manner, but finding it to be too close to the origin of the left subclavian artery he thought this would be technically impossible. Consequently, he ligated the stricture, dissected out the subclavian artery, divided it, rotated it to its new position and performed an *end-to-end* anastomosis to the aorta beyond the stricture – a feat only possible because the subclavian artery was so dilated as to be almost the same size as the aorta. The operation lasted four hours, but the patient's condition was good throughout and remained so; surprisingly the left arm (supplied with blood through the left subclavian artery) did not appear to have suffered[5]. During the next few years other surgeons, such as Gordon Murray[6], used this subclavian bypass operation as a routine in cases in which the ends of the aorta could not be brought together. However, it went out of favour when arterial surgery was sufficiently advanced for grafts to be used. The first to bridge the gap with a preserved human arterial graft was Gross on May 24, 1948; his patient was a seven-year-old boy[7]. Since then both arterial grafts and prosthetic tubing have been used, and surgeons made it a rule to have a graft at hand in case the unexpected was found.

In the early days it was hard to convince the medical profession that the aorta, the main artery of the body, could be joined by just one row of fine stitches and still withstand the pressure of the blood flow; yet it is so and the results of operation are good. The blood pressure in the upper part of the body falls, if not to normal certainly to less dangerous levels.

A few days after Crafoord's coarctation success, Alfred Blalock performed an operation on a 14-month-old baby girl with congenital cyanotic heart disease – the original 'blue baby' operation[8]. When the defect is such that the blood in the two sides of the heart becomes mixed, a variable proportion of unoxygenated (blue, venous) blood is pumped around the body and the patient is cyanosed – or 'blue'. A number of different defects can produce cyanosis but the classical one, and the commonest, that Blalock operated for, is known as Fallot's tetrad. As its name implies, four abnormalities make up the anomaly: stenosis of the pulmonary valve or some form of obstruction to the outflow tract of the right ventricle; a hole between the ventricles; a variable degree of shift of the aorta to the right so that it accepts blood from the right ventricle; and hypertrophy of the right ventricle. This formidable array was described in 1888 by Étienne Louis Arthur Fallot, a French physician[9]. Since then, however, the name has been applied to hearts with greatly varying grades of these deformities; the condition is not always full-blown, one component may predominate over the others. Nevertheless Fallot's tetrad, or tetralogy, continues to be a useful diagnostic label.

A patient with Fallot's tetrad may have yet more defects in his heart, and it was the presence of one of these that gave Helen Taussig an idea. At that time she was physician in charge of the Harriet Lane Home Cardiac Clinic at Johns Hopkins University, an appointment she had held since 1930; subsequently, in 1946, she became associate professor of paediatrics at Johns Hopkins University and, in 1959, professor. She had noticed that when children with Fallot's tetrad had an associated patent ductus arteriosus they fared better than their fellows. (The ductus joins the pulmonary artery with the aorta so that the lungs are bypassed before birth; after birth it normally closes spontaneously.) Apparently this persisting connection between the systemic and pulmonary circulations was being put to good use and some of the blood was flowing along it into the lungs and so having a second chance to pick up oxygen. Why not copy this principle, thought Helen Taussig, and create a channel from the aorta to the pulmonary circulation in those children with uncomplicated Fallot's tetrad. In this way some of the blue blood being circulated around the body would be drawn off soon after it left the heart and be sent to the lungs, bypass-ing the obstruction at the pulmonary valve.

She discussed the plan with Blalock who was an extremely experienced vascular surgeon – once again we see how cardiac surgery did not just appear out of the blue; all the leading protagonists in those early days had a solid grounding in some vital aspect of the subject without which satisfactory progress could not be made – and together they devised a suitable operation. On November 29, 1944, Blalock anastomosed the left subclavian artery to the left pulmonary artery in the baby girl. The result was dramatically satisfying. For the next two cases he used the innominate artery for the anastomosis[8]. Procedures of this nature, usually employing the subclavian artery, became known as the Blalock-Taussig operation.

In their report they mentioned joining the aorta directly to the pulmonary artery as a possible, and quicker, alternative, but they had only done it on dogs. It was Willis Potts of Chicago who first performed it clinically nearly two years later on September 13, 1946, after he had devised a special instrument for clamping off part of the aortic wall without interrupting the blood flow. His anaesthetist during the three-hour operation on a 21-month-old girl was William McQuiston whom we shall meet again when discussing hypothermia. The girl's condition afterwards was described as excellent. Within a fortnight Potts had operated twice more: on a girl of 11 who died 36 hours after surgery, and on a girl of eight who was much improved, having only slight cyanosis on walking[10].

Potts's operation could only be done on one side and was more trouble-some than the Blalock-Taussig if other abnormalities were encountered; against this it had a lower operative mortality rate, about 9 percent as compared with 12-18 percent, although these figures varied with the age of the patient. It must, however, be appreciated that these operations did nothing to correct the basic abnormalities of Fallot's tetrad; in fact they added yet another. In the early days some people were worried the operation might be responsible for added complications, but, as Blalock himself remarked, the fear of complications in the future was no justification for allowing a patient to die from lack of oxygen in the present. As it transpired these operations gave valuable respite and symptomatic improvement to a number of children and enabled them to live long enough to benefit from corrective operations when surgery on the open heart became possible. As Sir Thomas Holmes Sellors wrote in 1967: 'Of the considerable number of patients I operated on between 1947 and 1954 about a quarter or a third are capable of leading normal lives with minimal inconvenience. Of the remainder some have died and others are in need of more definitive corrective surgery.'[11] A shunt operation continued to be carried out when the child was too small for a corrective operation.

The Blalock-Taussig and the Potts shunting operations gradually gave way to direct but closed operations on the pulmonary obstruction and eventually to open surgery, in one or two stages – on the obstruction and the interventricular septal defect. But to avoid too many loose ends we shall continue with the Fallot story, jumping the details of the individual operations, with the first complete correction of all the abnormalities in 1954.

For several years before then, Walton Lillehei had done mock repairs postmortem on all patients at his hospital in the University of Minnesota who had died and who had been diagnosed as having a congenital heart defect. He was thus technically prepared for operating as soon as open heart surgery became possible, which it did in 1953. However, the early heart-lung machines did not satisfy him and for a short period he made use of a cross-circulation technique in which a human donor (a parent) acted as the oxygenating machine.

The first patient was a 19-month-old boy, intensely cyanotic and believed to be very close to death. With the 28-year-old father as donor, Lillehei operated on December 3, 1954. He closed the ventricular septal defect by direct suture, and resected the obstruction in the pulmonary infundibulum. All went well; the father was unaffected, and six months after operation the mother reported her child to be as active as her other unaffected children. Cardiac catheterization showed the boy to have a normal circulation and normal intracardiac pressures[12].

But what of the other components of the tetrad? The right ventricular hypertrophy can be dismissed as it is a response to trying to overcome the obstruction in the pulmonary valve area. It is treated by correcting the other defects. Shift of the aorta to the right, strangely enough, presented Lillehei with no serious obstacle to his corrective surgery. In fact he was inclined to believe that it was 'more illusory than real', the false impression being due largely to the presence of the septal defect[12].

Great work on the complete repair of Fallot's tetrad was also done by John Kirklin and his colleagues at the Mayo Clinic. They began shortly after Lillehei in April, 1955, and in 1958 reviewed their results[13]. Their first five patients had all died, so Kirklin, realizing the trouble lay in the technicalities of perfusion with the heart-lung machine, had called a halt while he and his team became masters of the situation. They resumed open heart surgery later that year and never looked back. In the next 69 patients the mortality rate was 23 percent, but in the last 10 of these there had not been a single death. In the discussion after Kirklin's paper, Lillehei said that in the three-and-a-half years since his first series of patients, there had been no late deaths among the survivors all of whom were proved to have a normal cardiac physiology with no symptoms of disability attributable to their heart[14]. The immediate operative mortality rate was 10 percent or less which, he said was comparable to, or even less than, that of the palliative shunt procedures.

Another participant in the discussion was Richard Rasmussen of Grand

Rapids, Michigan, who told how on April 24, 1958, he had bypassed the right side of the heart by anastomosing the superior vena cava to the pulmonary artery. The patient was a boy of 17 months who, since the age of four months, had been having spells of severe cyanosis with episodes of unconsciousness. The diagnosis was pulmonary stenosis with transposition of the aorta and main pulmonary trunk; the object of the exercise was to increase the flow of blood to the lungs. The immediate result was good and the strain on the child's heart was decreased[15].

Even though it was controversial, this operation was subsequently done in quite a number of centres for certain forms of cyanotic heart disease including patients with Fallot's tetrad in whom the risk of open correction was considered to be high. The procedure had its disadvantages but its proponents maintained it had advantages over the palliative shunt operations; these included the facts that it lessened the strain on the right heart, did not increase the load on the left heart, and shunted pure venous blood to the lungs, not a mixture of venous and arterial.

However, before open correction of all the defects in Fallot's tetrad was attempted, the two main components, pulmonary stenosis and ventricular septal defect, had been attacked individually. The first to be tackled was pulmonary stenosis, which can also exist on its own as indeed can the septal defect. The pulmonary valve lies in the outflow tract of the right ventricle and prevents venous blood from gushing back into the ventricle after it has been pumped into the pulmonary arteries and on to the lungs for oxygenation. In pulmonary stenosis the amount of blood reaching the lungs is reduced, oxygenation of the circulating blood is therefore deficient and in severe cases the patient is cyanotic and disabled. The right ventricle has to struggle to pump blood through the narrow opening and in consequence it dilates and eventually fails.

The term pulmonary stenosis is imprecise as it may refer to stenosis of the valve itself or to stenosis of the pulmonary infundibulum (the region leaving the right ventricle just before the blood flow reaches the valve) and the distinction is important as it affects the surgical technique. (Extremely rarely the obstruction may be beyond the valve.)

Surgeons contemplating operations on congenital stenosis of the pulmonary valve faced problems peculiar to that region. There was still the fear in the minds of some that relief of the stenosis might lead to secondary alterations in the cardiovascular mechanics which could prove to be disabling or even lethal. (There was also the erroneous belief that the stenosis was invariably infundibular.) But when Russell Brock of Guy's Hospital, London, examined these hearts postmortem and contemplated the minute size of the orifice through which the entire life blood of the body had to be forced, it was impossible, he said, not to feel that this simple mechanical obstruction must be amenable to surgery. 'Relief by direct attack must be our goal.'[16]

With an instrument specially made for him, Brock had for some time been studying the pulmonary valves during life. While operating for removal of the left lung he had, on occasions, taken the opportunity of passing this cardioscope along the cut left pulmonary artery and looking at the valve. This route seemed to be the best approach to the valve until three different experiences in three different patients – cardioscopy and more prolonged occlusion of the pulmonary artery than was usual contributed to the death of a 17-year-old man after a Blalock operation; a pulmonary artery too small to admit the cardioscope; and a cardiac arrest – made him decide to change and go in through the right ventricle attacking the valve in the direction of the blood flow. On February 16, 1948, he did just this and was able to pass a curved valvulotome effortlessly into the pulmonary artery of 18-year-old Miss DN. After withdrawal of this instrument he introduced a pair of specially made, gently curving, dilating forceps which he opened fully to relieve the stenosis. Three days later he repeated the performance on Gwenda B, aged 11, and on March 23 carried out his third operation, this time on Miss RC who was 23[16].

All were technical successes but vascular complications came as disappointments in the first and third cases. Both these girls were of an age when the outlook was usually poor and they were very severely disabled.

A fortnight after Brock's paper was published in the *British Medical Journal* in the summer of 1948, an account of what was in fact the first successful pulmonary valvotomy appeared in the *Lancet*[17]. Thomas Holmes Sellors of The Middlesex Hospital, London, had under his care a 20-year-old man with advanced tuberculosis of both lungs who was a typical example of Fallot's tetrad, cyanosed and short of breath. Although the man's tuberculosis was moderately stabilized, Holmes Sellors felt that little more could be done for his lungs unless the heart condition was improved. He decided to carry out a Blalock-Taussig operation on the left side, but when he entered the chest he found this to be impossible because of adhesions. He therefore opened the pericardium and when he put his hand over the pulmonary area he felt a firm structure being thrust with each heart-beat from the ventricle into the pulmonary trunk. This he interpreted to be the stenosed pulmonary valve. Several holding sutures were inserted in the right ventricle; then between these Holmes Sellors passed a long tenotomy knife through the ventricular wall and on until it engaged the valve where he made cuts in two directions. The patient's recovery was straightforward and he was markedly, though not completely, relieved of his cyanosis[17]. Nine years later he was dead from the spread of his tuberculosis[11].

These operations were all on congenitally stenosed valves which, as Brock said, were diaphragmatic in nature and eminently suitable for division. Nevertheless, though simple the technique called for experience to obtain consistently good results.

Infundibular stenosis, best thought of as a localized circular thickening of the outflow tract of the right ventricle, creates problems of its own[18]. If the thickening is too high, a 'blind' approach may damage the valve; if too low, it may damage other heart structures. For those stenoses that were suitably placed Brock designed a blunt-nosed punch which could be passed through an incision in the right ventricle and 'punch out' the obstructing tissue. He first used this in four patients in 1949 with success; in a fifth he found that dilatation with his finger was sufficient[19]. Not everyone was satisfied with this technique and some surgeons looked around for other ways of dealing with infundibular stenosis by increasing the circumference of the outflow tract, but without interfering with the circulation or requiring an open heart.

The solution had been reached almost 40 years previously by Tuffier and Carrel who, it may be remembered, had described how in dogs they had stitched a venous patch on to the outside of the heart in the area of the pulmonary valve. Then, with a pair of scissors slipped in beneath the patch they divided the valvular ring; the walls of the pulmonary artery fell back and took up the slack of about 1cm provided by the patch and so increased the circumference[20].

In 1950 Charles Hufnagel of Boston carried out essentially similar experiments, also in dogs, using patches of aorta and superior vena cava obtained from other dogs, and of the animal's own pericardium. The only slight difference was that he made the incision by pulling out a stainless steel suture he had inserted before applying the patch[21]. Although Hufnagel did not put the idea into clinical practice his experimental work gave John Kirklin a lead. Kirklin passed a doubled suture of stainless steel wire into the heart, through the orifice in the infundibular obstruction, and out again. He then proceeded to bury the outside part of the suture in a tunnel created along the length of the obstruction by gathering up the outer layers of the muscular heart wall on either side of of the wire and sewing them together. Under the cover he had thus arranged he sawed away with the wire until it cut through the obstruction. On May 30, 1952, he used the technique on a 17-year-old girl who was improved both subjectively and objectively[22].

Kirklin's operation nevertheless had the disadvantage of leaving a scar in the heart. So A Temesvári of The National Institute of Cardiology, Budapest, decided to cut a complete segment out of the wall of the outflow tract of the right ventricle and cover the defect with a full-thickness skin graft. Animal experiments showed the procedure to be safe and on June 15, 1956, Temesvári's colleague, Littmann, operated with success on a seven-year-old boy, disabled by Fallot's tetrad[23].

At that time other research workers were experimenting with a variety of tissues that might be suitable for enlarging the outflow tract; Robert Gross, for example, was successful with a patch of the patient's own pericardium in a case of Fallot's tetrad[24]. But by then hypothermia and the heart-lung machine were permitting operations on the open heart and, rather than wriggle under patches, surgeons could carefully excise the obstructing infundibular tissue and tailor a patch of synthetic material to increase the circumference should this prove necessary. Stenosis of the valve could also be operated on under direct vision when desirable, for instance if it was only one of a number of abnormalities.

We are now left with the ventricular septal component of Fallot's tetrad, but as this is just a 'hole in the heart', it can more conveniently be discussed along with the other holes.

17

HOLES IN THE HEART

Galen postulated the existence of pores between the two sides of the heart to explain his ebb-and-flow theory of the movement of blood in the body but, as we now know, the two sides are completely separate unless there has been an error in embryological development. Persistence of holes after birth sooner or later has a deleterious effect on the circulation, the seriousness of which depends on the precise nature of the defect and its size.

At a very early stage in the embryo a mass of cells differentiates into two tubes which gradually fuse to form a single heart tube. This in turn develops a number of bulges separated by grooves and eventually, by a rather complicated process, tissue grows in to divide the single tube down the middle into two sides, each with an atrium and a ventricle. While all this is in progress there is a considerable amount of give and take. For instance, as the dividing wall (septum primum) between the atria is taking shape the upper part decides to disappear and so more tissue (septum secundum) has to grow down to take its place. The oblique cleft between the two septa is termed the foramen ovale, and this persists during the remainder of fetal life so that oxygenated blood from the mother passing up the fetal inferior vena cava can directly enter the left side of the heart. After birth the situation is completely altered: the baby's lungs have to take over the task of oxygenation and so the hole closes. But sometimes the tissue is defective and the opening persists, maybe as a single hole, maybe as multiple fenestrations. This is the commonest type of defect between the atria and belongs to the group known as ostium secundum defects which are now treated quite routinely.

In its downgrowth, the remainder of the septum primum does not quite reach the upper border of the interventricular septum. The gap is normally closed by upgrowth of more tissue. When this fails there is another type of hole known as an ostium primum defect. This variety is more difficult to treat but fortunately is rare. The outlook in all these atrial septal defects when untreated depends on the size of the hole. If they are small the patient can have a normal life expectancy, but with large ones symptoms develop early and heart failure often occurs before the age of 30. Sometimes other abnormalities of the heart are present, but in these cases the atrial septal defect is usually of secondary importance.

The wall between the two ventricles develops in two parts: a muscular septum grows up from below and forms the major part of the division; it is met from above by a fibrous septum, which, because of some lack of symmetry also partly divides the left ventricle from the right atrium. Defects in the wall may occur in any part but are commonest between the muscular and fibrous septa. Untreated, more than half the babies with holes between the ventricles die before they reach their first birthday and only about a third of the survivors reach 20. Increased blood pressure in the pulmonary circulation is largely responsible for this poor outlook.

Patients with interventricular septal defects not uncommonly have other heart abnormalities such as a patent ductus arteriosus or deformities of the valves, and the condition is, of course, one of the major components of Fallot's tetrad. Errors in development are the commonest cause of these holes, but they may also result from penetrating injuries of the heart and from a myocardial infarction affecting the septum.

Basically, the surgical treatment of all holes in the heart (when this is indicated) is to close them by stitching the edges together when this can be done without tension, or by inserting a patch of plastic material in the larger ones. Some of the holes between the ventricles and ostium primum defects lie close to the nerves conducting the impulses of the heart-beat, and in these instances the repairing stitches may unavoidably damage the mechanism. However, in most cases where this occurs a normal rhythm is restored after two or three weeks by the use of a pacemaker and drugs. For the few patients in whom this does not succeed, artificial pacemaking has to be continued for life.

Nevertheless, to stitch or patch these holes deep inside the heart, the surgeon has to be able to get there through an incision, and this was impossible before the days of hypothermia and the heart-lung machine. But surgical ingenuity was equal to the challenge, and a number of remarkably clever techniques were tried. Atrial septal defects were the first to be tackled and the earliest attempts at closure in the human patient were made by Gordon Murray of Toronto. The septum runs in a fore-and-aft direction and, having thoroughly familiarized himself with the external landmarks, Murray passed sutures of silk, linen, or cotton on a needle, eye first, blindly through the substance of the septum, across the hole, into the septum again and out at the back of the heart.

Here he tied the two ends of the suture together, and then pulled the other ends taut at the front of the heart and tied them. In this way the sutures partially obstructed the hole, and also reduced its size by virtue of the tautness of the sutures pulling the front and back of the heart closer together.

Animal experiments had preceded clinical use, but Murray was unsure of the significance of the results, as he was impressed by the high pressure in the pulmonary artery in his human patients and did not know whether this was in fact due to the septal defect or to a congenital anomaly in the pulmonary vascular tree which would not be alleviated by closure of the hole. We now know that this high pressure in the vessels of the lung is due to the haemodynamic effects of the hole, yet Murray's perplexity illustrates most forcibly the lack of knowledge in those early days. He was faced not just with the tremendous technical problem of closing the hole, but with complete uncertainty about the effects of the operation even if this were to be successful.

In 1948 he reported on his use of the technique in a 12-year-old girl who had an enormously enlarged right atrium[1]. He inserted two silk sutures, and when these were drawn taut and tied, the atrium shrank to half its former size in two minutes. The girl made a good recovery and her health was much improved.

During the discussion of Murray's paper, Arthur Blakemore[2], a New York surgeon, said that some time before the war (1939, he thought) he had created, experimentally, holes between the atria in dogs. He had then proceeded to use two of nature's gifts to the surgeon in their repair. First he pushed the little pouch-like part of the atrium – the atrial appendage – through the hole from outside the heart and packed it with strips of fascia lata to make a self-retaining ball on the other side of the hole. (The fascia lata is a strong band of fibrous tissue on the outer side of the thigh which, in its time, has proved most valuable in the repair of hernias.) Blakemore did not comment on the results, and this form of treatment was not pursued. However, by the time of Murray's report the atrial appendage was already beginning to come into its own in the treatment of atrial septal defects in a different manner.

The idea originated in San Francisco, where Roy Cohn acted on a suggestion of his medical colleague, JK Lewis. A defect was made in the septum in dogs by inserting a curved clamp into the left atrium, pushing it through the septum, opening and closing it, and withdrawing it. The resulting hole was invariably circular and about 4-6mm in diameter. Two weeks later the right atrial appendage was invaginated on the defect and stitched round the edges of the hole, giving a doughnut-like appearance. As this invariably obstructed the superior vena cava, Cohn passed a doubled length of wire into the atrium in such a way that when it was pulled out it separated the part of the appendage covering the hole from the rest of the atrium. Before pulling it out, though, he had put in stitches to maintain the integrity of the atrium. Five of the eight dogs, recorded in Cohn's report in 1947, survived[3]. This 'de-doughnutting' was not put into clinical practice.

Despite the possibility that an invaginated atrial appendage might obstruct the inflow of blood to the atrium, most of the early operations, apart from Murray's, were designed on the invaginating principle. Henry Swan of the University of Colorado was the first to use it on a human patient. On October 27, 1949, he invaginated both atrial appendages on to the defect in a five-year-old boy, keeping them in place with plastic buttons held tightly together with strong silk. Regrettably, the operation failed and the boy died the next day. Swan's next essay was on another boy, aged nine, on May 6, 1950. This time he succeeded and there was subjective improvement, although the shunt from left to right through the hole was still present. He operated once more that year and twice in 1952 using the same technique and achieving satisfactory results[4], but this small number of cases gives an idea of the difficulties facing the surgeon. The aim was to get the appendages to adhere to the edges of the hole, but this did not happen and the operation was eventually abandoned as it was apt to obstruct the pulmonary veins. Realizing its deficiencies, especially in large defects, Swan in 1953 described an experimental modification in which the right atrium was opened and the button on this side placed directly against the hole; the left appendage was invaginated as before[5]. This gave 100 percent closure, but events were already on the move again and this particular line of approach came to a halt although buttons were used elsewhere with unhappy results.

Thus far no technique used clinically had succeeded in closing the hole completely, but on January 11, 1952, Charles Bailey achieved this in a 38-year-old woman who had a large ostium secundum defect. His method, which he christened 'atrio-septo-pexy', entailed invaginating the wall of the right atrium and securely fixing it to the edges of the hole by interlocking mattress sutures[6]. Later that year he operated on five more patients; three had very satisfactory results, but two with advanced disease died. Of an experimental operation on a cadaver Bailey wrote: 'There was no obstruction to the orifices of the venae cavae, and the atrial cavity, although much reduced in size, appeared adequate.'[6] Nevertheless, the procedure was suitable only for defects in the middle of the septum; for those elsewhere, which are in the majority, it was impracticable.

A modification of atrio-septo-pexy was devised by Harris Shumacker of Indianapolis. He fashioned a pocket out of pericardial tissue and then sutured it to the edges of an incision in the atrium. The object was to enlarge the atrium to make the invagination and subsequent stitching easier. The pocket was inverted and its bottom sewn to the edges of the defect in the atrial septum. After two abortive attempts, Shumacker operated on a 13-year-old boy on October 29, 1952. The lad was improved, but five months later he died suddenly, and at postmortem the graft was found to have 'melted away'[7].

In an attempt to overcome some of the difficulties of blind surgery, Robert Gross of Boston invented the atrial well. It was made of rubber and its base was sutured to the edges of an incision in the right atrium. Since the pressure in the atrium is relatively low, blood rose only partly into the well and Gross was able to put his fingers inside the heart and feel the defect. This device was a great step forward as it allowed the surgeon to work directly on the cause of the trouble, although he still could not see what he was doing. Gross reported his experiences on the first six patients, aged between four and 16 years, in 1952[8]. Most unfortunately the first three were failures as he had used Hufnagel buttons. These had recently been designed by his colleague, Charles Hufnagel, and were applied directly to the septal wall[9]. In experimental defects in dogs they had achieved considerable success as these defects were surrounded by a rim of tissue. But in the three patients there was a rim of tissue around only half the hole, and the buttons worked loose, with lethal results, in a few days. Thereafter Gross stitched the smaller defects and sewed patches of polyethylene sheeting into the larger ones, but even so his first success did not come until the fifth patient. Gross used heparin to keep the blood in the well fluid: in the first patient the well was in use for 12 minutes, but in a later case it was open for just over two hours.

Among other methods to be tried was the closed technique of Tyge Søndergaard of Copenhagen. After creating a surgical cleavage between the atria, he anchored a strong suture in the upper part of the ventricular septum and carried this round in the cleavage. Tension on the suture pulled the atrial septum down to the upper edge of the ventricular septum. His first patient was a boy of five who was much improved; but nine months after the operation on October 26, 1952, the boy died from whooping cough and bronchopneumonia. The defect was found still to be present but reduced to less than a third of its pre-operative size[10]. This technique became popular in Scandinavia for the short time that remained before the open heart became a reality.

The first operation successfully performed on an open heart (using hypothermia) was the closure of an atrial septal defect by F John Lewis of Minneapolis in 1952[11]. The astonishing progress made in cardiac surgery since the early days can well be judged by the fact that these defects were then major considerations, with the operation conducted by the chief surgeon and the outcome watched closely and not a little anxiously. Within not all that many years they were frequently handed over to the registrar with complete confidence in his ability to handle the surgical technique.

Defects in the septum between the two ventricles posed much greater problems for there is no convenient appendage and the walls of these two great pumping chambers could not be stitched down onto the hole. Then there are the purely anatomical hazards presented by the bundle of nerve-impulse conducting tissue, the cusps of the heart valves, and the chordae tendineae and papillary muscles (the structures concerned with the action of the valves), all of which can get in the way with awkwardly placed holes. But Gordon Murray overcame all these difficulties – and the additional one of the presence of the coronary arteries – by a technique essentially similar to the one he had used for atrial septal defects. In his paper, read in 1948[1], he told a spellbound audience how he had passed strips of fascia lata through the septum, across the hole and out at the back. The strips of fascia were cut about three-quarters of an inch wide and had a blob of muscle at one end to serve as the anchor at the front of the heart. When the strips were pulled taut from the back, the heart was compressed antero-posteriorly. Murray reported on three patients – a girl of 17 months, and two children of 11 and 13 – all of whom were improved.

Charles Bailey was also concerned with the problem and experimentally he tried two methods. One was patching the hole with a sheet of pericardium, but as this degenerated to nothing it was not pursued. The other was a 'corking' method suitable for small to medium-sized holes: the defect was plugged by a tapered tube, fashioned from pericardium, which was pulled through and the ends sewn into place on each ventricular wall. The end result was thus like a sling across both ventricular cavities. Bailey first put this idea to use on February 6, 1951, in a 26-year-old man who, at the time of the report the following year, was in excellent health[12]. His second case eight months later was that of a youth of 18 with Fallot's tetrad. A Brock operation was done on the pulmonary infundibular obstruction and a pericardial sling inserted. However, the outflow tract of the right ventricle was narrow and as the sling only made it narrower, it had to be removed, but the patient did well.

Attempts to close interventricular septal defects were thus few, sporadic, and not persevered with. The problems really were too great unless the surgeon could operate under direct vision, and the wherewithal for achieving this, they realized, was not far off. It was better to wait.

18

MITRAL STENOSIS

'I have been asked this question:' wrote Claude Beck in 1954[1], "'Why did Cutler stop the operation for mitral stenosis?" There were several reasons. The valves we examined were calcified and rigid, and it looked as though a piece of valve should be cut away in order to relieve the stenosis. It is probable that the pathology of mitral stenosis has been changed by the use of sulfonamides and antibiotics, for we did not then see soft, pliable valves that could be opened by finger dilatation. Furthermore, I cannot recall any words of encouragement for Cutler after he operated on his seventh and last patient with mitral stenosis.'

Beck's comments are extremely valuable because of the link he provides between Cutler's work and the modern era. However, they give more insight into the state of mind that led to the work being abandoned than into the technical reasons for failure. Even today, with all the help given by antibiotics, a number of patients who come to surgery have calcified valves and many can be operated on successfully without the need for valve replacement. So, of itself, calcification need not have been an insuperable barrier. Where, then, did the trouble lie?

Beck gave a hint in his 1954 paper by remarking that the creation of the valvulotome probably delayed the development of operation for mitral stenosis by some 20 years. In a sense this is true, yet he was being less than fair to himself. Cutler's experimental work and clinical observations had conditioned his followers into believing that mitral incompetence was less serious than stenosis. Therefore, if blood could be made to flow freely through a stenosed valve by cutting a hole in it, the ensuing incompetence would be acceptable.

Unfortunately, the results of his operations did not show the fallacy of this belief – there was always some other reason to account for failure. In Cutler's and Beck's concluding paper in 1929[2] they had pondered on the ill-effects of suddenly creating incompetence, but by then they had already given up the struggle. The truth of the matter is that a hole is a hole is a hole and if it is created in a place where nature never intended, she objects. The mitral orifice is indeed a hole, but it is a hole protected by a *competent* valve. When this simple truth was realized, surgeons were able to forge ahead.

Mitral stenosis has had a particular appeal surgically, because it is the commonest form of valvular disease and is nearly always rheumatic. Thus it strikes down previously healthy persons, often children or young people at the outset of their careers, and, in more cases than is realized, inexorably advances to an early and unpleasant end. In the 1930s physicians were still complacent. They could keep the patients alive – rather, they could delay the coming of death. The surgical challenge was there in full measure and, despite Cutler's experiences, the determination to prove conclusively that life could truly be given to these patients continued to burn in the hearts of a few men.

It is a common belief that surgery for mitral stenosis was forgotten during the 20 years between Cutler's last operation in 1928 and the successes in 1948. But this is not so. William Wilson in Edinburgh published a paper in 1930 on the experimental creation and relief of mitral stenosis[3]. Then, in 1936, Gordon Murray of Toronto began a series of experiments on intracardiac surgery in which 'resected valves were successfully replaced by venous grafts'. His report appeared in 1938[4].

The technique was most ingeniously Murray's own and, in concept, not unlike that which he was later to use in the repair of interatrial and interventricular septal defects. He accepted the truth about regurgitation and this worried him greatly since the only way he could see for relieving the stenosis was to cut out a piece of the valve (Cutler's influence was still preventing a new line of thought). But, Murray reasoned, if he could do this and then in some manner counteract the regurgitation, all should be well. In his animals he resected the posterolateral cusp of the mitral valve and inserted a sling made of an inverted segment of external jugular vein across the valve opening. The two ends of the sling, thrust in blindly from outside, were sutured to the left ventricular wall under very slight tension. The animals withstood the operation well and subsequently had no regurgitation; the longest survivor died naturally after seven years and its valve replacement showed no signs of deterioration.

As the new valve had to survive and not contract into scar tissue, it had to get its nutrition from the blood stream flowing past it. So the material Murray used was a length of cephalic vein (from the arm) pulled inside out, with a strip of palmaris longus tendon (from the forearm) within its lumen to give it substance. Two of these lengths were inserted through an incision in the left ventricle and guided into place by a finger invaginating the left atrium. In some instances he used a cardioscope to assess visually the adequacy of the holding sutures. The valve was suspended on the ventricular side of the mitral orifice so that the blood could flow through from the atrium to fill the ventricle, but when the ventricle contracted the strips were forced back against the orifice and so prevented regurgitation into the atrium.

Although he did not date these clinical essays precisely, Murray stated that he operated on his first patient, an Indian, in 1945. This man was known to have done well for some time, but later he moved away up North and was lost to follow-up. Nine more patients, aged between 23 and 47 years, had this form of surgery, probably in 1947 and 1948, and seven had fairly satisfactory outcomes. Little or no attention was given to this work and by the time Murray published his results in 1950[5] the method of valvotomy was already well on the way to becoming established.

For some reason Murray's claim to priority has been ignored in many historical surveys. Who knows why the Fates choose to smile in one direction and not in another. It may have been due to the delay in publication, but it seems more likely that the profession was even then not ready to accept the situation. His technique inclined to the unorthodox as it entailed inserting material into the heart, but in reality Murray was again ahead of his time. Not for another 10 years were surgeons prepared to cut out a severely diseased valve and replace it with one obtained from a cadaver. Admittedly Murray did not do precisely that, but the underlying principle was the same.

At all events, in 1948 four different surgeons successfully operated for mitral stenosis and their achievements are usually bracketed together as marking the start of modern mitral-valve surgery. This also is strange because the technique of two of the men represented not the beginning but the end of an era.

If you ask why Cutler's technique should at last be crowned with success when all the arguments are against it, there can be no satisfactory answer – fortunate choice of patients, adaptability of the human body, luck. Who knows? Nevertheless, Horace Smithy's magnificent efforts were the last brilliant flickers of a dying fire. Cutler's technique was doomed as alas! was Smithy himself. Throughout the papers he read and wrote during 1948[6] can be sensed an urgency as though each one might be his last. Indeed, the article describing the details of his eight operations on seven patients was not published until after his death[7] – from rheumatic aortic stenosis at the age of 34.

Horace Smithy of Charleston, South Carolina, was initially concerned with laboratory experiments on the aortic valve in dogs and with problems of irregularity of the heart action during surgery. But Cutler's shadow lay over him and he turned his attention to 'mitral valvulectomy', the objective of which was the 'excision of a segment of scarred valvular leaflet from the margin of the constricted orifice so as to permit a greater flow of blood from the auricle to the ventricle through the affected valve.' He seemed untroubled by the inevitable regurgitation.

He repeated Cutler's experiments and found that he, too, preferred the ventricular approach as access through the atrium was more difficult and the haemorrhage harder to control. He also found it easier to reach the valve with his special biting valvulotome through the ventricle. Nevertheless, in the eight operations he used each approach four times.

His first patient was a 21-year-old woman who had had scarlet fever at the age of 10. This had damaged her heart; then at 18 she had an attack of acute rheumatic fever. By 1948 she was seriously ill and in chronic congestive heart failure. Inevitably, for a reason not explained, she came to Smithy from several hundred miles away in an aeroplane. She was carried from the plane on a stretcher, propped up on pillows and breathing with difficulty. The operation took place on January 30, 1948. Smithy went into her greatly enlarged heart through the apex of the left ventricle and removed a segment of valve tissue about 0·8cm long. The procedure was without untoward incident, although the piece of valve was lost on its way to the pathology laboratory![7]

Some while after operation her congestive failure gradually returned and she died 10 months later. The postmortem showed, incidentally, an aneurysmal dilatation at the ventricular apex where the valvulotome had been introduced.

In his second operation on March 1, Smithy was unable to excise a segment because the valve was too hard and calcified; the 25-year-old man died 10 hours afterwards, probably because his myocardium had been too severely damaged by the disease to withstand surgery. The third patient died of pneumonia 48 hours after operation on March 8. Smithy's last four patients all survived, the greatest success being a 39-year-old woman operated on on April 20. She was admitted with a chronic exhausting cough, severe palpitations, constant fatigue, severe shortness of breath on exercise and paroxysmal attacks of shortness of breath at night. After operation, performed through the atrium, she had no more disturbing symptoms and was able to return to work as a laboratory assistant. When she was seen by one of Smithy's colleagues a year later her condition was excellent and she was most enthusiastic about the result.

Smithy's last patient, a 36-year-old woman, had two operations. The first on May 26 was unsuccessful, as the atrial approach was tried but the chamber was friable and he was unable to locate the valve. So the attempt was abandoned, and 19 days later he went in again, this time through the ventricle. Afterwards the patient could take moderate exercise without becoming short of breath.

When we seek the long-term results in these patients we find, as so often happened, that most were lost to follow-up[8]. The only information we have is that five years later one patient was known to be alive and improved, and another was believed to have been so.

All Smithy's operations were completed before anyone else of the modern era (except Murray) accomplished success. He died on October 28, 1948. His obituary notice in the *Journal of the American Medical Association* on December 25 contained the doubting phrase: 'is said to have performed the first successful heart valve operation.'[9]

Charles Bailey was the next surgeon to operate on a patient who survived. His work merits the highest praise since he was the first to tackle the problem in the truly modern manner by realizing that it was possible to restore fairly normal mobility to the fused valve and so make it function again without too great a danger of regurgitation[10]. His story began in 1940, when he started a series of 'diverse and repeated' operations on the mitral valves of some 60 mongrel dogs which led him to several important conclusions. These included: (1) An approach through the left atrium was the most satisfactory. (2) The production of a sudden degree of mitral incompetence was poorly tolerated. (3) Whenever a cutting instrument was used it was necessary to palpate the valve. And (4) the palpating finger was well tolerated.

Bailey was particularly insistent on the need to develop an operation for mitral stenosis, emphasizing the lack of appreciation of the frequency and horrors of the disease, and the poor quality of the lives of those who were 'successfully' treated medically. His first four clinical cases were failures, but his determination to succeed was eventually rewarded.

A man of 37, severely incapacitated for 16 years, was brought to the operating table at the Hahnemann Hospital, Philadelphia, on November 14, 1945, but he died from haemorrhage from his extremely friable atrium before surgery on the valve could be attempted. A woman of 29, a cardiac invalid for 11 years, was operated on on June 12, 1946. Her mitral orifice was too small to admit a punch instrument, so Bailey used his finger to make tears at the fused commissures. The woman was improved for 30 hours but then went into a decline and died in another 18 hours. The postmortem showed that the tears had not extended into the normal valve tissue at the edges; as a result, the torn surfaces had hardly separated, and fibrin had accumulated which gummed them up and made the orifice smaller than it had been at operation.

For his third patient on March 22, 1948, Bailey used a commissurotomy knife – a thin, curved blade that fitted into a sheath fixed to the palmar curve of his index finger – and nearly succeeded. The patient was a 38-year-old man who, a year previously, had had part of a lung removed elsewhere in the mistaken belief that his haemoptyses were due to bronchiectasis from which he suffered. In reality they were caused by his mitral stenosis. The initial response was good, but in view of the fibrin coagulation in the previous patient, Bailey administered an anticoagulant in a continuous drip after operation. Regrettably, there was a misunderstanding over the orders for fluid intake, and the man developed pulmonary oedema from which he died. In addition, he bled into a pleural cavity; this had been exacerbated by the anticoagulant therapy which, in retrospect, Bailey reckoned had been unwise. Postmortem examination showed that again the splitting of the commissures had been inadequate.

Bailey's fourth patient was really too bad a risk for surgery and the man died on the table before the proposed finger dilatation could be attempted.

Then on June 10, 1948, after an 80-minute operation in which the fused commissures were split with a hooked finger knife, CW, a woman of 24 with severe mitral stenosis, was restored to almost perfect health. She was out of bed on the third day, walking on the fourth and not long afterwards was taken 1000 miles to a medical convention without ill effect[10].

Hard on Bailey's heels came the second follower of the Cutler technique, though with a difference. Dwight Harken of Boston realized the importance of a functioning valve and chose the site of excision of valve tissue with this in mind. Before the war he had carried out a variety of intracardiac manoeuvres to see whether any might have surgical value until such time as the heart-lung machine was perfected – even then, when the machine was scarcely more than an idea he foresaw its future[11]. His experience during the Second World War had served him well and on his return to civilian life he resumed his experiments making use of a modified Cutler valvulotome. He operated on his first patient, a man of 26, on March 22, 1947, passing the instrument into the heart though the left superior pulmonary vein[12]. Apart from this approach the operation followed the Cutler pattern and segments of valve were excised. Unfortunately, during the manipulations tachycardia developed, which had a 'devastating' effect and led to the man's death after 24 hours from respiratory collapse and pulmonary oedema.

Harken's next step was in the right direction, though the result was a mixture of ancient and modern. He saw the importance of restoring mobility to the valve cusps, but was still sufficiently bound to the Cutler school of thought that he believed the removal of tissue was a necessity. The mitral valve has two cusps, giving the orifice a slit-like appearance; in mitral stenosis these fuse inwards from the two extremes of the slit, and what Harken decided to do was to cut out the fused tissue as two wedges, one from each end of the slit. Regurgitation was bound to follow, but Harken considered this the price to be paid for success – he termed it 'selective insufficiency'. The first patient he operated on in this manner was a man of 27; the date, June 16, 1948. This time he used the atrial approach. The patient, who had had six attacks of rheumatic fever since the age of eight years, felt he was dramatically improved, although objectively there was little improvement in cardiac function[12].

Harken carried on with this techniqne of removing wedges from the commissures, accepting the selective insufficiency[13], but when, after operating on a small series of patients, he saw that the mortality rate was prohibitive compared with that of finger or instrumental dilatation, he changed to these other techniques.

In England, Souttar's operation was remembered, and Russell Brock. of Guy's Hospital, working independently of the Americans, used his finger to 'split' the stenosed mitral valve in a 24-year-old woman. The result was most encouraging. In six of his first eight patients, reported on in 1950[14], Brock was able to separate the valve cusps adequately with his finger alone; only twice had he to resort to the use of a finger knife. His second and third patients died – from cerebral embolism and the consequence of heparinization, respectively. The cerebral emboli were clots of blood reaching the brain, and heparin is an anticoagulant drug given to prevent the blood from clotting. As this may seem a trifle confusing, a brief diversion is in order.

Blood clots that form in the atrium or atrial appendage are a recognized hazard in mitral stenosis, particularly when the condition of atrial fibrillation is present, but an enlarged heart and calcification of the valve are also predisposing conditions. Pieces of clot may dislodge spontaneously and shoot off into the systemic circulation and lodge, for instance, in the brain; they may also be disturbed by surgical manipulations. This is appreciated, and steps, such as allowing blood to gush from the initial atrial incision and clamping the carotid arteries if clot is suspected, became routine practice. In the early days of mitral surgery, systemic embolization, sometimes lethal, was a complication in somewhere around 5 percent of cases.

One important feature of Brock's work concerned the troublesome problem of regurgitation. He clearly showed that with his technique the complication did not occur; in fact, when there was an associated regurgitation before operation, it was improved. Nevertheless, regurgitation remained a possibility after surgery.

Thus, by the end of 1948 the pattern for the future progress of surgery for mitral stenosis was set. The Cutler era had been brought to a glorious close by Horace Smithy. Almost exactly a quarter of a century separated the first operation and the last – both qualified successes. Cutler himself did not live to see the end – he died in 1947 at the age of 59, spared the knowledge that the moment of triumph was also that of ultimate failure.

However, while these few surgeons were attacking the valve itself, others considered the time was not quite ripe for this direct approach to the source of the trouble and were scouting around for methods of relieving the symptoms by reducing the pressure behind the valve in the pulmonary circuit. Two different techniques were practised for a short period, but it must be emphasized that they were only intended to be palliative, and could do little more than bring a temporary easing of the patient's lot. This is because the high blood pressure in the left atrium in mitral stenosis has a purpose, namely, to force blood through the narrow valve. When this pressure is lowered, less blood passes through; the pulmonary circuit obviously benefits but not the systemic, which becomes increasingly congested.

Both techniques originated from the observation in 1916 of a French physician, René Lutembacher, that patients with a tight mitral stenosis who also had a hole between their atria did not usually suffer from paroxysms of pulmonary oedema[15]. (Needless to say, the association of the two conditions is now known as Lutembacher's syndrome.) The first person to suggest deliberately creating the atrial septal defect was Alexander Jarotzky of Moscow in a paper published in 1926[16]. On November 23, 1925, his colleagues had carried out the operation experimentally on a dog, but this could only have been an exercise in creating the defect; the effect on the symptoms of mitral stenosis could not be assessed as no one had yet produced the condition in an experimental animal.

The idea went into cold storage until after the Second World War, when it was resurrected by Alfred Blalock and Rollins Hanlon of Johns Hopkins and by Richard Sweet and Edward Bland of the Massachusetts General Hospital, Boston. But they had differing views on the best way of lowering the pressure in the left atrium.

Blalock and Hanlon thought that creating an atrial septal defect might balance the work of the two sides of the heart[17], and the operation was performed clinically by Bailey[18] and Harken[12] even though they were working on the direct approach. Harken's two patients derived short-lived benefit, but their symptoms returned. In practice the idea failed to live up to expectations.

Sweet and Bland did not favour going inside the heart and their technique was based on their observation that in patients with tight mitral stenosis the bronchial veins (which drain through the azygos system of veins into the venae cavae; that is, they are part of the systemic circulation, not the pulmonary – the azygos system of veins returns blood to the heart from the chest wall and contents other than the lungs) became enormously dilated and provided a limited outlet for the congested pulmonary vessels. This gave them the idea of deliberately linking the pulmonary and systemic circulations.

Their first patient was Mrs Olivia CB, a 17-year-old mulatto girl who had had rheumatic fever when she was five[19]. Mitral stenosis was diagnosed at 14, and in one attack of pulmonary oedema she nearly died. Sweet decompressed her hypertensive pulmonary circulation on March 23, 1948, by anastomosing a branch of her right inferior pulmonary vein to her azygos vein. In Olivia's favour was the fact that her heart was strong and only slightly enlarged; it was well able to deal with the altered strain put upon it. She later became pregnant twice but on both occasions the pregnancy was therapeutically terminated to avoid any further strain on her heart.

When successes with the direct operation on the mitral valve had been achieved, Sweet and Bland continued with their anastomotic operation as they were worried about the unfavourable effects of regurgitation and the mortality risk. In their paper published in 1949[20] they reported on six patients, all of whom had been seriously ill. The first three were enormously improved, but eventually deteriorated owing to thrombosis in the anastomosis – the reason why Blalock preferred to create an atrial septal defect.

A similar operation to Sweet's was devised independently in France by François D'Allaines[21] and first employed on January 29, 1949; the 31-year-old woman showed clinical improvement 12 weeks after operation. Although in his paper D'Allaines mentioned he had operated on nine other patients with three postoperative deaths and six successes, the tide had moved on and these operations were no longer needed.

Besides these pressure-relieving measures two other techniques were discussed at the time; one was used and one was only proposed. During attacks of pulmonary oedema the hearts of some patients with mitral stenosis beat extremely rapidly and when this could not be controlled medically Harken thought it might be a good idea to denervate the heart. He did this on one patient, reported on in 1948[12], with some benefit.

The second technique was to bypass the valve, and in the discussion of Sweet's and Bland's paper in 1949 Blalock[22] said that Robert Gross was then using '(at least experimentally) a graft of aorta connecting the auricle and the ventricle'. The principle dates back to 1910 when Carrel[23] experimentally bypassed the aortic arch. He was followed in 1913 by Ernst Jeger[24] who described a technique for bypassing the mitral valve itself, the graft joining the pulmonary veins to the left ventricle. And in 1924 Strickland Goodall and Lambert Rogers[25] took a fleeting glance at the relief of mitral stenosis by a graft of tubed pericardium extending outside the heart between the left atrium and ventricle. But as far as can be discovered the principle was never used in mitral-valve surgery; by the time surgeons were ready to put it into practice it had already become part of history.

Mitral valvotomy by the finger, aided or not by a knife as demanded by circumstances or the surgeon's preference, flourished. The practice spread to centres all over the world and before long hundreds of operations had been performed. With experience the results improved and the mortality rate fell, though rates were obviously unfavourably influenced by the patients with severe disease and gross calcification of the valve.

In 1962 Clifton Lowther and Richard Turner, physicians at the Western General Hospital, Edinburgh, analysed the results in the first 500 cases of mitral valvotomy in Edinburgh[26]. Over 11 years the operative mortality rate had remained at 6 percent; the chief hazard throughout had been systemic embolism, accounting for 13 of the 31 deaths. One year after operation 84 percent of patients had good results; five years after, the figure had fallen to 72 percent; and nine years after only 20 percent of 37 patients still had a good result. 'It is concluded from this analysis', they wrote, 'that, although most patients with severe mitral stenosis are improved by valvotomy, surgical treatment is but an incident in the relentless progress of rheumatic heart disease, whether from activity of the rheumatic process or from the progressive fibrosis which follows activity.'

Patients often had second operations when their stenoses recurred. Although many surgeons considered the cause of restenosis – it occurred in about 5 percent of patients five years after operation, and in perhaps 50-70 percent 10 years after – to be an inadequate first operation[27], the Edinburgh group were not so sure believing the natural progress of the disease to be an important factor. Even so, when a new dilating instrument appeared the Scots were among the first to adopt and popularize it.

This instrument was devised by Charles Dubost of Paris who reported on its use to the French Society of Cardiology on December 20, 1953[28]. He had grown dissatisfied with the usual valvulotomes as he had never been able to do more with them than with his finger alone. His new instrument had two parallel blades and was guided through the atrium and into the valve orifice by a finger. When in place, the two blades were carefully separated. In his successful cases Dubost achieved a good anatomical result with no evidence of regurgitation.

In May, 1954, one of the Edinburgh team saw Dubost using the instrument and came home filled with enthusiasm. Hitherto, Andrew Logan would have used the atrial route but the handle of the dilator he possessed was so shaped that he had to go in through the anterior wall of the left ventricle. He used this route sporadically during the next year until Dubost's instrument became available. But when he introduced this through the atrium he found it was inclined to become entangled with the chordae tendineae[29]. So back he went to the ventricular route and there he, and eventually the majority of other surgeons, stayed. The operative mortality rate among his first 438 patients was 5 percent compared with 6·4 percent before this technique was adopted, and more patients were improved[29].

The dilator had considerable advantages over other methods largely because the two blades provided counterpressure for each other and there was no dragging on the heart as could happen when the finger alone met with resistance. The force and amount of opening could be carefully controlled with the dilator but the finger was still needed to assess the situation at the start (when the finger itself might sometimes quite easily achieve all that was necessary), after each opening of the dilator, and to separate any adhesions in the ventricular structures attached to the underside of the valve.

The remaining episode in the story of the stenosed mitral valve is its replacement by another valve taken from a dead body, from an animal, or manufactured in a factory. But for this to be possible surgeons needed to be able to operate on the open heart. The wherewithal was just around the corner.

19

MITRAL INCOMPETENCE

Surgical treatment for incompetence of the mitral valve got away to a slow start and made rather a dismal tale until all the conditions were right for neat reconstructive plastic operations or replacement of the valve, either with a graft of one sort or another, or with a mechanical prosthesis. The technical problems facing the surgeons who first tried to relieve the incompetence were immense; in comparison mitral stenosis was a simple condition.

For most practical purposes mitral incompetence is caused by rheumatic fever. It may be associated with greater or lesser degrees of mitral stenosis which add to the difficulties of accurate pre-operative diagnosis and may make it necessary to treat the stenosis as well.

When the mitral valve is incompetent it does not close properly and allows blood to regurgitate through its orifice into the left atrium as the left ventricle contracts. To complicate matters the valve may be deformed in a number of ways: the valve cusps may be fused giving a mixture of stenosis and incompetence, the cusps may have clefts in them, the chordae tendineae (the 'guy ropes') may be contracted, and the periphery of the valve may be dilated.

Cutler[1] based his operation for mitral stenosis on the observation that patients with incompetence lived longer and withstood their disease better than those with stenosis. Indeed, these patients do go for a long time with only slight disability, though they are inclined to become severely fatigued. Heart failure is inevitable sooner or later and once it develops the patient usually goes quickly downhill. For many years doctors had viewed mitral incompetence rather complacently but the improved techniques for mitral stenosis brought the true nature of incompetence into focus; it was a vicious disease.

The large number of different procedures tried in the 1950s gives an idea of the extent of the problem and also shows that none was satisfactory, although individual surgeons were sometimes able to get good results with their own operations. Interestingly, too, most of the techniques were introduced after the arrival of hypothermia and extracorporeal circulation but were still designed to be carried out 'blind' – this gives an insight into the early lack of confidence in the methods for obtaining an open heart when the patient was seriously ill and with heart muscle of poor quality.

In a previous chapter we saw that one of the difficulties in working out a suitable operation for mitral stenosis was the inability to produce the stenosis experimentally in animals. This was decidedly discouraging as the obvious way to correct an incompetent valve seemed to be to 'stenose' it. But human ingenuity was equal to the challenge and the starting point was Murray's early method of treating mitral stenosis[2]. In this, you will recall, he deliberately created incompetence of the valve to relieve the stenosis, and then slung a graft of tendon and vein beneath the valve opening to correct the incompetence.

Now for a diversion which is not really irrelevant since it concerns the choice of material for later work. In 1949 John Templeton and John Gibbon of Jefferson Medical College, Philadelphia, experimented with the reconstruction of the tricuspid valve (between the right atrium and ventricle)[3]. They studied the literature and decided that vein or pericardium would be the most acceptable tissue for inserting into the heart – plastics they rejected because they thought the heart would do likewise. First they resected a portion of the tricuspid valve and then spent about 45 minutes cutting the chosen material to shape on a board. This they put in place with a rather complicated system of sutures and so reconstituted the valve cusp to its natural shape. Five of their 19 dogs survived for more than seven months although some of those that recovered were killed at intervals to study the progress of the graft. Pericardium was found to give better results than vein, but in a postscript to their paper, Templeton and Gibbon had to record evidence of shrinkage of the grafts at a later stage[3].

This work influenced Charles Bailey, who was then in the same city of Philadelphia. He had repeated Murray's work, but with the difference that his interest lay in mitral incompetence. To his disappointment all the slings soon became shrunken, fibrotic bands, so he turned to Templeton's and Gibbon's preference for pericardium. But slings of this tissue also shrank. Right, thought Bailey, if free grafts are not going to work, we will just have to leave the sling attached to its blood supply. And when he did this the grafts showed no tendency to contract. The pericardium was mobilized and part of it folded into a tube, with the smooth surface on the outside; this was passed through the heart from front to back beneath the mitral orifice. A finger in the atrium guided the tube accurately across. The front end was anchored by the pedicle containing the blood supply and the rear end by sutures after the tension had been adjusted. In December, 1950, Bailey and his colleagues reported on seven patients who had had this operation (two had also had a commissurotomy at the same time for stenosis). They considered six to have had successful results, but in the seventh there was little or no control of the regurgitation. Their paper was published the following year[4].

In Scotland Andrew Logan and the physician Richard Turner of Edinburgh had the same idea and in 1952 they reviewed 11 patients they had treated surgically[5]. All had incapacitating symptoms and were deteriorating. The first case was a woman of 37 who developed a severe haemoptysis and was operated on on October 1, 1951. A sheet of pericardium was mobilized on a pedicle and a free corner sutured to the eye of a seven-inch (17·5cm) silver probe. Logan then opened the left atrium and, having confirmed the presence of regurgitation, he passed the probe through the anterior wall of the left ventricle, guided it across the underside of the valve orifice with his finger in the atrium, and brought it out at the back of the heart. He pulled the sheet of pericardium through after it and, by feel, showed that the sheet filled the valve orifice when the ventricle contracted. All that remained was for him to adjust the tension to allow a free flow in diastole and to suture the sheet to the back of the heart. The woman made an uninterrupted recovery and 10 months after her operation she had had no further haemoptyses and could do more without becoming short of breath.

The other 10 of Logan's patients all had similar operations, except that in the last five the graft was pulled through from back to front which made the technique easier. Nine patients claimed they were improved.

We now return to Bailey who, by 1954, had really got his teeth into the problems of mitral incompetence. Increasing surgical activity inside the heart had shown that most incompetent mitral valves were incompetent predominantly at their posterior end. Instead of the valve cusps coming together in a smooth curve, they left a pear-shaped gap between them with the bulge of the pear at the back. So why tackle the whole valve? Why not concentrate on the guilty area alone? Bailey did.

He first tried to obliterate the broad end of the gap with a suture made from a strip of pericardium (strengthened sometimes by threading it through another, concertinaed, strip of pericardium). This was passed through the wall of the left ventricle at a distance below the level of the valve and guided with a finger in the atrium blindly through the valve substance on both sides of the gap. The long end of the strip went through a hole in the short end – thus giving a tight loop that drew the edges of the valve together – and came back to the ventricular wall where it was sutured in place. In a series of 72 patients there were 20 hospital deaths which, as Bailey said, obviously indicated that the procedure was inherently too dangerous[6]. The reasons for this were the

166

poor state of the heart muscle which readily fibrillated during the manipulations and the proneness to an oozing haemorrhage which was uncontrollable. Postmortem examination showed too, that, in many cases, the strip had cut through the valve tissue because it had had to be put in under tension to bring the valve leaflets together. Add to this the degeneration of the strip and it becomes apparent that, besides being dangerous, the technique didn't work.

Bailey's next idea came from a finding in one of the patients on whom he had done the tubed, pedicled pericardial sling-type operation four years previously – the sling had sealed the orifice. An instrumental 'commissurotomy' on this unique form of mitral stenosis gave a good result with no regurgitation and set Bailey wondering whether he could suture some material or other to the valve itself to fill in the gap. One of his colleagues, Henry Nichols, then came up with the suggestion that a non-mobile pericardial tube placed diagonally across the posterior half of the valve orifice close to the cusp would have the same effect and would be technically easier. Finally, another colleague, William Jamison, in 1953 developed an instrument on the principle of the looper used in the hosiery industry for sewing the toes on ladies' stockings. This was attached to a finger and allowed all the stitching to be done through the atrium. By a rather involved technique the looper put in nylon stitches which were then tied to the pericardial strips and pulled them into place. The looper method of inserting pericardial strips across the gap in the valve was used in 25 patients with four deaths[6].

While all this was going on in Philadelphia, Dwight Harken was pursuing a different approach at Harvard[7]. He did not always see eye to eye with Bailey and their reported discussions at meetings were often acrimonious. The thought of pericardial slings made Harken unhappy as he said they offered a framework on which clots could form, and anyway they did not survive – opinions with which many agreed. But, even if they did survive, they might become jammed in the orifice of the valve or, if they did their job and the dilated heart became smaller, they would cease to be effective.

Harken placed great stress on the importance of valve-leaflet mobility, so in three patients with incompetent but mobile valves he inserted nylon sutures across the valve in such a way as to distort the periphery (annulus) of the valve into an elongated elipse and so make the cusps close on each other. The sutures were anchored outside the heart with buttons. One patient died soon after operation and another after six weeks from cerebral embolus; but the third was improved and maintained the improvement when seen more than a year later[7].

This technique was also adopted by Earle Kay and Frederick Cross of Cleveland who in 1955 reported on their experiments[8] and on four clinical cases[9]. Their first patient was a woman of 26 who was operated on on May 28, 1954, and at a check-up three months later was much improved. Their fourth patient died 16 days after operation from a suspected pulmonary embolus.

But back to Harken who next tried to achieve an artificial leaflet mobility by inserting a moveable baffle made of plastic. His first baffles were ball-shaped; they were passed into the left ventricle through an incision in the atrium; a suture was inserted through the wall of the ventricle, just below the valve, through a hole in the middle of the ball and back through the ventricular wall. Thus slung, the ball moved into the valve orifice with each contraction of the ventricle. Unfortunately it also caused obstruction, so Harken designed a new baffle shaped like a bottle and used it on 24 patients. Seven died in the immediate postoperative period and seven later. Nearly all the patients were in an advanced stage of their disease but eight of the 10 survivors were substantially improved[7].

Still, Harken was dissatisfied. There was risk of clot formation and consequent emboli; he found it difficult to place the baffles accurately and they did not always stay in the desired position. To overcome these problems and lessen further the possibility of obstructing the orifice, he produced a spindle-shaped baffle in a variety of sizes. Of the 17 patients reported on in 1954, three had died in the postoperative period and one later[7].

The next idea came from Robert Glover and Julio Davila, members of the Philadelphia team[10,11]. They were unimpressed by the operations on the valve leaflets themselves and reckoned that little could be done in this direction. But how about another component of incompetence – the dilated periphery of the valve? This seemed something well worth tackling because, they said, when the left ventricle began to give up the unequal struggle it dilated and the atrioventricular ring also became enlarged. This produced a relative loss of valve substance, a greater degree of incompetence and consequently more strain on the ventricle which dilated further. If they could put a constricting ligature around the atrioventricular ring they believed they could break this vicious cycle. Far from being discouraged by the inability of others to produce experimental stenosis in this manner, they regarded the failure as a good sign for the treatment of incompetence.

Glover and Davila carried out anatomical studies to assess the problems likely to be met, and then moved on to animal experiments. The coronary vessels were saved from injury by tunnelling under them, the 'effective' myocardium was undamaged, and provided the purse-string suture was properly placed it did not cut through into the left atrium or lead to 'appreciable' conduction defects.

In May, 1956, the two men reported on 27 patients who had been operated on. They were aged seven to 52 years; in all the disease was a result of rheumatic fever and all were in an advanced stage of congestive heart failure. The first operation took place on January 20, 1955, and the patient was living a normal life 16 months later. The purse-string suture consisted of umbilical

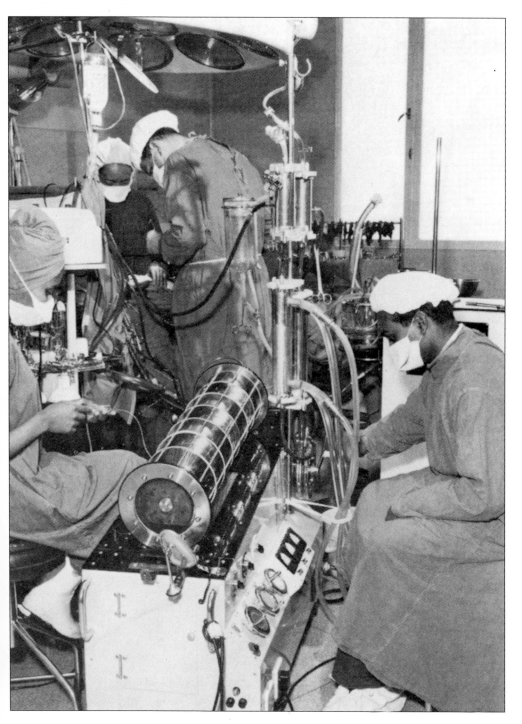

Extracorporeal cooling during open-heart surgery. The heat exchanger is behind the pump-oxygenator in the foreground. (By courtesy of the Department of Medical Illustration, Royal Postgraduate Medical School.)

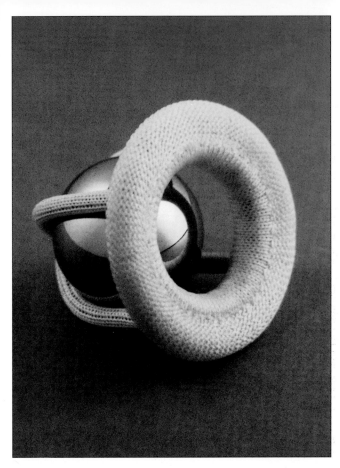

Starr-Edwards prostheses: (a) cloth-covered mitral valve; (b) aortic-valve (not cloth covered). (These photographs were kindly lent by Dr Albert Starr.)

(b)

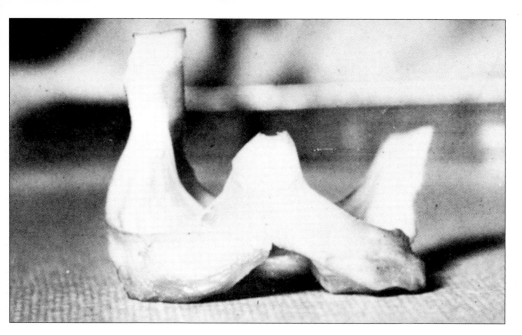

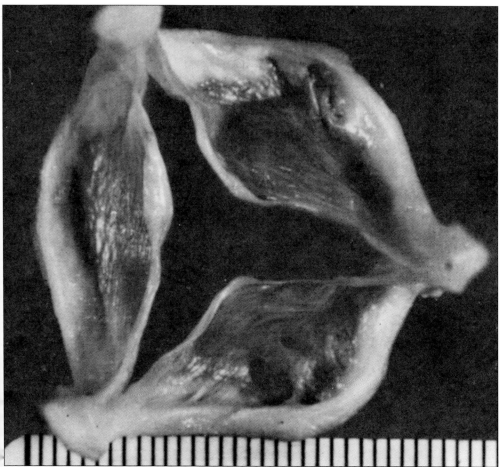

Homograft aortic valve trimmed and ready for insertion. (a) From the side. (b) From above. (These photographs were kindly lent by Mr AJ Gunning.)

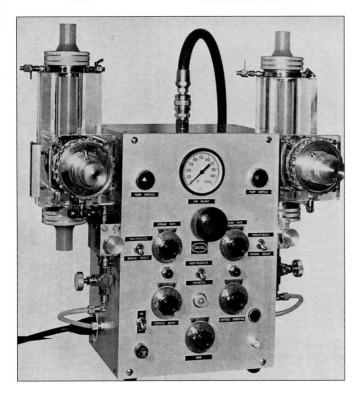

The electronic control box of Dwight Harken's arterial counterpulsator, with actuator and ventricles assembled. (Clauss RH, *et al.* (1961). By courtesy of Dr Harken and the Editor, *Journal of Thoracic and Cardiovascular Surgery.*) [Chapter 28; ref. 6.]

BELOW: Adrian Kantrowitz's intra-aortic cardiac assistance balloon. A balloon of this nature was first used clinically in the case of a 45-year-old woman on June 29, 1967; she was discharged from hospital recovered from her cardiac infarction (Kantrowitz A, *et al.* (1968). By courtesy of Dr Kantrowitz and the Editor, *Transactions. American Society for Artificial Organs.*) [Chapter 28; ref.11.]

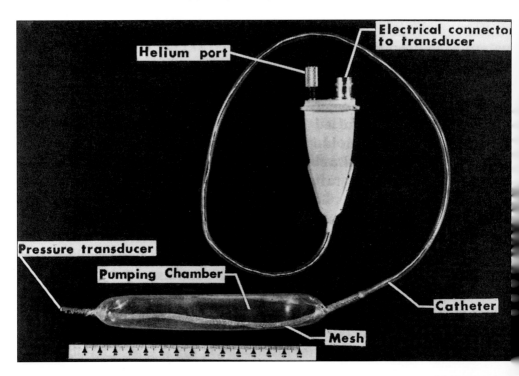

The blood-vessel connections made when Charles Guthrie and Alexis Carrel grafted the heart of a small dog into the neck of a larger one. The arrows indicate the direction of the blood flow. R.E.J.V. = right external jugular vein; L.C.C.A. = left common carotid artery – diagram by Charles Guthrie. [Chapter 29; ref. 1.]

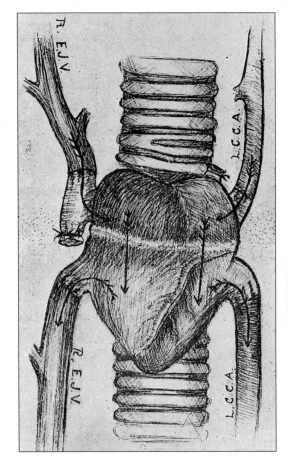

Borzoi, the dog that was given a second heart by Vladimir Demikhov on October 4, 1956. The dog was sacrificed on the 32nd day when the heart started to fibrillate. (Demikhov V. (1962). By courtesy of the publishers, Consultants Bureau Inc.) [Chapter 29; ref. 12.]

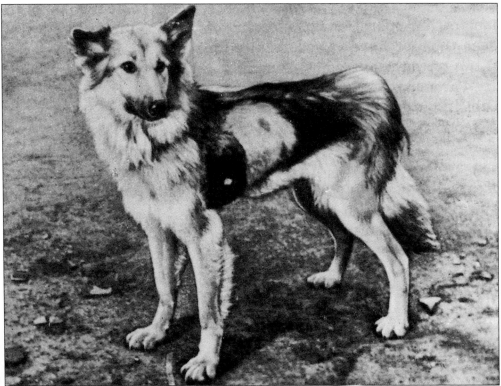

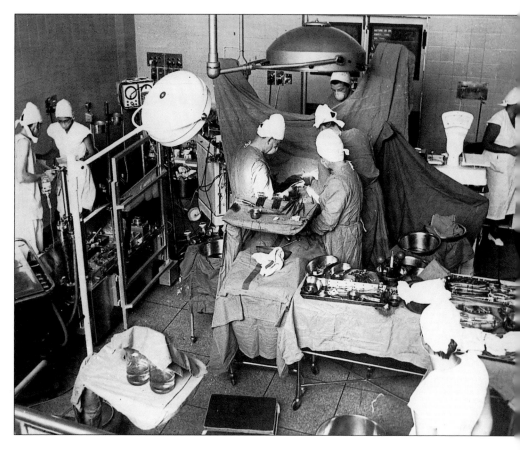

The operating theatre at Groote Schuur Hospital, Cape Town, in which the world's first human cardiac homotransplantation was carried out on December 3, 1967. (This photograph of an open-heart operation was taken on the following day.) (Photo: Associated Press.)

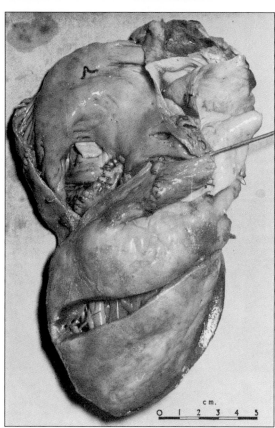

(a)

The first homotransplanted human heart: (a) anterior view; (b) posterior view. (Thompson JG. (1968). By courtesy of Professor Thompson and the Editor, *British Medical Journal*.) [Chapter 30; ref. 10.]

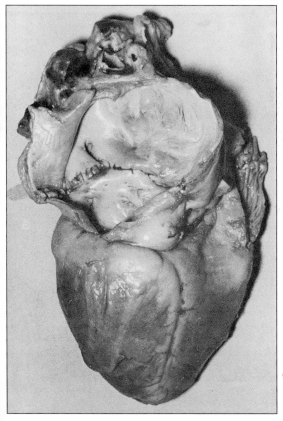

(b)

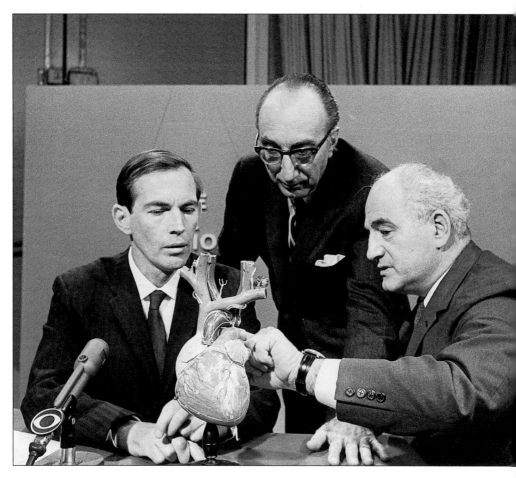

From the left, Christiaan Barnard, Michael De Bakey and Adrian Kantrowitz discussing a model of the heart before giving a television interview in the USA on December 27, 1967. (Photo: United Press International (U.K.) Ltd.)

tape or a narrow strand of cotton with a sleeve of pericardium stitched over its mid portion – this part was designed to lie in the transverse sinus. A finger inside the heart guided the needle. When the suture was in place it was pulled tight while the finger assessed the effect on the regurgitation.

The heart failure in 14 of the patients was intractable; medically, nothing could be done to improve their symptoms before surgery. In this group the results were 'most disheartening', but those who survived the operation were made more comfortable for most of their remaining days and one lived for as long as eight months. Medical measures enabled the other 13 to come to the operating table temporarily freed of symptoms, and the 10 who were living at the time of the report were all vastly improved[11].

Later in 1955, on August 16, Henry Nichols attacked the dilated valve ring by what he called his polar cross-fusion or cross polar plication technique[12]. This amounted to taking a tuck in it. He used a strip of pericardium to encase a non-absorbable suture and, with a finger passed through the atrium to assess the situation, he placed a plicating stitch in such a way as to lessen the gap at the incompetent (usually the posterior) pole of the valve. In 1958 he reported on 93 patients; all those over 50 years succumbed and the total mortality was 27 percent. Nichols, however, concluded that polar cross-fusion represented a satisfactory surgical approach[13].

Thus far no one had attempted open-heart operations for mitral incompetence and even the surgeon who first used a heart-lung machine in this disease began his animal experiments without its aid. Plastic materials for use in the human body had been improving by leaps and bounds so Walton Lillehei of the University of Minnesota decided to experiment with polyvinyl sponge. When he used this to straddle the posterior commissure of the mitral valve in dogs he found the material would contract and become shaped in response to the pressures applied by the mitral leaflets. It would thus tend to fill any deficiency of valve tissue[14].

By 1956 Lillehei had developed an improved heart-lung machine and on August 29 of that year he carried out a successful open operation on a boy of 15 years. The following May he reported on five patients; they were, he said, among the sickest on whom he had ever undertaken surgery. The method he used was an extension of Nichols's plication of the valve. Under direct vision Lillehei inserted interrupted mattress sutures of heavy silk into the annulus fibrosus of the valve. The stitches were put in over small 'pillows' of compressed Ivalon sponge to prevent their cutting out. On occasion as many as eight stitches were needed to reduce the orifice to a reasonable size. In the fifth patient, a woman of 43 years, the posterior leaflet had virtually disappeared owing to contraction of scar tissue. Lillehei made good the deficiency with a carefully placed cylinder of compressed Ivalon sponge. This turned what was left of the leaflet into a firm buttress against which the other leaflet could close effectively. All Lillehei's patients did extremely well; the 15-year-old boy returned to school and one woman said she had been given 'a new life'[15].

In 1956 Gordon Murray published his account of an operation quite breath-taking in its ingenuity[16]. He actually inserted an *aortic* valve taken from one dog into the mitral orifice of another dog as a closed technique. He started by removing the aortic valve and an attached length of aorta from the donor animal. Having removed the excess of muscle tissue from around the annulus of the valve, he proceeded to split the aorta into two or three strips which he trimmed neatly to a width of about a quarter of an inch (0·6cm). Then he stitched strong silk thread along the margins of the strips, leaving lengths free as tails at the end. Three sutures placed at intervals round the annulus of the valve completed the preparation of the graft.

Murray's next task was to put the valve where he wanted it to go in the recipient dog. He entered its heart through the safe doorway of the left atrial appendage, threaded the silk tails on needles and passed these one at a time through the mitral orifice, taking a sharp bend to pierce the ventricular wall just below the valve at evenly spaced intervals. By gentle traction on the threads, he pulled the aortic strips through the wall and thus manoeuvred the new valve into the mitral orifice and anchored the strips to the ventricular wall. He fixed the new valve itself by catching the sutures in the annulus with a crochet hook inserted from outside, pulling them through and tying them off. The experimental period lasted for more than eight months after operation and during this time the grafted tissues in his animals survived well.

This operation was performed clinically, though the details were meagre. To make sure that the mitral orifice would accommodate the new valve (obtained postmortem) Murray widely lacerated the patient's incompetent valve cusps. The regurgitation was relieved and 'the effect postoperatively was quite satisfactory'[16].

Although the open heart was a long time coming to mitral incompetence, surgeons were all too aware of how badly they needed it. For instance, Bailey began his 1950 report on mitral incompetence by saying that since 1940 he had been actively engaged in trying to devise a practical pump-oxygenator, and had, in fact, achieved complete occlusion of venous inflow to the hearts of experimental animals for as long as 70 minutes with a portable machine[4]. But when the means to an open heart arrived in the theatre surgeons were caught in a cleft stick. It was unacceptable to operate on early incompetence as there was no reliable technique available. And by the time operation was really needed the patients were seriously ill with their hearts and other organs in such a bad state that hypothermia or extracorporeal circulation would be too hazardous. Surgeons had to bide their time until pump-oxygenators were improved and satisfactory techniques of valve replacement were worked out – only in patients in whom the valve tissue had been destroyed, by subacute bacterial endocarditis for instance, were the cusps still sufficiently supple for plastic operations to be satisfactory. In the meanwhile they had to do the best they could with 'closed' operations. For this reason there was no continuity of development; the varied techniques had short lives and were rarely adopted by others apart from their originators. Their deficiencies were apparent and it is small wonder that surgeons disagreed about their relative merits. But all credit must go to the men who refused to stand by and watch their desperately ill patients die when they believed there was a chance – perhaps only a remote one – of saving them or making them more comfortable. Their dedication increased our knowledge of mitral incompetence and so brought victory that much closer.

20

AORTIC STENOSIS

D isease of the aortic valve, severe enough to produce symptoms, is utterly without mercy. Stenosis of the valve has a number of possible causes and it may not always be easy to decide which is the responsible one. The valve is, after the mitral valve, the next most frequently affected by rheumatic fever, and when the aortic valve is involved it is not uncommon for the mitral to be diseased as well. But for the moment we shall consider aortic stenosis in isolation. Apart from rheumatic fever, it may be a degenerative condition due to calcium forming in the cusps or it may be congenital, in which case, like pulmonary valve stenosis, the obstruction may be in the valve itself, below it or, very rarely, just above. Then there is another congenital condition in which the valve has only two cusps instead of the normal three; this predisposes to calcific changes and stenosis. Indeed, a diseased or abnormal aortic valve is extremely prone to calcification which varies in extent; sometimes it is so extensive that the cusps are all joined together and it may be impossible to locate the commissures. This is of practical importance since splitting the valve other than at the natural commissures produces a lethal incompetence.

Surgeons were, at first, faced with much the same problem as they were with mitral incompetence. With no really satisfactory operation to offer, they had to wait until the patient was going downhill, and by that time the dice were very heavily loaded against them. Like those with mitral incompetence, patients with aortic stenosis may go for a long while before symptoms develop, but once these appear there is usually little time left. Angina pectoris is frequently the first symptom, to be followed by fainting attacks and progressively severe shortness of breath. When congestive heart failure appears, the patient may well be beyond the aid of surgery. In view of the fact that some patients with mild aortic stenosis never develop symptoms, surgeons, mindful of the operative risks, were reluctant to operate before symptoms appeared; when they did appear, though, the decision had to be made quickly. Help in predicting which patients were going to deteriorate did, however, become available in the shape of electrocardiographic changes and other special tests.

Technically, the aortic valve posed some brutish problems. Because the mouths of the coronary arteries lie just above it, a constant danger in the early days was air getting into the coronary circulation. Incisions in the grossly hypertrophied ventricular wall bled freely and this was difficult to control by sutures. The ventricles were also highly irritable and thus prone to fibrillate; often this could not be reversed. The arrival of extracorporeal circulation and hypothermia did not help with this problem as much as might have been expected, since hypothermia (in particular) was liable to increase the ventricular irritability in the older patients, who constituted most of those with aortic stenosis. Add to all this the not infrequent association with aortic incompetence and the difficulty of judging whether relief of the stenosis would aggravate the incompetence, perhaps lethally, and we have some inkling of the tremendous obstacles to be overcome. Fortunately, surgeons appreciated that the only way to help these desperately sick condemned patients was in the operating theatre; it was no use twiddling their thumbs, waiting for a miracle.

Nothing happened between Tuffier's memorable 1912 operation[1] and 1946, when Russell Brock was looking, in the Guy's Hospital postmortem room, for a simpler and safer route to the aortic valve than through the left ventricle. He found that an instrument passed through the innominate artery or one of its branches would go straight there. In March, 1947 – remember this was more than a year before his first operation on mitral stenosis – a suitable patient appeared and on the 27th Brock exposed the 40-year-old man's right subclavian artery by a small incision in his neck. Without any difficulty he passed a cardioscope through the artery right down to the aortic valve. This gave him a good view of exuberant masses of calcified material with no valve orifice detectable. Wisely realizing that an attempt to cut the valve semi-blindly with the retractable blade at the end of the cardioscope was unlikely to be successful, he withdrew the instrument and no harm was done. During the next year or two Brock operated on a few patients by a retrograde approach (arriving at the valve from above, in the opposite direction to the blood flow) through the innominate artery, but the results were so bad that he abandoned the technique[2].

Way back in 1925, Henry Souttar had suggested the possibility of reaching the aortic valve with a finger inserted through the left atrium and hooked through the mitral valve[3]. Brock tried this approach in 1950, but even though he was extremely gentle he felt something go and as he withdrew his finger he became aware of severe regurgitation through the mitral valve. The patient died some 48 hours later, and the postmortem examination showed that a papillary muscle had been ruptured[2]. Brock's distress at this unfortunate accident is apparent between the lines of his paper. But by 1952 he was dilating the valve with a special instrument passed through the wall of the left ventricle. Five years later he reported an average mortality rate of about 5 percent, though in the severe cases and particularly in the early ones of his series it was between 25 and 50 percent. Seventy percent of the survivors had a good result[4].

Most of the work was, however, done in the United States of America where, also in 1947, Horace Smithy, so soon to die of rheumatic aortic stenosis, reported on experimental operations on dogs in which he used a thin sheathable barbed valvulotome inserted from above through the aorta to divide one or more of the valve cusps. More than a third of his dogs died, either during operation or later from severe loss of blood from the aorta – though closing this incision with stitches over a pad of gelatin sponge helped to control the haemorrhage. Nevertheless, lesions of the valve were found in only 12 of the surviving 14 animals. After he had finished these experiments, Smithy said he believed an approach through the left ventricle would be preferable to the aortic one on account of better healing of the incision, but this belief was based on experimental findings in healthy dogs and would not necessarily be applicable in sick human beings[5].

Charles Bailey[6] was meantime puzzling away at the problem, and in his laboratory tried various methods. First he followed Murray's principle in treating mitral stenosis: he excised part of the aortic valve to relieve the 'stenosis' and treated the ensuing incompetence by slinging a length of the dog's external jugular vein – turned inside out – across the valve orifice to act as an artificial valve. He placed the graft by pushing a hollow cork borer through the aorta from one side to the other and passing the vein through its lumen[7]. Unfortunately, the aortic valve is seated too deeply in the heart and the borer could only be used some way above it. Consequently the vein graft had to be on the long side and was inclined to flap about ineffectively.

Next, Bailey tried using direct grafts of small sections of aorta or pulmonary artery bearing their respective valves. But, although he believed these would one day be satisfactory, at that time (1950) they failed, owing primarily to massive haemorrhage[7].

Bypassing the valve was another possibility. To achieve this Bailey dissected out, postmortem, a long segment of aorta with the aortic valve at the end of it. This gave him the material for the bypass which he grafted between the left ventricle and the descending aorta in another animal. The graft was first divided and reconstructed so that the valve came to lie in the middle of the bypass. Various complications, including ventricular fibrillation, bedevilled this idea, and Bailey's final attempt was to lengthen the graft with a polythene tube and put the ventricular end of the bypass into the left ventricle through the left atrium and mitral valve (which was big enough to take it) . But this also failed[7].

Bailey then came back to thinking about punching a piece out of the valve. Never one to take other people's experimental work on trust and, in this instance, worried about Smithy's apparent belief that some degree of aortic incompetence would be acceptable in the human being, Bailey partly repeated Smithy's work but used a backward cutting punch. This gave him a mortality rate of 75 percent, from which he concluded that the sudden production of a fair degree of aortic regurgitation was intolerable to the normal ventricle[7]. So when it came to operating on a diseased valve, care would be needed not to create incompetence.

Bailey's first essay on a patient was a disaster. On March 9, 1950, he operated on a 26-year-old woman. He made a small stab incision in the left ventricle through which he passed a knife, but was unable to get it into a position where it could be used. He removed it and in its place introduced a dilating instrument. This went through the valve orifice all right, but when he tried to pull it back again it seemed to be stuck, and he had to overcome great resistance to get it free. The woman's heart immediately failed and she died 15 minutes later[7].

But Bailey was not to be put off. He still believed that if he could divide the cusps along their lines of fusion all should be well. He therefore set to and devised an instrument with an umbrella-like tip that could be expanded by a screw at the end of the handle. On April 6, less than a month after his previous attempt, he passed this device through the right common carotid artery into the left ventricular outflow tract, and after expanding it, pulled it forcibly back through the aortic valve. The patient recovered from the operation, although it was doubtful whether he derived any benefit, for he had suffered considerable regurgitation pre-operatively. Two more patients were submitted to the same operation; one appeared to be improved, but the other died because a false passage was created[7].

On June 22, 1950, Bailey used the instrument through the left ventricle and over the next two years operated in this manner 11 times. Although a third of the patients died, some of those who survived were greatly improved. Nevertheless, Bailey was dissatisfied, believing that it should be possible to achieve a more accurate and agreeable dilatation. This time he had made for him an expandable triradiate instrument that would adjust automatically to the residual aortic orifice. With it he could be reasonably certain that the three blades expanded along the lines of the commissures. He first put it into operation, by the ventricular route, on April 4, 1952[8]. All went well, and the technique was subsequently employed many times. Four days later, on April 8, Bailey carried out the first combined mitral and aortic valvotomy.

All the methods mentioned so far had one great drawback. Of necessity they were blind, but truly blind, as the surgeon had to operate with no idea of the state of the valve. So the next stage in the proceedings was to devise some means of assessing this before the instrument was inserted. A finger had to be got to the valve. As it was impracticable to put a purse-string suture in existing structures, Bailey isolated a segment of aortic wall close to the valve with a Potts clamp. He could then safely make an incision in this and attach a pouch of pericardium to the edges. When the clamp was removed he invaginated the pouch into the aorta with his finger and, with only pericardium and glove intervening, could feel the valve. The triradiate instrument was then used to dilate the valve through the ventricle with appreciation of what it had to achieve. Subsequently, on March 3, 1953, both finger and instrument were inserted at the same time to give even greater control, and in his report later that year Bailey and his colleagues recorded 11 such operations with three deaths[9]. Other surgeons also adopted a similar technique; for instance, Dwight Harken used a small cylinder of plastic material stitched to an aortic incision through which he could safely insert a finger[10].

The first attempt at direct-vision surgery of the aortic valve was reported in 1954 by George Clowes and William Neville of Cleveland[11]. Their patient was a man of 55 suffering from severe aortic stenosis, moderate mitral stenosis and regurgitation, and hemiparesis from a previous cerebral infarct. They used a heart-lung machine, but the man died an hour after closing the chest.

Despite its risks, hypothermia provided the means to the first successful open operation. On November 17, 1955, Henry Swan improved the health of a 29-year-old man with calcific aortic stenosis by attacking the valve directly through an incision in the aorta and dividing the fused commissures[12]. He was followed by Brock[4] on January 26, 1956, and on January 31 by Walton Lillehei, who used his improved heart-lung machine (with bubble oxygenator) and retrograde perfusion of the coronary sinus – the reasons for perfusing the coronary system were to give more blood to the contracting heart muscle and to eliminate the hazard of coronary artery air embolism. Lillehei's patient was a 37-year-old woman with calcific aortic stenosis. Besides opening the commissures to the annulus with stout dissecting scissors, he also trimmed off some of the calcium deposits which helped to restore mobility to the cusps and improve the anatomical result. The patient made an uneventful recovery[13].

Bypassing of the aortic valve was resuscitated when suitable synthetic materials became available. In 1955, Stanley Sarnoff of Bethesda reported his successful experiments on dogs in which he had used a plastic tube containing a Hufnagel ball-and-cage valve to connect the apex of the left ventricle with the thoracic aorta[14]. Unfortunately postoperative complications, such as destruction of the red cells by the valve and clot formation (with risk of emboli) at the anastomoses, prevented any possibility of using the bypass on human patients. But by the time the problems had been ironed out to an acceptable degree, it was possible to remove the diseased valve itself and put a relacement in the anatomically correct place.

21

AORTIC INCOMPETENCE

The remarkable ingenuity and technical dexterity of Charles Hufnagel of Georgetown University, Washington, made the early stages of the surgical correction of aortic incompetence quite his own province. Prosthetic valves came into prominence only in the early 1960s, yet Hufnagel was using them – admittedly not where nature intended the valve to be – 10 years earlier. He succeeded in this most difficult field, although other surgeons who inserted his valves could not match his results.

His experiments with ball valves began in 1946 and were sufficiently advanced for clinical trial in 1952[1,2]. The ball-and-cage was put in the descending aorta where it prevented 70 percent of the reflux. At first the valve clicked and could be heard opening and closing across a room; this was later remedied by employing silicone-covered balls. The dynamics of blood flow in the area of the new valve and its attachment were most complex, and a tremendous amount of work was put into the construction of the valve and the method of its fixation in the aorta. About 10 percent of the first patients to have the valve inserted suffered from clotting and embolism, but with improved techniques, including multiple-point fixation rings, that Hufnagel described in 1958[2], these problems had almost been eliminated.

In this paper Hufnagel also said that if clamping the aorta while inserting the valve would be undesirable, a temporary bypass could be constructed between the subclavian artery and lower down the aorta or to the femoral artery (though in the latter case a pump would be needed to keep the blood flowing). It was even possible, he said, to make the bypass permanent by including in it the valve and resecting the intervening length of aorta.

Hufnagel was not alone among surgeons in the attack on aortic incompetence. Nevertheless the difficulties were so formidable that only a few took up their scalpels – and by now it should be fairly easy to guess who they were and what methods they chose. Charles Bailey in 1955[3], wrote that he had used a strip of nylon fabric tied around the outside of the aorta; this was controlled by a finger inside but was a practicable possibility only when the valve cusps were virtually normal. In a few cases since 1952 he had used balls suspended in the aorta by one or two tails and designed to fall back into the aortic orifice between contractions of the ventricle[4]. Neither of Bailey's methods was satisfactory, though the constriction procedure was the better and was employed more frequently.

Gordon Murray[5] came next. He tried a number of techniques with animals, including bypassing the valve with a valve-bearing length of aorta taken from another animal, in much the same way as Bailey had attempted a bypass for aortic stenosis. At the same time, Murray also experimented with bypassing the mitral valve from the left atrial appendage to the left ventricle. In both cases, though, he found difficulty in getting a satisfactory suture between the graft and the muscular wall of the ventricle. So he turned his attention to inserting a cadaver valve into the aorta.

He took the aortic valve from a dog cadaver and oversewed the stumps of the coronary arteries to give a smooth internal surface. Then, with clamps in place, he excised between a half and one inch (1·25-2·5cm) from the aorta of the recipient dog just beyond its left subclavian artery. The donor valve was stitched into the gap. In some of the early experiments Murray passed a plastic tube through the valve orifice while the stitching was going on, to allow the circulation to continue to the lower part of the animal's body.

When the dog's own aortic valve was perfectly competent and functioning normally, the transplanted valve stayed open and eventually became stuck in that position. But if Murray damaged the animal's own valve to produce a strong regurgitation, the transplanted valve began functioning at once and was seen to continue working well for at least nine-and-a-half months.

Greatly encouraged by these results, Murray operated on a man of 22 in October, 1955. The donor valve had been taken at necropsy from a 33-year-old man and preserved in physiological saline solution at 4°C for 36 hours; it was inserted into the patient's aorta on a level with his sixth thoracic vertebra. The suture line was completed in 37 minutes, and Murray had no need to use a plastic tube to allow blood to flow while he was stitching. The immediate result was good and the patient's enlarged heart became considerably smaller. Eighteen months later the man was doing heavy manual labour, and when seen six years after operation he was well and free of symptoms[6].

By 1960, Murray had operated on three other patients with severe regurgitation; all were clinically improved[7]. He believed the technique had a place when narrowing the aortic ring or sewing the cusps (which we are coming to next) was impossible. However, despite the good results, the cases were too few to ensure this place and valve replacement was coming ever closer.

The heart-lung machine came into the picture of aortic incompetence on May 23, 1956, when Walton Lillehei operated on a woman of 52 who had a mixture of aortic stenosis and considerable regurgitation. The extracorporeal circulation was augmented by retrograde perfusion of the coronary sinus. Lillehei freed the adhesions between the valve cusps but then found that the cusps did not meet in the midline. He therefore inserted two mattress sutures to turn the valve from an incompetent tricuspid one into a bicuspid one that closed effectively. The patient was greatly improved[8]. (With his experimental experience, Lillehei had planned to use polyvinyl sponge to restore deficient valve tissue, but it was not needed in this case[9].)

Lillehei's first operation on pure aortic insufficiency took place on January 8, 1958. The patient was a 45-year-old man, and again a pump-oxygenator with retrograde perfusion of the coronary sinus was used. With sutures, Lillehei made the valve bicuspid. This operation, for the appropriate patient, became quite popular.

The big problem, though, was replacement of the valve itself, and in his 1958 paper[2] Hufnagel mentioned that a number of ingenious methods had been devised to put the prosthesis in the proper place. These included helical springs and ball valves which had been shown to work in dogs for at least six months. In the subsequent discussion, William Scott[10] said that two surgeons, Adams and Lance, had shifted, by grafting, the origins of the coronary arteries to a higher point in experimental animals. This highlighted a major difficulty, because it is vitally important to ensure that the coronary circulation is in no way impeded by any technique of aortic-valve replacement. An efficient valve in this site is valueless if it blocks the adjacent mouths of the coronary arteries.

22

TUMOURS OF THE HEART

Until the 1950s the presence of tumours inside the heart was of interest only to pathologists in the postmortem room, and even in pathology textbooks intracardiac tumours seldom received more than passing mention. Their diagnosis during life, let alone their surgical removal, was unheard of. Nevertheless, an operation that has borderline relevance to our theme was carried out in 1907. Cast your mind back to the chapter on pericardial disease and Alexander Morison's plan to give an enlarged heart more room to work in by removing part of the bony rib cage. The principle obviously had great appeal for him and for his surgical colleague at the Great Northern Central Hospital, Ewen Stabb. Morison had in his ward a girl of 13 with a large glandular tumour in the upper part of her chest which was pressing on her trachea and oesophagus and 'crowding' her heart. After Stabb had removed about two inches (5cm) of the second and third left rib cartilages she was able to breathe and swallow more easily[1].

We now move on to June, 1934, when Claude Beck of Cleveland drained a pericardial cyst in a young man who was relieved of his symptoms for four years. But in March, 1938, a second operation was needed. This time Beck decided to do more than simply drain off the fluid; he dissected out the cyst (which proved to be teratomatous – that is, composed of tissues foreign to the part in which it occurs) and the man made a complete recovery[2].

On the occasion of the first removal of a tumour from the heart itself, the surgeon was once again Beck. The date was September 7, 1940, and the patient a 39-year-old man with a 'tumour' in the wall of his left ventricle. Beck first of all used a curette to remove the contents and then by sharp dissection excised the calcified wall of the growth. There was no connection with the cavity of the heart, and the operation did not weaken the ventricular wall. The man was apparently cured, though the identity of the lesion was never established[2].

Reports then began to appear of the successful removal of intrapericardial tumours, but no one went further because no one could realize there was further to go until it was too late. That the diagnosis of an intracardiac tumour during life was a significant achievement is shown by the title of a paper published in 1952: 'Myxoma of the left atrium. Diagnosis made during life with operative and postmortem findings.'[3] The paper also records the tragedy that was inevitable until open-heart surgery was possible. Written by Henry Goldberg, Israel Steinberg, and their colleagues from the New York Hospital-Cornell Medical Center, it describes the case of a boy of three-and-a-half years who came to them apparently suffering from mitral stenosis with peripheral emboli. The investigations included angiocardiography which revealed the correct diagnosis of myxoma – a benign form of tumour that often produces the symptoms of mitral stenosis by acting as a ball valve. Goldberg operated on October 11, 1951, 19 months after the onset of symptoms.

During the next two years a few more attempts were made to remove tumours from the heart but they all failed.

The first surgeon to be successful was Clarence Crafoord of Stockholm in 1954. His patient was a middle-aged woman with a large myxoma in the left atrium. Crafoord used a heart-lung machine and had his assistant compress the atrioventricular ring and ventricular chamber while he was excising the tumour to prevent pieces from breaking off and producing emboli[4].

Shortly after Crafoord's operation. Alfred Blalock of Johns Hopkins was operating on a 57-year-old woman for what was thought to be advanced mitral stenosis. In reality, she had a left atrial myxoma and during the exploratory manoeuvres this became stuck in the mitral valve and her condition suddenly deteriorated. Blalock dislodged the tumour and wisely closed her chest. Three weeks later, on April 3, after discussing the problem, his colleague, Henry Bahnson, removed the tumour while the patient's circulation was temporarily taken over by a heart-lung machine. Six months after surgery the woman could do anything she wanted; her heart appeared normal and was free of murmurs[5].

In April, 1955, Wilfred Bigelow of Toronto, whose basic research work was largely responsible for the introduction of hypothermia to cardiac surgery, was exploring the heart of a 56-year-old woman suspected of having mitral stenosis. But instead of a valve lesion, he found a large myxoma in the left atrium. What was to be done? On the face of it, the tumour had to be removed, and Bigelow's way of attaining the open heart was by hypothermia. There was no time for surface cooling so he lowered the woman's temperature to 31°C by flooding the open chest with cold saline solution. He then stopped the circulation for two periods of a minute each, during which he cut the tumour into three pieces and removed these through the open atrium. More than a year later the woman was in excellent health[6].

But Bigelow was lucky; impromptu removal of tumours was usually lethal. Aware of this, Gordon Scannell of Boston retired gracefully when he operated for mitral stenosis in a man of 33 on May 23, 1955, and found a myxoma in the left atrium. Then, knowing the disposition of the enemy, he prepared for a successful attack. On June 15, he operated again, this time with the patient's temperature reduced by surface cooling to 26·4°C – rather lower than he had intended. All went well, and the patient was fit when seen 22 months later[7,8].

Not every cardiac tumour is a myxoma in the left atrium, as shown by Scannell's next case, a seven-year-old girl with a low-grade fibrosarcoma (a malignant tumour) in the wall of the right atrium and projecting partly into the cavity, partly outside the heart. The tumour together with a wedge of atrial wall, was successfully removed on March 18, 1956; one year later the little girl was alive and well[8].

Although removal of an unexpected myxoma was hazardous, Libero Fatti of Johannesburg believed that abandoning a mitral exploration was in itself a danger, and since the induction of hypothermia required reorganization, he put forward his technique as an alternative in an emergency. On November 7, 1955, he was operating on a 43-year-old woman suspected of having a tight mitral stenosis. When he discovered the myxoma he removed his exploring finger and clamped the incision in the left atrium. He then put a purse-string suture in the left ventricle and made an incision in its centre through which he raised the tumour into the atrium with his right index finger. The atrial incision was unclamped, and with the gloved nail of his left index finger he divided the stalk of the tumour. With his finger pushing from below, the tumour popped out of the atrial incision. During this manoeuvre the anaesthetist was compressing the carotid arteries in the neck in case pieces should break from the tumour and become emboli. The woman was discharged nine days after operation, but two days later she had a pulmonary embolus associated with pain in her left calf. This was treated with anticoagulants, and when she was seen 18 months later she was completely well[9].

Owing to the friability of most of the tumours and the consequent risk of embolus, Fatti's alternative was not received with wild enthusiasm and 'reorganization' was considered thoroughly justified. But by this time tumours of the heart had made their mark and increasing numbers of successful operations were reported with, at first, hypothermia usually the means to the open heart[10,11]. Surgeons were alert to the possibility of intracardiac tumours and so despite sometimes incredible difficulties in diagnosis – for tumours of the heart can mimic an array of other conditions besides mitral stenosis – the unexpected was met less and less frequently on the operating table.

23

HYPOTHERMIA

The dream of a few inspired investigators since the beginning of the 20th century and of surgeons at large since heart surgery became a reality was to have a dry, motionless heart to operate on. Techniques could be worked out with these ideal conditions in the postmortem room but it was quite a different proposition to put them into practice in the operating theatre where the patient's heart had to continue pumping its blood and life-giving oxygen around the body. That the dream was realized, unlike so many of mankind's aspirations, was due, not to chance, but to hard work and perseverance.

By 1953 surgery of the heart had well and truly established itself. It was no longer an occasional or experimental event, for in the years since 1945 a number of operations had taken their place in the repertoire of clinics all over the world. However, they suffered one outstanding disadvantage: the techniques were 'blind' or limited to those that could be performed without entering the heart. The need for better conditions had become desperate if cardiac surgery was to progress. Thus, when hypothermia and the extracorporeal circulation made their appearance in clinical practice, the impact was tremendous. At first the two methods developed side by side and it seemed as though a race was on to see which would emerge victorious. Yet neither was perfect. Physiologically both had drawbacks and uncertainties. Surgeons had to wait until hypothermia was effectively united with the heart-lung machine before they had adequate flexibility to meet the needs of the individual patient on the operating table. But for 10 years after the first use of hypothermia in 1952 various forms of surface cooling were popular – and it is these, and others that shared the same disadvantages, that we shall be talking about in this chapter.

Oxygen is at the centre of all the difficulties facing the person who wishes to bypass or stop the heart. Every cell in the body must have oxygen to live; it must have sufficient and it must have it in a form that it can use. Both hypothermia and extracorporeal circulation bristle with anoxic dangers and even if the major ones are overcome, little ones, of themselves perhaps innocuous, may start a biochemical or pathological chain reaction of other little events which together overwhelm the whole organism.

Experimental surgeons in the opening years of the 20th century simply stopped the blood flow for as long as the animal's body would tolerate the insult, which was about a minute or two. On one occasion, however, a dog belonging to Rudolf Haecker of Griefswald survived after the venous inflow to the heart had been occluded for 10 minutes. In his paper, written in 1907[1], Haecker described a special clamp he had devised for temporarily occluding the venous inflow (usually for only a minute-and-a-half) while he experimented with heart wounds and operations. Earlier that same year and in the same German surgical journal Sauerbruch[2] and Rehn[3] independently reported that they were also using methods of inflow occlusion. Sauerbruch illustrated how he gripped the vena cava and right atrium between his middle and ring fingers, a simple technique that was sometimes adopted by later surgeons either in experiments or while suturing heart wounds, despite the fact that even temporarily shutting off the circulation was regarded as most hazardous. Rehn's paper, as might be expected, was mainly concerned with the treatment of heart wounds, but he recorded the experimental compression of the right atrium for one-and-a-half minutes on March 4, 1907, by Professor Rudolf Magnus at Heidelberg.

Carrel and Tuffier found clamping of the whole pedicle of the heart a useful technique during their experimental operations. The clamp could be left on for two-and-a-half to three minutes. At the end of these open operations they took no special care to empty the right ventricle of air and had no case of emboli affecting the lungs. But they did make sure that no air remained in the left heart, for this could kill the animal if bubbles entered the coronary circulation or reached the brain. In 1914 Carrel wrote: 'It may even be regarded as extremely doubtful whether this class of operations may ever be applicable to human surgery.'[4] For once, his vision failed him.

Unknown to him, or perhaps unappreciated, clues as to how the difficulties might be overcome were even then scattered throughout the world's scientific literature. Physiologists wanted to study function and pharmacologists the effects of drugs on organs in isolation from the rest of the body, and so they had contrived pumps and crude oxygenators. And in 1912 Ernest Starling[5] had devised the isolated heart-lung preparation by means of which he could examine the behaviour of the heart in all kinds of circumstances – including variations in the temperature of the blood.

In 1914 Jean François Heymans[6] of the University of Ghent had begun his work which he continued for four years isolated from libraries and colleagues and even prohibited the use of his own university laboratory during the demoralizing occupation of his country by German troops. In experiments on 340 rabbits, he passed heated or cooled blood up to the brain or down to the heart through a glass cannula connected to a shunt between the internal jugular vein and the common carotid artery. Outside the body the cannula led through a water jacket for producing the temperature changes; there was no pump and the flow of blood was directed up or down, as required. With this primitive apparatus Heymans laid the foundations for the subsequent definitive studies on extracorporeal cooling.

But these and many other physiological experiments were not designed with the needs of some future surgeon in mind; they were solely to find out how the body worked. The information was there, growing all the time, and it was up to the surgeon or anaesthetist in need to recognize the significance of the physiological data and then to apply the findings to his own work. That in so doing he unearthed a whole barrow-load of problems emphasizes the gulf that so often exists between the experimental laboratory and the sick human being.

Disappointingly another gulf is found between the behaviour of hibernating mammals and other mammals when cooled. For more than 100 years hibernators have been a great source of interest to physiologists. When the environmental temperature drops, the body temperature of these animals wavers for a few days and then falls slowly over a period of hours; they do not shiver (which would use up great quantities of oxygen), their hearts beat slowly and they continue to have a capillary circulation (albeit reduced). Experimentally, the reactions of their hearts and nerves are not abolished by anaesthesia. When they warm up, they do so from the inside out, so that their 'engines' (their hearts) can cope with the task of getting the rest of their machinery going again. Unfortunately none of this happens when non-hibernating mammals are artificially cooled by, for example, plunging them into a bath of ice-cold water. They shiver (though this is preventable by anaesthesia), and somewhere around 26°C the human heart begins to fibrillate and the capillary circulation stagnates. The choice of anaesthetic agent has a considerable influence on the amount of oxygen consumed and warming is from the outside in. Despite all this, it is important to understand what happens in hibernating mammals when they are cooled as the process is physiological and provides a model which the surgeon can strive to imitate. It was only approached when hypothermia and extracorporeal circulation came together.

The reason why hypothermia was chosen as one of the methods of achieving an open heart is deceptively simple: At low temperatures the demands of the tissues for oxygen are reduced. The brain is the organ most sensitive to lack of oxygen and at normal body temperature can only be cut off from its blood supply for two or three minutes before it is irreversibly damaged. Lower the body temperature and the brain could withstand a few extra minutes deprived of oxygen during which the surgeon could operate on the open heart. If only it were as simple as that; but the moment one starts to cool the body one begins to move away from the physiological into the pathological. Fortunately, by keeping careful control on the depth and duration of hypothermia it was possible to keep from wandering too far along the path of danger.

Nevertheless, the dream was far from complete. The heart was still beating slowly even while the circulation to the body was cut off. Ten minutes inside the open heart was all the surgeon could expect at the safe limit of 28-30°C. Longer than that and irreversible damage, first in the brain then in other organs, would occur. Lower the temperature still further and as likely as not the surgeon would have all the time he needed to finish his operation – in the postmortem room.

At temperatures a degree or two below the 'safe' level the ventricles start fibrillating; this would give better operating conditions, but unfortunately at these low temperatures a normal heart-beat can rarely be restored. Even at the 'safe' levels the heart is abnormally irritable and operating on the ventricles sometimes caused fibrillation.

But besides the beating heart the surgeon had to contend with the blood from the coronary (and bronchial) circulation obscuring his field of vision. If he found he had to stop this as well to see what he was doing he ran the serious risk of increasing the irritability of the heart still further.

The problem was tied up with the methods of cooling and rewarming then available; all of these were from the outside. This meant that the fibrillating heart – useless as a pump – was one of the last organs to benefit from the warmth. By the time it was warm enough to be defibrillated, all the other warmed tissues had used up the oxygen in the stagnating blood. Resuscitation was impossible. The heart had to be kept beating at all costs, so that when the period of occlusion was over there was an effective pump capable of circulating the blood.

Cooling by surface methods was also imprecise as it had to stop before the desired temperature (measured in the mid-oesophagus where the temperature is almost the same as in the heart) was reached owing to the phenomenon of 'after-drop'. This fall of a few degrees occurs with surface cooling owing to the internal organs losing heat to the colder outer tissues after active cooling has ceased.

But the disadvantages were swept aside by the overwhelming benefits of an open heart. Nevertheless the risks were appreciated and one surgeon, an outstanding exponent of surface cooling, expressed his feelings in an incredibly honest comment.

'We have limited our work entirely to what one might call acute hypothermia,' said Henry Swan[7], of the University of Colorado, when the technique had been in use for just over two years. 'I have always been scared to death of it. My philosophy has been that I do not know what is going on; I have some definite purposes for it, and I would like to induce it and get the job done and get the patient back up where I believe I can understand him a little better, as quickly as possible.

'This is a purely emotional approach, as you can see.'

Initially, deliberate use of the slowed metabolism of the cooled body had nothing to do with cardiac surgery. Instead Temple Fay of Philadelphia, at the end of the 1930s thought it might be of value in treating patients with cancer. He had noticed that metastases tended to develop in areas of high body temperature and by applying cold locally he was able to relieve pain. The nutritional state of the patient was also improved[8]. Next he decided to cool the whole body to about 30°C for up to eight days in an attempt to stop the growth of the cancer. This did not happen although, again, pain was relieved[9]. His work served mainly to attract attention to the possibilities of adapting physiological findings on cold to clinical practice.

Hypothermia was first used in cardiac surgery not to obtain an open heart but to lower the metabolic demands of seriously ill children while they were being operated on. William McQuiston, anaesthetist to Willis Potts in Chicago, had read widely on cold therapy in adults and concluded this to be safe. But there was nothing about its use in critically ill infants. In fact the literature abounded with reports of the need to conserve bodily heat in children about to undergo surgery. Yet, so deeply concerned was he for the 'blue babies' who, with the added stress of the operation, sometimes just could not circulate enough oxygen to keep themselves alive, that he felt he had to put his belief in cooling to the test.

In May, 1948, he surrounded a boy of three months and 25 days with ice bags and brought the rectal temperature down to 96°F (36°C). During the next few months he 'refrigerated' 25 children out of a series of 123[10]. Subsequently he lowered the temperature further, to 92 or 93°F (33 or 34°C), by running cold tap water or ice-water into a mattress on the operating table as soon as the child was asleep[11]. By reducing the demand for oxygen McQuiston saved many of these children from an anoxic death, and also enabled surgery to be performed successfully on others who would otherwise have been refused operation.

At about the same time Wilfred Bigelow and his colleagues in Toronto began their investigations into the effects of lowering body temperature[12]; their valuable experimental work laid the foundations for the widespread adoption of hypothermia into cardiac surgery. The mortality rate among their dogs was rather heavy but they were exploring the unknown with the deliberate intent of seeing how far it would be possible to go if the technique of immersion in a bath of ice-cold water were to be applied in the theatre. They showed that ventricular fibrillation or cardiac arrest occurred if the temperature fell too low, but more troublesome was the death of a number of animals from shock within 12 hours of rewarming.

Bigelow's work was published in 1950; for once the seed fell on fertile ground and a number of surgeons in different centres were inspired to try their luck. Brian Cookson, Wilford Neptune and Charles Bailey of Philadelphia studied Bigelow's results and decided to repeat the experiments[13]. After 10 preliminary operations they evolved a procedure that allowed them to occlude the venae cavae for 12 minutes and open the right ventricle in 11 consecutive dogs, nine of which survived. They managed to prevent ventricular fibrillation in all but one of the animals, and by their careful, meticulous technique avoided postoperative shock. But to their consternation four of their first six patients died, three from ventricular fibrillation. A woman of 30 had had a previous operation at which a persistent ostium primum unsuitable for repair by Bailey's closed atrio-septo-pexy technique had been found. So, as her symptoms were progressing, on August 29, 1952, she was lightly anaesthetized and cooled in a cold chamber until her rectal temperature was 27°C. Her chest was then opened, her circulation arrested and the hole repaired. But at this point her ventricles began fibrillating, and in spite of efforts to restore a normal beat, her heart eventually stopped.

Their next patient, a boy of 11, was cooled to 31°C on September 19, but when the surgeon explored the interatrial defect he decided that an atrio-septo-pexy was feasible and this was done without circulatory arrest. The result was good. Ten days later this same team operated on another 30-year-old woman who suffered with progressive mitral insufficiency; although they deliberately repaired the valve cusps by a closed technique, they used hypothermia because they argued that lowering the temperature was equivalent to speeding up the operation. But she too went into ventricular fibrillation and died. The second success was with the relief of a pulmonary infundibular stenosis, again by a closed technique and without stopping the circulation. The last two cases in this series, reported at the end of 1952[14], were baby boys with transposition of the great vessels; the circulation was stopped in both. The first died on the table; the second, operated on on November 10, 1952, was cooled to 22°C and the vessels transected and sutured into their proper places during 22 minutes of circulatory arrest. Ventricular fibrillation then developed but a normal beat was fortunately restored and the boy went on to make a rapid recovery. A short while after, he was undergoing a routine bronchoscopic procedure when his heart stopped; it could not be restarted. The authors believed that but for this misfortune he would have been cured of his congenital heart defect.

As a result of their experience, Cookson and his colleagues believed that hypothermia was best suited to young children with congenital defects, although not those with holes between the atria for there was too great a danger of systemic and coronary air embolism when both atria were open. They were also unhappy about using the technique in adults with long-standing disease, as they felt the heart muscle was often in too poor a state to tolerate the cooling.

The first operation in which hypothermia was successfully used took place on September 2, 1952, and confounded the Philadelphia team's prognostications[14], for the patient had an atrial septal defect which was only the first of many treated with the help of hypothermia. The death knell of atrio-septo-pexy was sounded.

F John Lewis and Mansur Taufic of the University of Minnesota had carried out animal experiments in which they had created and repaired interatrial septal defects under hypothermia. When they were ready to operate on a patient, their colleague Richard Varco found them a girl of five years with an atrial septal defect who was a suitable candidate for the new procedure. On that September day she was anaesthetized and wrapped in rubberized blankets through which flowed a cold alcohol solution. After two hours and 20 minutes her rectal temperature had fallen to 28°C and the operation began. It lasted 58 minutes; the cardiac inflow was occluded for five-and-a-half minutes during which the actual repair took place. After the surgery was completed the girl was put in a bath of hot water at 45°C for 35 minutes[15].

Another type of cooling was to immerse the patient in a tub of ice-cold water. This was practised by Henry Swan and his anaesthetist, Robert Virtue, who were instrumental in popularizing hypothermia. Their first patient was an 11-year-old boy who was immersed on January 9, 1953, for 37 minutes. He was removed when his temperature had fallen to 34°C though, due to the after-drop, it continued to fall to 28°C. After a standard transventricular pulmonary valvotomy he was rewarmed in a tub and went on to make an uncomplicated convalescence. In his first series of 15 patients Swan stopped the circulation for two to eight-and-a-half minutes and had one operative death[16]. Hypothermia had arrived and its simplicity (a collapsible canvas bath on the operating table, for instance) contributed greatly to its appeal.

Some time before surface cooling had been introduced to the operating theatre – in fact, in 1948, the same year that McQuiston cooled his babies and Bigelow began his research, thus demonstrating that when there is need for a bright idea it often strikes a number of minds independently – Ite Boerema of Amsterdam had started his research into the direct cooling of the blood stream. With dogs as his experimental animals, he cannulated a femoral artery and led the blood through a spiral glass tube in a bath of ice before returning it through a cannula in the femoral vein of the same leg. After studying the effects of cooling alone, he progressed to opening the chest and successfully performed intracardiac experiments while the circulation was interrupted for 10-15 minutes. This work was published in 1951 in a Dutch journal[17]; just over a year later the *Lancet* carried a report of the basically similar work done in Edinburgh by Edmund Delorme, who had started his experiments in 1949[18].

This method, however, did not catch on as it had serious disadvantages; in particular the cooling itself became progressively more inefficient as the output of the heart gradually decreased with the fall in temperature. Also the use of a peripheral artery with the possible hazard of spasm did not add to its charms. But before long another method of cooling the blood came on the scene. This was known as veno-venous cooling and was devised in 1954 by Donald Ross of Guy's Hospital, London, to avoid the disadvantages of arterio-venous cooling. Ross took the blood from the superior vena cava and, with the help of a mechanical pump, passed it through a cooling apparatus and back into the body through the inferior vena cava[19]. Obviously, the chest had to be opened before the cooling could be started and this gave the technique one advantage over surface cooling – the decision whether to lower the temperature or not was deferred until the surgeon had had a look at what was wrong and had made up his mind on the choice of operation[20].

Veno-venous cooling had, as Ross pointed out[19], other advantages over surface cooling. The need to expose the body surface to about 0°C could damage the skin and underlying tissue and nerves; this was avoided. Unlike cooling by surface methods, with which control of the rate and depth was difficult, the temperature fell quickly and smoothly; as soon as the desired level was reached the cannulae were removed and the entire apparatus cleared from the operating field. There was no after-drop, as the cooling was from the inside out. However, veno-venous cooling still relied on the heart to pump blood round the body. Yet, despite its apparent superiority, it never achieved the popularity of the surface methods.

The techniques we have been describing produced what is known as moderate hypothermia. They were simple and reduced the internal (core) temperature to a relatively safe level of about 28-30°C which allowed the surgeon some 10 minutes or so inside the heart. This was sufficient for uncomplicated procedures such as repair of interatrial defects, but when a longer time was needed moderate hypothermia alone was found wanting. And as time was desperately needed it looked as though the rapidly developing heart-lung machines would win the day.

24

EXTRACORPOREAL CIRCULATION

I t is no easy matter to withdraw the blood from the body, oxygenate it and return it without damaging its properties. Consider what nature achieves in the lungs. Over millions of years she has evolved an incredibly thin membrane (the alveolar walls) so vast that if spread out it would cover an area the size of a tennis court. On one side of this membrane is the air we breathe, on the other, evenly distributed, are 10 pints (5·68 litres) of blood. Carbon dioxide passes out of the red cells, across the membrane into the air and is breathed out. Oxygen passes the other way into the cells. Entering through the inflow pipes (the pulmonary arteries) the 10 pints take about a minute to pass over the membrane, then they are gathered into the outflow pipes (the pulmonary veins) and returned under pressure to the heart. And man wished to reproduce this miracle.

The names heart-lung machine and the medically preferred pump-oxygenator, indicate clearly what is required to produce the extracorporeal circulation – a pump to replace the heart and an oxygenator to replace the lungs. As with hypothermia, basic scientists had paved the way and both components had been used in their experiments.

The pump has to move the blood in the correct direction, at the chosen speed and without contamination or damage. These requirements were met in varying degrees by diaphragm, piston or roller pumps with a system of valves where needed and operated mechanically, hydraulically or electrically. An early model was built by Johann Carl Jacobj, an assistant in the pharmacological institute at Strassburg (*sic*), in 1890 for perfusing isolated organs with a mixture of blood and air[1].

Extracorporeal circulation

In 1905 Edward Embley, honorary anaesthetist to the Melbourne Hospital, and Charles Martin, director of the Lister Institute of Preventive Medicine in London, concocted a pump for their investigation on the action of chloroform on the blood vessels of the kidney and bowel[2]. It was made from the bulbs of small Higginson syringes compressed by adjustable rotating cams. The principle was developed in 1927 by Henry Dale at the National Institute for Medical Research, Hampstead, who constructed rapidly adjustable, diaphragm types of pumps. He intended that separate pumps should take over the systemic and pulmonary circuits and support the complete circulation of a heartless animal, but at the time of his report in 1927-28[3] they had not yet been used for that purpose. Nevertheless, pumps of this nature kept the physiologists happy until the demands of cardiac surgery led to an almost explosive improvement.

For a long time the pumps reproduced the natural action of the heart by giving a pulse to the flow, but with their practical development for heart surgery physiologists began to wonder whether this was necessary. For instance, in 1955 Sigmund Wesolowski and his co-workers at the Walter Reed Army Medical Center, after carrying out a series of controlled experiments, wrote: 'the entire systemic circulation appears to be maintained equally well by the use of pulsatile and nonpulsatile flows for periods up to six hours'[4]. There were, nevertheless, many questions remaining unanswered, and five years later the matter was still undecided[5]. Fortunately, the delicate red cells stand up remarkably well to carefully designed pumping, though subsequently their life span, normally about 120 days, is reduced by half or two-thirds – thanks to the body's recuperative powers, this is not of major practical significance. The clotting properties may, however, be more seriously damaged and the transfusion of fresh blood may be required.

The really big problem is oxygenation, and possibly the obvious solution is to bubble oxygen through the blood. Certainly the idea occurred in 1882 to Waldemar von Schröder, another assistant at the Strassburg pharmacology institute when studying the function of isolated dog kidneys. He dripped the blood into a bottle and bubbled air through it. Admittedly he produced some nice red blood but he got far more foam, and each experiment had to stop when all the blood was turned to froth[6]. The method was grossly inefficient although Embley and Martin also had a crack at it before deciding that the only satisfactory method was to use the animal's own lungs[2]. Success had to await the discovery of antifoaming agents which, fortunately, are harmless and can remove all the little bubbles so that the blood can safely be returned to the body without risk of air embolism.

Another way of usurping the lungs' functions is to expose a thin film of blood to an atmosphere of oxygen. This can be done by filming the blood over a number of stationary vertical screens, like rain streaming down window panes, or by having a series of 40, 50 or more discs rotating vertically on a central spindle, and half-submerged in a trough of blood. As the discs turn, they bring up a thin coating of blood that picks up the oxygen. Max von Frey and Max Gruber of Leipzig, in 1885, used a tilted rotating cylinder to supply oxygenated blood for their physiological researches on isolated organs[7]. The blood flowed into the upper end of the cylinder (which was kept filled with oxygen) and spread out thinly over the whole inner surface as the cylinder revolved on its long axis. The apparatus failed to inspire either their colleagues or their successors, who found it much more convenient to link up their physiological preparations to the blood supply of another animal. The 'filming' principle was, however, revived and used in the first clinically successful heart-lung machines.

The first man to suggest that an extracorporeal circulation could have a place in cardiac surgery was the Russian, Sergei Brukhonenko, another pharmacologist interested in the effects of drugs on the heart and other organs[8]. In the early 1920s he had been using a roller type of pump for blood transfusion work, but when, in 1926, with his colleague in Moscow, S-I Tchetchuline, he designed an extracorporeal pump for canine experiments, he used a diaphragm type with valves. For the oxygenator he employed the isolated lungs of another dog rhythmically inflated by hand. Venous blood was pumped from the experimental animals into the pulmonary circuit of the isolated lungs; the oxygenated blood was then pumped back by a second pump into the animal's arterial system. In various experiments over the next two years he kept dogs 'alive', sometimes for several hours, after stopping their hearts. On three occasions he managed to get the hearts beating again, although only for a short while.

Brukhonenko was fully aware of the technical deficiencies of his apparatus but the clarity of his vision was most unusual – there was none of the airy-fairy quality so common in predictions, none of the 'One day such and such may be done, but don't ask me how' attitude. At the end of 1928, when cardiac surgery was at one of its lowest ebbs, he wrote: 'If this method were perfected would it not be possible to use it in medicine, in particular when it is necessary to replace, if only temporarily, an inadequately functioning *human* heart? Without going more deeply into the matter, we accept, on the basis of our present work, that *in principle* the application to man (in certain cases, and perhaps even for the performance of certain operations on the temporarily arrested heart) of the method of extracorporeal circulation is capable of realization, but for this to come about an adequate technique must be worked out in detail…. The solution to the problem of the artificial circulation of the whole organism opens the way to the problem of operations on the heart (for example on the valves).'[8]

Indeed, a machine based on Brukhonenko's principles was used by another Russian, N N Terebinskii, between 1935 and 1940, for animal experiments in which he produced valvular lesions in the heart and then treated them successfully by surgery[9].

Whether Brukhonenko foresaw mechanical oxygenators as part of the perfected apparatus or whether he believed isolated lungs to be the answer, we do not know. Lungs were in fact used clinically for a brief period in the early days of open-heart surgery, but the bulk of research was directed towards the machines.

The story of the pump-oxygenator as a force to be reckoned with in cardiac surgery began on May 10, 1935, when John H Gibbon Jr of Philadelphia artificially maintained the circulation of a cat while experimentally occluding its pulmonary artery[10]. Gibbon's vision of the future was backed by an unswerving determination to overcome the difficulties and produce a machine suitable for human use. His perseverance was rewarded 18 years after his first experiment, although he was nearly pipped at the post.

His early experimental mortality rate was high, and even in 1950 Gibbon was losing 80 percent of his dogs. But by then events in cardiac surgery were moving swiftly and, as if sensing the growing need, the canine mortality rate rapidly began to drop and at the time of his report on four patients in September, 1953 (published in 1954[11]), stood at 12 percent. Only one of these patients survived, yet Gibbon attributed the failures to human errors of one sort or another and not to the machine. The first operation took place in 1952; a 15-month-old baby was believed to have an atrial septal defect, but at operation no hole was found – the postmortem disclosed a large patent ductus arteriosus. The other two failures were both five-and-a-half-year-old girls, one with five atrial septal defects and the other with multiple anomalies.

Gibbon's moment of triumphant realization came on May 6, 1953. A girl of 18 was connected to the machine – consisting of a roller-type pump and vertical mesh screens of stainless-steel wire in a plastic chamber as the oxygenator – for 45 minutes and was dependent on it for 26 minutes while an atrial septal defect was closed. All went well, and at the follow-up examination there was no evidence of any hole remaining. In the discussion after Gibbon's paper Forest Dodrill of Detroit[12] mentioned that over a year previously he had successfully operated on a mitral valve using a left side bypass only (meaning that the patient's pulmonary circuit had been left intact to oxygenate the blood).

The surgeon who almost deprived Gibbon of his well-earned priority was Clarence Dennis of the University of Minnesota[13]. On April 5, 1951, he used a modified Gibbon machine during the repair of a persistent ostium primum defect in a girl of six years. She was dependent on the machine for 40 minutes. Regrettably, owing to a human error, air embolism occurred and despite several hours of partial support by the machine she died from the effects of the embolism.

At the Mayo Clinic, John Kirklin[14] had extensive experience of operating with a Gibbon-type machine and was able to treat complex congenital defects, though as we saw when discussing Fallot's tetrad, he had to stop for a while in 1955 to train his team thoroughly in all the minutiae of the technique. His work undoubtedly was instrumental in improving and making safer the use of the extracorporeal circulation.

Oxygenation by filming the blood over stationary screens has one or two practical disadvantages. Rivulets tend to form which reduce the surface area exposed to the oxygen; once started, the machine has to be kept going as the screens cannot be allowed to dry; and there are difficulties over controlling the rate of flow since the faster this becomes, the more blood is held on the screens. However, even while Gibbon was still experimenting, Viking Olov Björk of Stockholm was working on the rotating disc principle[15], and in 1948 reported on its reasonably efficient performance in animals[16]. The idea was subsequently taken up by Denis Melrose at the Postgraduate Medical School (now the Royal Postgraduate Medical School) in London who produced a clinical version which was first used on December 9, 1953, though only to assist the circulation, not to take it over[17].

The feeling towards pump-oxygenators at this time can best be appreciated by two quotations. The article describing the operation just mentioned began: 'Interest in the clinical application of the various forms of pump-oxygenator (extracorporeal circulation or artificial heart-lung machine) is growing so rapidly, and the use of this type of apparatus in man has so seldom been followed by recovery, that it is customary for isolated examples of its use to be reported.'[17]

And in November, 1953, André Juvenelle of Paris and his Swedish colleagues stated: 'To the present time no such machine or method has been found; at their best their use is limited in duration and any minimal dysfunction is paid in terms of death or irreversible damage.'[18]

Yet progress was not to be denied. Towards the end of the 1950s Melrose worked for a time with Frank Gerbode at the Stanford University Hospital in America, where his rotating disc machine was used alternately with John Osborn's Stanford machine which had a plastic screen oxygenator. Thus the two methods of oxygenation by filming were compared, and in 70 cases no real differences were found. However, on the grounds of convenience, cost per infusion and other administrative considerations, the Melrose machine was finally adopted at the hospital but with one important modification – all parts that came in contact with the blood were changed so that they could be sterilized in an autoclave and thrown away after use. The comparison, more than anything, underlined the similarities between the two machines, and Gerbode and Melrose concluded that teamwork was all important now that the apparatus was efficient. Morbidity and mortality, they said, depended chiefly on case selection and surgical management[19].

The other popular method of oxygenating the blood – by bubbling the gas through it – was resuscitated in 1950 by Leland Clark and Frank Gollan of Yellow Springs, Ohio, who found that coating all the glass parts with a silicone resin prevented frothing and made the tiny bubbles coalesce into larger ones which escaped into the atmosphere[20]. The following year on August 7 the Turin surgeon, Mario Dogliotti, used a bubble oxygenator while removing a massive mediastinal tumour that was compressing the right side of the patient's heart. The machine maintained the circulation for about 20 minutes[21].

Many modifications of this type of oxygenator were designed with the oxygen and blood flowing in the same or opposite direction, with large bubbles of oxygen and small defoaming surfaces or small bubbles and larger surfaces, but credit for the development of an apparatus most suited to cardiac surgery must go to the team of Walton Lillehei and Richard DeWall at the University of Minnesota. Because of expense and difficulties with sterilization, they set themselves the task of finding a cheap, disposable oxygenator. It did not take them long, and in early 1955 they began using one made of plastic the size of which could be chosen to suit the patient[22].

Thus the design of heart-lungs incorporating the two main principles of oxygenation – filming and bubbling – was continually improved, always with simplicity, disposability of the parts in contact with the blood and gentleness to the blood's components as major considerations.

Extracorporeal machines, however, require priming before use and in the early years pooled heparinized blood (about 2 litres) was used. Unfortunately, this could be troublesome; complications from incompatibilities of the blood and biochemical upsets from the citrate in the banked blood soon became known as the 'homologous blood syndrome'. The Lillehei-DeWall disposable oxygenator improved the situation because its size and hence the volume of blood for priming was adjustable[22], but some other fluid was badly needed and various blood substitutes and physiological solutions were tried; the worry was the effect they would have by diluting the blood. David Long and Lillehei experimented with low molecular weight dextran and found that it prevented or minimized thrombosis and aggregation of the blood cells inside the small vessels. In their report in 1961 they said they were then using it for all open-heart operations in their clinic[23].

Nazih Zuhdi and his colleagues[24] at Oklahoma City settled for 5 percent dextrose in distilled water with a moderate degree of internal hypothermia (to cut down the oxygen requirements and so compensate for the dilution of the blood); other surgeons followed suit with considerable success. Denton Cooley of Houston, Texas, picked up the idea from Zuhdi's early reports in 1960, but the need for rapid uncomplicated priming was really brought home to him when one day he was faced with an emergency pulmonary embolectomy. By 1962 he had used the dextrose solution with a disposable plastic oxygenator at normal temperature in 100 patients[25]. Cooley replaced the blood lost at operation by transfusion with compatible blood and noted that recovery of his patients was more normal and that postoperative bleeding was reduced as was the incidence of cerebral, renal, and pulmonary complications. Fourteen of the 100 patients died but in no case was death attributable directly to the perfusion technique. Five percent dextrose prime rapidly became popular and gave the heart-lung machine the added benefit Cooley had needed of being readily available in emergency situations.

A third type of mechanical oxygenator – using a membrane to separate the blood from the oxygen – was discussed in 1958 by Melrose, Gerbode and other members of the Stanford University team[26]. In many respects this should be the ideal oxygenator since it imitates nature's way of doing things; yet even when chemical engineers produced a suitable semipermeable membrane, a vast number of problems still remained. Melrose's and Gerbode's experiments underlined 'the importance of the character of such membranes in regard to the transport of carbon dioxide' and suggested that it might prove advantageous to use two different membranes to get the greatest efficiency in oxygenation and carbon-dioxide removal.

Writing on the subject in 1960, Melrose said that it was necessary to give a pulsing effect to the artificial lung to achieve full efficiency. If this could be done, the 'lung' itself might be used as the circulating pump. Then, 'with the addition of accurate heat control a heart-lung machine very close to the ideal would be available.'[27]

The technique of extracorporeal circulation was essentially the same whichever type of pump-oxygenator was used: catheters were placed into the two venae cavae, usually through the right atrial appendage. When the bypass was to start, tapes were tightened around the cavae to grip the catheters and ensure that all the blood flowed into them. The venous blood was pumped into the oxygenator, oxygenated and pumped back into the body through a catheter inserted into either the subclavian or femoral artery. The aorta was clamped across just above the heart and there were then upwards of 30 minutes in which the surgeon could operate on the open heart. But there was far more to it than this simplified statement would seem to imply as the whole perfusion had to be kept as near the physiological normal as possible – blood volume, pressures, flow rate, biochemistry, all had to be monitored and many methods were devised for this, some rather tedious, some highly automated.

In the first year or two of its clinical use the pump-oxygenator suffered the same drawbacks as did moderate hypothermia – the heart was still beating and the coronary and bronchial blood was returned into the field of operation. Could the heart be stopped? More important, if it was, could it be started again? Once again the pharmacologists and physiologists had given a clue. As long ago as 1878, Rudolph Boehm of the Pharmacological Institute at the University of Dorpat had studied the resuscitation of cats whose hearts had been stopped by overdoses of chloroform, by asphyxiation or by the use of potassium salts – little could he have realized that one day these last would be used for deliberately arresting the human heart. In his successful experiments he noted that the circulation really had been restored because of the pink colour of the blood[28]. Five years later the professor of medicine at University College, London, Sydney Ringer (of Ringer's solution fame) showed that excess of potassium salts in the fluid bathing an isolated heart would stop it beating[29]. And in 1904, E G Martin of Johns Hopkins University carried out extensive experiments on the isolated hearts of terrapins (quite popular laboratory animals in those days). He arrested the hearts for periods up to 35 minutes by infusion of potassium chloride solution; when the solution was washed out the heart-beat came back[30].

But there is a world of difference between stopping an animal's heart in the laboratory and stopping a human heart on the operating table. To take the step demanded courage of the highest order. Denis Melrose possessed that quality. After experimental work on dogs and on isolated hearts at normal temperatures and down to 26°C he was thoroughly convinced that the heart would in fact start beating normally again after it had been stopped by an injection of potassium citrate. So, in 1955, two or three months after his preliminary paper reporting his animal experiments had been published[31], he carried out the first elective cardiac arrest on the operating table[32]. When the heart-lung machine was connected to the patient and working, he injected the drug into the aorta on the heart side of the aortic clamp. The potassium citrate was carried into the coronary circulation and the heart stopped in the relaxed phase of diastole. At the end of the operation inside the dry, motionless organ, the aortic clamp was released, blood flowed through the coronary vessels washing out the potassium citrate, and the heart-beat was restored.

During this period of elective arrest, which can last 15 to 20 minutes, the heart is not 'dead'. Its metabolism continues though at an incredibly low level. Nevertheless, before the heart is stopped the surgeon must be sure that it is well oxygenated and while operating must treat it with great respect.

A year later, in America, Conrad Lam of the Henry Ford Hospital in Detroit introduced acetylcholine for producing elective cardiac arrest. This drug (whose action on the heart had also previously been studied by physiologists) was not a competitor to potassium citrate but rather an alternative. With it the heart can be slowed very markedly without actually producing arrest, and this Lam claimed to be an advantage in certain cases. For example, when stitching near the conducting mechanism of the heart, as in interventricular septal defects, the surgeon can see immediately whether he has accidentally included part of this mechanism in his stitches. Lam's paper in 1956[33] recorded eight children who were operated on for ventricular septal defect with the aid of a pump-oxygenator and acetylcholine arrest. Two died on the table from ventricular fibrillation but Lam was uncertain whether the arrest or the pathological state and operation was to blame. Two others died in the immediate postoperative period but from causes outside the heart.

The bitter realization that the heart-lung machine alone could not give a dry heart prompted another line of thought and small ancillary pumps were designed to keep the coronary circulation out of sight, as it were. Walton Lillehei and his team investigated the possibility of direct cannulation of the coronary arteries through their aortic orifices, but this proved technically difficult and was liable to damage the lining of the arteries besides creating the danger of coronary air embolism while doing the cannulation. They then remembered the work of Frederick Pratt[34] in 1898 and of Joseph Roberts[35] in 1943, on the ability of the heart muscle to pick up oxygen from oxygenated blood flowing backwards through the veins to the arteries. (We dealt with this when discussing the Beck II operation for the treatment of angina pectoris.) So they decided to perfuse the coronary system in a retrograde direction by cannulating the coronary sinus and using a small pump to deliver 125ml of oxygenated blood per minute. This was first done during an operation on the aortic valve on January 31, 1956. The perfusion lasted 11 minutes and the heart remained pink and healthy[36]. The technique proved particularly valuable in operations on this valve as it eliminated the risk of coronary air embolism – a bugbear in surgery of this region because the mouths of the coronary arteries lie closely above the valve. Coronary perfusion with blood of normal or reduced temperature was subsequently developed but is a later part of our story.

We have thus far trodden the path of extracorporeal circulation following the route dictated by the main signposts but, as you probably realized, we hurried past one or two sidetracks to avoid complicating the issue. Now we can retrace our steps to have a look at biological oxygenators and the cross-circulation technique.

The early difficulty of finding a mechanical oxygenator that worked properly led to experiments with nature's own device. William Mustard in Toronto began his research on dogs in the late 1940s. The oxygenator was the isolated lung of another dog of the same species; he obtained his first survivor in March, 1949. An entire lung was used initially, but later he found that a single lobe ventilated with 100 percent oxygen would suffice. The donor lobe could be successfully used for up to five hours after death. His attempts to use the animal's own lungs were foiled by technical problems and because of pulmonary oedema he found himself forced to follow the experiment with a lobectomy[37,38].

At the beginning of 1952, before anyone had succeeded with any sort of pump-oxygenator, Mustard decided to put his experiments to clinical test in patients whose outlook was hopeless. Between January 17 and November 18 he operated on seven infants, all of whom had transposition of the great vessels – we shall be dealing with this congenital abnormality in a later chapter; all we need to know now is that most affected babies are dead before they reach their first birthday if nothing surgical is done for them, and in 1952 surgery had practically nothing to offer. The operation was well thought out and a theoretical step forward, but success did not come. The babies survived the extracorporeal perfusion which used monkeys' lungs as oxygenators and lasted from 10 minutes to as long as three hours, but they all died within a few hours of the end of the operation[39]. At the postmortems there was no sign of gross biological damage resulting from the use of the monkeys' lungs and one can only wonder what the outcome would have been had Mustard given himself a better chance and chosen a patient with a condition more amenable to surgical correction. Nevertheless, he persisted until 1958 with experiments on dogs in the attempt to use their own lungs as the oxygenator, since he believed in keeping as close to the normal state of affairs as possible[40].

In the discussion of Mustard's 1958 paper Charles Bailey spoke about 13 patients in whom he had employed their own lungs as oxygenator – though he had always had a bubble-type mechanical oxygenator standing by, and had needed it several times. The technique had been developed by Gumersindo Blanco, the head of their research laboratory, after some three-and-a-half years work; Bailey's reason for adopting it was that less damage would be done to the blood than with mechanical oxygenators. The 13 patients had aortic-valve disease with normal lungs, which made them suitable candidates. The longest perfusion lasted for two hours and 20 minutes. Bailey, who did not say when these operations took place, was uncertain why five of the 13 died, but he thought it was probably owing to lack of oxygen in the heart muscle or conducting system during surgery[41].

Although we have not quite finished with biological oxygenators, we must make an apparent digression to the subject of rates of flow during perfusion. In the early days of heart-lung machines, two different avenues were explored. One was to imitate nature as closely as possible and provide a rate of flow that approximated the normal cardiac output. This principle was adopted in the majority of machines we have been discussing, but it had its problems – expense, sterilization, serious damage to the blood components and so forth. The other was to see how low a rate of flow one could get away with. This principle was used by the group at the University of Minnesota, but by about 1958, when the design of disposable oxygenators could be said to have been perfected, low rates of flow were gradually abandoned except when the extracorporeal circulation was combined with hypothermia. At normal temperature low flow rates often meant that working time inside the heart was dangerously shortened.

The low flow idea originated with Anthony Andreasen and Frank Watson at the Royal College of Surgeons of England between 1949 and 1953[42]. They showed how dogs could withstand up to 30 minutes of vena caval occlusion, provided the blood returned to the heart by the azygos system (from the chest wall and chest contents, other than the lungs) was allowed to circulate – this amounted to about 10 percent of the resting cardiac output. Having established the 'azygos flow principle', Andreasen and Watson then used it in cross-circulation experiments. In these, the circulation of one animal (the donor) was connected to that of another and acted like a heart-lung machine already primed with compatible blood. The necessary pumps between the two animals were set to deliver the blood to the 'patient' at a low rate of flow[43]. Unfortunately, this work at the Royal College was brought to a premature close, largely through lack of funds.

But it was not wasted, for we now move once more to Minnesota where the truly fantastic team of Walton Lillehei and his associates took it up and brought it to completion. At a time when most other research workers and surgeons were struggling with single methods of extracorporeal circulation, these men turned their hands to many methods of oxygenation and succeeded with them all. Everything they touched seemed to turn to gold. And although the azygos flow principle eventually fell by the wayside, it provided the means whereby this group were able to lift the heart-lung machine out of shaky infancy to competent maturity.

Lillehei repeated the experiments of Andreasen and Watson[44,45]; his only important modification was to introduce a single motor for the pumps of the pulmonary and systemic circuits to achieve a better balance[44]. Then on March 26, 1954, he used the cross-circulation technique for the first time[46,47]. In all, during 1954 and 1955, he operated on 45 children using a parent for the donor circulation. The parent's blood was taken through a cannula in a superficial femoral artery and pumped into the infant's aorta through the left subclavian artery. It was returned from the infant's venae cavae into the parent's great saphenous vein in the same leg. The period of bypass could last safely for up to 40 minutes, which gave time for reflection and on-the-spot improvisations should the unexpected be encountered. There were 19 deaths, an excellent record considering that all the patients had complex anomalies, including ventricular septal defects and Fallot's tetrad, which previously were considered either incurable or suitable only for a palliative procedure. The method, he said, was 'physiologically superb for those seriously ill patients' as the blood was constantly undergoing homeostatic adjustment in the donor. Not one of the donors died[47].

In 1953 Lillihei reported on experiments using a lobe of a dog's own lung left *in situ* as oxygenator. Again the azygos flow principle was adopted. Gaseous exchange was efficient and in only a few of the early cases did oedema of the lobe necessitate its removal[44]. Perceptively, he suggested that the use of hypothermia would reduce still further the amount of blood pumped per minute, would provide greater safety and would prolong the period of bypass. Later, his colleague at the medical school, Gilbert Campbell, made some important modifications in his experiments with isolated lung lobes. Instead of cannulating the pulmonary veins of the isolated lobe, he allowed the oxygenated blood to drip into a container from which it was pumped back into the experimental animal. This prevented back pressure in the isolated lobe and thus lessened the risk of its becoming oedematous. Campbell also introduced a depulsator between the pump and pulmonary artery of the lobe to prevent high pressures. His dogs recovered satisfactorily from 30 minutes of inflow occlusion with this form of oxygenation[48].

Early in 1955 Lillehei put the method into clinical practice. Using a specially prepared dog's lung as oxygenator, he bypassed a man's heart and lungs for 15 minutes while repairing a traumatic ventricular septal defect[47]. In the following months of that year a dog-lung oxygenator was used for 15 patients, but its value was limited because it could quite unpredictably become oedematous.

Finally, Lillehei used a reservoir of arterialized venous blood in five cases; this proved practicable only in babies because their requirements of blood are small and once the reservoir was empty, perfusion had to stop[47].

Lillehei began using the simple, disposable, bubble type of oxygenator at the beginning of 1955 and as soon as the team was trained in its operation and it was giving good results, the other methods were abandoned. They had served their purpose admirably and the cross-circulation technique in particular had shown that extensive repairs in seriously ill patients were no longer a dream.

In 1957 the Minnesota group reported on their results in 305 patients aged from six weeks to 66 years; 204 (67 percent) survived which was an outstanding achievement considering their enthusiasm for accepting extra-bad-risk cases. These results were comprehensive; in the early days the mortality rates were comparable regardless of which method of oxygenation was used[47].

But the success of pump-oxygenators was more apparent than real, and as surgeons demanded more than they were capable of delivering, so their deficiencies restricted their value. As hypothermia alone failed, so too did the pump-oxygenator.

25

HYPERBARIC OXYGEN AND EXTRACORPOREAL COOLING

B asically, both hypothermia alone and extracorporeal circulation alone failed because of lack of oxygen and the inability to adapt them to the precise needs of the patient on the table. Their failure was honourable, for in a limited sense, they did succeed and opened up the diseased or malformed heart to a whole new range of surgical procedures. But each by itself was found wanting when time – and safe time – was needed. Hypothermia gave a maximum of 10 minutes which was suitable for the correction of simple defects such as holes between the atria and stenosis of the pulmonary valve area. There was no margin for manoeuvre should the diagnosis prove wrong or the unexpected be found. If ventricular fibrillation developed (and this might happen at a relatively high temperature in a diseased heart) there was little hope of resuscitation. The pump-oxygenator gave more time, but even with elective cardiac arrest or the use of retrograde coronary perfusion, the biochemistry began to go wrong in the oxygenator if the surgeon was tempted to stay too long in the open heart.

Before moving off on the story of how the two techniques came to be combined we will make one of our now customary diversions and describe a method that demonstrates how desperately surgeons were seeking to improve the oxygenation of their patient's bodies.

Chambers in which the atmospheric pressure can be increased have a medical history going back some 300 years, but they really came to the fore in the middle of the 19th century. Hyperbaric chambers were to be found in many of the important cities of Western Europe; courses of 'treatment' were offered, much as they were at spas, for the same multitude of vague complaints and with much the same results. (A more respectable variant was the compressed-air diving caisson that made its first appearance at this period.) After a few decades the novelty began to wear thin, although one or two enterprising gentlemen continued to exploit the chamber's supposed benefits. For instance, in 1928 a Dr Orval Cunningham built a six-storey 'chamber', with 72 rooms in Cleveland, Ohio. It was fitted out like a first-class hotel and promoted to attract a clientele who suffered from high blood pressure, cancer, diabetes mellitus and syphilis[1]. The real trouble was that no one had made any systematic study of the physiological effects of increasing the atmospheric pressure; this only began in the early 1930s with investigations of caisson disease in industry.

Hyperbaric therapy was brought into the fold of orthodox medicine by Ite Boerema of Amsterdam in 1956 with his suggestion that it might be of value in cardiac surgery. Since then it has also been used in the treatment of a wide variety of conditions including myocardial infarction, cancer (to reinforce the effects of radiotherapy or chemotherapy), carbon monoxide poisoning, head injuries, and gas gangrene and tetanus infections. These applications of hyperbaric oxygen are outside our story; so far as we are concerned raising the atmospheric pressure in cardiac surgery has a ring reminiscent of the time 50 years previously when Sauerbruch built his low pressure cabinet to overcome the problems of the open thorax. And the outcome was very little different: hyperbaric therapy lacks the simplicity needed for general adoption; the apparatus is bulky and expensive and suitable for installation only in major centres.

In 1956 Boerema was working on hypothermia and puzzling out ways and means of increasing the operating time. As the Dutch had been prominent in hyperbaric research, it was perhaps natural that Boerema should look in that direction for help. With rabbits as his experimental animals, he showed that saturating the body with oxygen doubled the time during which the venous inflow to the heart could be clamped. Some animals recovered even after 45 minutes of circulatory arrest[2].

His work started inside a small caisson belonging to the Royal Dutch Navy. The pressure was increased to three atmospheres absolute, and the animals were given oxygen to breathe. Under these conditions, oxygen goes into physical solution, and at 27°C Boerema found the animals' requirements for oxygen to be reduced by half. The operators also had to be inside the caisson breathing air at the high pressure, but this caused them no trouble – in fact they were working under conditions similar to those of caisson workers in industry and like them had to undergo slow decompression to avoid the 'bends' once the experiment was ended.

Boerema's reports to two European congresses in 1956 were received with 'tremendous enthusiasm', but virtually no attempt was made to follow on with the good work in other surgical centres. Despite this, he pressed ahead, and by 1960 had installed at the Wilhelmina Gasthuis in Amsterdam a large caisson containing an operating theatre. His results, mostly in treating patients with anaerobic infections (gas gangrene and tetanus), finally succeeded in whipping up practical enthusiasm in other clinics.

In 1960 he used this large caisson to perform Potts's palliative anastomotic operation on a few children severely incapacitated by Fallot's tetrad. The patients were cooled and operation was carried out at a pressure of three atmospheres absolute. Anaesthesia was maintained with intravenous agents and for the 10 minutes before and during the actual anastomosis 100 percent oxygen was given[3]. Surgeons at the University Department of Surgery, Western Infirmary, Glasgow, in 1963 reported that they had operated on four children, using hypothermia at two atmospheres absolute. Three of the children were under eight weeks old (two had large ventricular septal defects and one had transposition of the great vessels), the fourth was a boy of two years with Fallot's tetrad. All died, the infants from profound falls in blood pressure and biochemical alterations, and the boy from collapse of his left lung a day after operation[4].

Boerema also experimented on dogs with the use of pump-oxygenators in the caisson. His main objectives were to avoid the homologous blood syndrome by priming the apparatus with dextran and to make safe a low rate of flow.

However, despite all this research by Boerema and others in clinics in different parts of the world, one is driven to the conclusion that those who used hyperbaric oxygen in cardiac surgery were intrigued more by the hyperbaric side of the work than by the cardiac surgery. So we shall leave this subject with the words of Robert Gross of Harvard Medical School, one of the great paediatric cardiac surgeons of his age. In 1963, after experimenting in dogs with both hypothermia and cardiopulmonary bypass, he concluded: 'it is doubtful whether the benefits derived under pressure are of sufficient magnitude to warrant the routine application of this technique in the surgical correction of the more common cardiac defects.'[5]

Now we can return to the events leading to the union of hypothermia and extracorporeal circulation. They make rather a disjointed story; no one woke up one morning after the two methods had been in use for some years and said, 'Let's combine them.' In fact research on the combination in its own right had been going on before either method was introduced to clinical practice. The chief problem lay in the cooling side of affairs, though in saying this we are not overlooking the importance of a perfected pump-oxygenator.

We must first go back quite a long way in time to the physiology institute of the University of Belgrade in 1940 where Jean Giaja was endeavouring to reproduce artificially the characteristics of hibernation in hibernating mammals. This he achieved by lowering the barometric pressure as well as the temperature. Then he turned his attention to rats. It had been known since the days of

Claude Bernard that rats died when their temperatures fell to 20°C, but by his careful control of the environment Giaja showed how they could be made to 'hibernate'. He put them into a chamber at 13°C and lowered the pressure slowly over three hours to 230mm of mercury (atmospheric pressure at sea level is 760mm of mercury). Their respirations slowed markedly to once every three or so minutes, and they consumed extremely small quantities of oxygen; their hearts continued to beat. They had lost the normal mammalian reaction to cold of increasing heat production by shivering, and were in a state of asphyxia[6]. Giaja improved on the rat's performance by increasing the carbon dioxide tension of the atmosphere, and it was later shown, in 1943, by James Barbour and Maurice Seevers of the University of Wisconsin, that the carbon dioxide was the important factor, not the lowering of oxygen tension[7]. Giaja revived his rats by currents of warm air after two hours in the asphyxiated state[6].

In 1951, 11 years after Giaja had published his work in a French journal, Radoslav Andjus, also from the Belgrade institute of physiology, reported, in the same journal, how he had resuscitated rats after cooling them to 1°C. This was an outstanding piece of research because, despite Giaja's work, a body temperature of 15°C was believed to be the lethal limit. Andjus adopted Giaja's technique of cooling with gradual lowering of the atmospheric pressure in a confined chamber; the rats became progressively hypoxic and carbon dioxide accumulated in their bodies. At the low temperatures he reached, the rats showed no sign of life – no respiration, no heart-beat, no reflexes. But his major achievement was in his method of rewarming. This was done in stages.

First the heart was warmed, and when it was beating at 50 to the minute Andjus began artificial respiration, from time to time insufflating a jet of carbon dioxide. Then the neck was warmed in water at 40-50°C. By the time the animal's temperature had reached 15°C spontaneous respiration and movements began. In general, Andjus said, he could obtain prolonged survival in rats cooled to 7-9°C, but when he cooled them to 1°C this was not so certain, though he had succeeded after one-and-a-half hours of suspended animation at that temperature[8].

Thus, experimentally, at any rate, there was seen to be no barrier to cooling below 15°C and a state of suspended animation with subsequent recovery was a theoretical possibility. It remained to adapt theory to the practical demands of cardiac surgery.

André Juvenelle, a Frenchman, was, in 1952, working in Stockholm with John Lind and Carl Wegelius. Two years previously, in Buffalo, New York, Juvenelle had been the first man in the Western world to replant the lung of a dog; the animal stayed in good health with normal respiratory function until it was sacrificed 35 months later[9]. (He had been preceded by the Russian, Vladimir Demikhov, in 1947 although the world outside Russia did not learn of these experiments until 1962[10]). But in Sweden Juvenelle's interests turned to deep hypothermia combined with an artificial circulation. Preliminary studies convinced the three men that 'the gross biochemical changes taking place during refrigeration were reversible and comparable in many respects to what is seen in the hibernating animal.' Their technique was to cool the dog in a cold bath until its heart began to fibrillate, at a little below 20°C. The dog was then connected to a Björk pump-oxygenator and cooling continued down to 12°C. After a variable time, rewarming was started – still continuing with the perfusion – and when the dog's temperature had reached a suitable level, between 20 and 24°C its heart was electrically defibrillated through the closed chest. The first report of Juvenelle and his Swedish colleagues, in 1952[11], drew attention to the enormous importance of the method of anaesthesia to be adopted before inducing hypothermia and noted that the duration of the period of fibrillation was irrelevant; destruction of the blood elements was the restricting factor. As their experience widened, they increased the period of fibrillation to more than two-and-a-half hours, during which the volume of blood flow could safely be reduced to one-tenth to one-twentieth of normal. They found they could always defibrillate the hearts, although at an early stage of their experiments the animals did not always survive.

Juvenelle was aware of the complexity of the method (equipment for both surface cooling and extracorporeal circulation was needed) and realized that it would have to be simplified; but for the time being it was valuable for physiological studies.

In 1954 the three authors reported on their progress[12]. The longest period of fibrillation with survival of the animal was three hours and five minutes, and one dog had been revived from 9°C , although it died 24 hours later. But the significant feature of this series of experiments was opening the chest and carrying out operations, for they encountered almost no bleeding and the coronary blood flow was very greatly reduced – a most valuable observation, since the reaction of the heart to anoxia is to increase the coronary flow, as we saw when Beck introduced the technique of coronary sinus ligation in the treatment of angina pectoris, and as surgeons found to their cost when the coronary flow obscured the sight of what they were doing in the open heart.

It was in this paper that Juvenelle made the comment, quoted in the last chapter, about the failings of pump-oxygenators, so as well as a small machine operating with a considerably reduced flow, it is not surprising that he also used isolated lungs as oxygenators. These could satisfactorily oxygenate the small amounts of blood required for several hours, and at these low temperatures, the appearance of oedema in the isolated lung was never a nuisance.

The big danger was 'stress' during rewarming as this could lead to death from irreversible ventricular fibrillation or acute heart failure. But it could be avoided, they discovered, by being extremely careful over the rewarming so as not to produce marked temperature gradients between different parts of the body.

This paper[12] carried a brief postscript stating that since it was written (in November 1953) human application had been started in association with Olivier Monod, the Parisian thoracic surgeon. Unfortunately, further information on these cases seems not to have been published.

An early practical attempt to overcome some of the operative hazards associated with surface cooling was taken by Brian Cookson, a British graduate, and J Costas-Durieux working in Philadelphia, who added an arterial transfusion to the technique. In their experiments they cannulated the right carotid artery and transfused the animal's own red cells suspended in a Ringer-Gelatin solution during the operative procedure. The idea was to prevent air getting into the coronary arteries when both sides of the heart were opened through a septal defect; also, by providing extra arterial blood, oxygenation was helped and the risk of shock diminished.

On March 13, 1953, the plan was put into operation on a 15-year-old girl with an interventricular septal defect. She was cooled to 24·4°C, her venae cavae occluded, and the transfusion given directly into her aorta. A continuous flow of blood through the coronary arteries was thus ensured[13]. Nevertheless, although successful, the technique did not catch the popular imagination.

In the United States, Frank Gollan, of Yellow Springs, Ohio, and later of Nashville, Tennessee, was working on combined hypothermia and extracorporeal circulation before either was adopted by surgeons – as indeed also was Juvenelle on the other side of the Atlantic. His papers, published in 1952, for instance in the *Journal of Applied Physiology*[14], told how he employed the principle of extracorporeal cooling first used by Heymans[15] in his experiments during the First World War. Gollan's oxygenator was of the bubble type and cooling took place in a heat exchanger that formed part of the apparatus. In dogs he demonstrated that the volume of flow could be reduced to meet the diminished cardiac output as the temperature fell. He succeeded in perfusing the animals for up to 47 minutes, though below 29°C the mortality rate began to rise, and no animal survived a temperature below 27°C.

By 1955 he had made considerable progress and could point out that the combination overcame the difficulties of hypothermia alone (anoxia and irreversible ventricular fibrillation) and extracorporeal circulation alone (air embolism and an operating field obscured by coronary blood). His apparatus was small and simple, and essentially the same as in his earlier research. Gollan's experimental animals were large mongrel dogs and he set up the extracorporeal circuit in such a way that the site of operation in the heart was not obstructed – venous blood from the venae cavae was drawn off by a catheter inserted through a femoral vein, and oxygenated blood was returned to the aorta close to the heart through another long catheter inserted in the femoral artery of the same leg. When the dog's mid-oesophageal temperature had reached about 20°C the respirator was turned off and the lungs allowed to collapse. The temperature was allowed to fall further and at about 13°C the heart action ceased completely. Out of 17 dogs, 13 survived. and the four that died did so from postoperative complications such as haemothorax, infection or thrombosis[16].

In 1959 Gollan wrote: 'It is my conviction that hypothermia of 0°C is compatible with life of adult, large, nonhibernating mammals if adequate perfusion of the vital organs is maintained.'[17] By that time, as he said, satisfactory pumps were available and the problems were physiological, not technical. But he warned that below 15°C high flow rates and perfusion pressures had to be avoided as they could dilate the heart and lead to irreparable myocardial damage.

Thus far we have dealt only with experimental work, but during this period operations on human patients with the aid of extracorporeal cooling had already been carried out, though not at the low temperatures Gollan had been using. The first occasion (*pace* Juvenelle and Monod) was on June 21, 1956, when Will Sealy of Duke University School of Medicine, Durham, North Carolina, successfully repaired an atrial septal defect in a seven-year-old girl; including refrigeration and rewarming, the whole procedure lasted seven hours and 15 minutes. Sealy's reasoning was impeccable: extracorporeal circulation at normal temperatures and low rates of flow allowed only a limited time inside the heart; the flow rate should therefore mimic the normal cardiac output. *But* the machines giving high rates of flow were complicated to run, expensive to acquire and maintain, and difficult to clean and sterilize. So he reasoned that the low oxygen requirements in hypothermia could be supplied by a simple low-flow pump and diffusion-type oxygenator; this would also cause less damage to the blood than the high-flow machines[18].

In 1958 Sealy and his colleagues reported on 49 patients with a variety of cardiac defects who had been operated on using the combined technique[19]. The first 40 were cooled by the surface method of packing the patient in ice – this needed one to two hours to reach the operating temperature (measured in the oesophagus) of 29-31°C. For the last nine, Sealy incorporated a heat exchanger in the extracorporeal circuit and reached the same temperatures in five to 12 minutes. From the operating point of view, conditions were good as bleeding created no difficulties and ventricular irritability was never a problem; in fact at about this time Gollan commented: 'During cardiopulmonary by-pass ventricular fibrillation has lost its deadly scare and is not more than a cosmetic defect of the electrocardiogram.'[20]

On a number of occasions Sealy electively arrested the patient's heart, and in these cold conditions was able to keep it at a standstill for up to 17 minutes; experimentally in a dog the period of arrest had been as long as 31 minutes without ill-effect.

By now many groups were working on extracorporeal cooling to low temperatures. For instance, Thomas Shields and F John Lewis of Northwestern University Medical School tried to simplify things by eliminating the extracorporeal oxygenator. They cooled mongrel dogs rapidly to below 20°C and rewarmed them in 10-15 minutes[21]. Unfortunately, the method was unsatisfactory as it caused differential cooling of organs.

The great advance came at the Westminster Hospital, London, in January 1959: Charles Drew operated on two children after lowering their body temperatures to 15°C. The first was seriously ill and died after operation; the second, aged four years, had holes between the atria and between the ventricles successfully repaired. Drew first of all exposed the left femoral artery; then he opened the chest, heparinized the blood to prevent risk of clotting and inserted catheters into both atria and a cannula into the exposed femoral artery. About 20-25 percent of the left atrial flow was led into a reservoir, through a heat exchanger and returned to the femoral artery. The object of this was simply to start the body cooling. When the temperature reached 25°C the heart could no longer act as a pump, owing either to its beat becoming feeble or to the onset of ventricular fibrillation. So at this point Drew established separate and complete bypasses of both sides of the heart – he used the patient's own lungs as oxygenator. The whole of the venous return to the heart was drained by the right atrial catheter into a second reservoir and pumped from there into the lungs through a catheter inserted into the pulmonary artery. Likewise, all the blood flowing into the left atrium (not just a part of it) was led through the heat exchanger and cooling continued to below 15°C; in the infants this took just under the half-hour, but when, later, adults were operated on, the time for this stage needed to be doubled. Anyway, at a temperature of 12-15°C (measured in the nasopharynx) the pumps were turned off, artificial respiration discontinued, the venae cavae closed by tapes, the heart drained, the aorta clamped (to prevent air embolism), and the operation performed. This state of complete circulatory arrest was maintained for 45 minutes: Drew had no problems with fibrillation or myocardial anoxia and the heart began beating of its own accord on rewarming, which was done by gradually slowing the pumps as the heat from the now warming heat exchanger began to have effect, and by making the bypasses partial before stopping them completely[22,23,24].

By the next year Drew had operated on more than 60 patients, aged from three months to 55 years, and with results that bore favourable comparison with other methods of open-heart surgery. He was aware that the long period of arrest might possibly damage the brain, but in two patients who showed very slight mental aberration for a day or two after operation there were other feasible explanations. Both were about 50 years old and both had calcific aortic stenosis, so air embolism or embolism of small pieces of calcium were possibilities[24]. Nevertheless, as other surgeons took up the technique, reports of brain complications such as phobias and temporary or permanent paralyses began to appear. Although these could be attributed to errors of technique, as they tended to appear in the early cases of a series, they were a disturbing feature, and the initial enthusiasm that had greeted deep hypothermia (also known as profound hypothermia) waned for a period.

However, the benefits conferred by deep hypothermia were too good to lose. Hypothermic arrest of the heart was preferable to elective arrest produced by chemical means, and time inside the heart was all-important to the surgeon now that even more complicated procedures were possible. So machines were designed and built that pumped, oxygenated and cooled the general circulation with a separate system for the coronary circulation. With these, the surgeon could suit the extracorporeal circulation and the depth of hypothermia to the needs of his patient. For instance, he could choose to operate without cooling the patient at all, but if he decided on hypothermia he could keep the body temperature at 25-30°C; at this level the vascular responses are still intact and a good arterial blood pressure can be maintained by a low flow of approximately 50 percent of normal. Then, if he so wished, he could cannulate the coronary arteries and separately perfuse the heart at a much lower temperature, thereby producing hypothermic cardiac arrest. Or he could produce complete deep hypothermia, perhaps recirculating cooled blood every 20 minutes or so during a long perfusion.

Thus, by 1962 or 1963 hypothermia and the pump-oxygenator had come together. Unlike their separate arrivals on the clinical scene 10 years previously, the marriage was a quiet affair, but one of the deepest significance.

26

TRANSPOSITION OF THE GREAT VESSELS

All the heart conditions we have discussed so far had at least a modest surgical history before the open heart came to their rescue. Some, of course, such as certain cases of mitral stenosis, were still best treated by closed operations, but a number of complex congenital anomalies needed all the benefits of experience and technical progress before any real impression could be made upon them. One of these, and the only one we shall consider, is transposition of the great vessels. True, work of fundamental and lasting importance was done before the open heart arrived, but it concerned palliation; the bulk of the work and attempts at correction came after.

Transposition of the great vessels means that the aorta and the pulmonary artery are in each other's place. The aorta leads out of the right ventricle (instead of the left) and the pulmonary artery out of the left (instead of the right). The net result is that oxygenated blood is returned to the left side of the heart (as normal) but is promptly pumped back to the lungs, and venous blood returned from the body to the right heart is simply circulated again throughout the body without so much as a look at the lungs. Thus we have two entirely separated circulations which are utterly intolerable and incompatible with life. However, some babies with the condition manage to survive because they have associated anomalies (holes between the atria or ventricles, or a patent ductus arteriosus, or these in combination) which allow some mixing of the circulations.

In early embryonic life the two great vessels are a single tube, known as the bulbus cordis. Growth and fusion of ridges produce a spiral septum which divides this bulbus cordis into the two arteries; if the septum fails to spiral we are left with transposition. The condition was at one time thought to be extremely rare, but as surgeons and pathologists became more aware of its existence, the diagnosis was made more frequently (both before and after death), and we now know that it occurs almost as often as Fallot's tetrad, which accounts for about 8 percent of all congenital cardiac abnormalities. Affected babies are severely incapacitated and live only a short time, though there are recorded instances of patients reaching adult life (even their 50s) when the associated anomalies were exceptionally efficient.

Surgical treatment is far from easy. For a start these babies are poor surgical risks; they are grossly anoxic and require extremely careful handling. Then there is the problem of 'balancing' the two circulations: whatever procedure is undertaken to mix the blood or direct it along its proper route, fine judgment is needed to avoid overloading one side of the heart or the other. The two sides are delicately poised, and either will fail at the slightest excuse. The obvious way of correcting the abnormality might perhaps seem to be to swap the two vessels around after cutting them off where they leave the heart. This unfortunately has two major snags. First, the closeness of the origins of the coronary arteries to the aortic valve makes it difficult to take these arteries with the aorta, even assuming they are so placed that the journey would be possible; if they are left behind, the heart will be supplied with venous blood from the pulmonary artery – though it has been argued that the oxygen content of this blood would be higher than that of the blood reaching the heart from the aorta before operation took place. Secondly, if the arteries are swapped over, the powerful right ventricle (powerful because it had been doing the work of the left ventricle) would be pumping blood into the lungs at an uncomfortably high pressure. Let us see how events worked out.

Alfred Blalock of Johns Hopkins was acutely conscious of the deficiencies in the early stages of modern cardiac surgery and devoted a good deal of his time to devising reasonably safe and efficient palliative operations that would fill the bill until corrective procedures were a practical proposition. The best known, the Blalock-Taussig operation for Fallot's tetrad, was introduced in 1944; this consisted of an extracardiac anastomosis between the aorta and pulmonary artery. Blalock's initial approach to transposition of the great vessels was governed by a variety of factors: his skill and experience as a vascular surgeon, the wish to keep outside the heart, and the difficulty of creating transposition in experimental animals – indeed, the impossibility of doing this as a first operation, for it would immediately be lethal.

Working with Rollins Hanlon, he anastomosed the pulmonary veins to the superior vena cava in one set of dogs, and the pulmonary veins to the right atrium in another. The plan was next to transpose the great vessels and see whether the previous operation brought sufficient oxygenated blood to the aorta, in its new position, to keep the animal alive. Unfortunately, by the time of their report in 1948[1], they had been unable to carry out the second part of the experiment. Nevertheless, the anastomosis between the pulmonary veins and the superior vena cava remained patent for up to three-and-a-half months in more than three-quarters of the dogs, and Blalock thought this might be a feasible operation in human patients. (The anastomosis to the right atrium was generally unsatisfactory.)

Thus, right at the beginning, we see the possibility of attacking the normally placed veins while leaving the transposed arteries alone.

In 1950 Blalock and Hanlon reported on 33 children, aged between eight days and eight years, who had had a variety of operations performed on them[2]. In all cases the diagnosis (not an easy matter in those days) was made by Helen Taussig, and only four of the children died during the operation. None of these deaths appeared to be due to the anaesthetic and for her fine achievement Blalock paid a well-deserved tribute to his anaesthetist, Miss Olive Berger – a nurse anaesthetist.

The 33 patients can be divided into three major groups. In the first were nine children who had an extracardiac anastomosis (such as pulmonary veins to vena cava or pulmonary artery to vena cava) – some of these also had their subclavian artery joined end-to-end to their main right pulmonary artery – but in every case this unbalanced the circulation and all the patients died in hours or days.

For the second group, Blalock made use of the observation that children with septal defects tended to have a better prognosis than those with some other form of compensatory anomaly, and also of his recent experimental experience in creating atrial-septal defects. Twelve children had a hole made between their atria. Nine died as a result of technical faults; the three survivors were improved but not dramatically so – the first of these was a girl of eight months operated on on May 24, 1948.

The third group also consisted of 12 children, and these had an anastomosis created between their subclavian and pulmonary arteries as well as the hole between their atria. Eight survived, and Blalock felt that they really did seem to be improved. He also contemplated operating on the veins as well but was dissuaded by the complexity of the task and the poor results of previous venous anastomoses.

Now we come to two procedures already mentioned in the chapters on hypothermia and extracorporeal circulation. The first of these was designed by William Mustard of Toronto who, you remember, decided to try monkey lungs as biological oxygenators in hopeless cases; the cases he chose were babies with transposition. The first operation took place on January 17, 1952, on a three-month-old girl and by November 18 of that year he had operated on seven babies. He attacked the transposed vessels directly as he found they were mostly of similar size and even if there was some disparity it was insufficient to interfere with the anastomosis – not all surgeons later agreed with this view. Anyway, Mustard divided the pulmonary artery about half an inch (1·25cm) beyond the valve and then cleverly cut the aorta obliquely, leaving the right coronary artery on the proximal stump, but taking the left coronary artery so that it was moved with the aorta. This was possible because the left artery was conveniently placed close to the original pulmonary artery. When he had divided the aorta, he perfused the left coronary artery with oxygenated blood[3]. But, as we saw, none of the babies lived for more than a few hours, although they all survived the perfusion.

On November 10, 1952, Charles Bailey and his team at Philadelphia carried out a 'switch-over anastomosis' of the two arteries on a seven-month-old Negro boy. They thought they had succeeded until 30 hours after operation the child's heart stopped beating during a routine investigation[4].

It will surely come as no surprise to learn that Walton Lillehei was also bringing his talents to bear on the problem. He reckoned the aim should be complete correction of the transposition, but the obstacle to this was the origins of the coronary arteries. So he thought instead about switching the veins over. Beginning on March 21, 1952, he anastomosed the right pulmonary veins to the right atrium in four babies with two successes. The chances of complete cure, he said, were likely to be greater the more severely ill the patient, as this implied the absence of serious intracardiac defects – but surgery could easily unbalance the circulations and was hazardous unless large shunts already existed[5].

Lillehei decided, therefore, to create a second anastomosis between the inferior vena cava and the left atrium to try to keep the balance. He soon found, though, that fatal unbalancing could develop within minutes after completing the first anastomosis. So to counteract this he inserted a temporary shunt between the superior vena cava and the left atrium which was opened as soon as the first anastomosis (between pulmonary veins and right atrium) was completed. This shunt was removed after the second anastomosis was completed. Lillehei admitted that the whole series was a matter of trial and error and that knowledge came slowly with experience[5]; yet there was no other way to tackle the problem. When, in 1955, he and his co-workers reported on 20 boys and 12 girls, seven were still alive and progressing 'modestly well' between 15 and 36 months after operation[6].

The next attempts at correction went back to operations on the transposed great vessels themselves. In 1954 Viking Olov Björk of Stockholm used arterial grafts obtained from babies dead at birth to join, end-to-side, the aorta to the pulmonary artery and the pulmonary artery to the aorta. He then divided the two arteries and stitched the cut ends so that all the blood flowed through the grafts in the correct directions. Björk, who gave no results, said that this operation was suitable only when the pressure was high in the pulmonary artery[7].

Earle Kay and Frederick Cross of Cleveland, Ohio, in 1955 reported that they had devised a series of anastomoses which produced complete correction. Instead of a direct swap-over they used the two main branches of the pulmonary artery. First they joined the right pulmonary artery to the aorta, then the pulmonary conus to the arch of the aorta just beyond the innominate artery, and finally they bridged the gap between the left pulmonary artery and aorta with a homologous arterial graft. When all the necessary dividing of vessels and stitching was completed the result looked like the normal anatomy except that the coronary arteries came off the pulmonary artery[8,9]. Kay and Cross had considered transposing the coronaries, but decided against it. Three infants were operated on; all died. One, four weeks old, died because the graft became kinked[9].

The last direct attack on the great vessels carried the assault right into the heart. Åke Senning had been in America in 1954 working on the idea that it was possible to dissect both aorta and pulmonary artery all the way down into the ventricles to below valve level. On his return to Sweden he operated on a six-month-old child with Clarence Crafoord assisting him. A ventricular septal defect was created and the aorta (already dissected out) was turned over and sutured to the hole. The pulmonary artery was then stitched into the opening in the right ventricle from which the aorta had come[10]. This incredible operation was performed under hypothermia and, said Crafoord, with practice could be done in half an hour. Regrettably, the bundle of His (part of the nerve-conducting mechanism) got caught in a suture and the child died. Two other patients recovered from the operation but died because they were unable to maintain their systemic arterial pressure owing to the sudden change in the demands made on the left ventricle[11].

After a great deal of experimental and clinical work, Thomas Baffes, a colleague of Willis Potts in Chicago, concluded – like everyone else, he said – that most arterial operations to correct transposition inadvertently imposed severe surgical trauma on the patient. So it was back to the veins again, but Baffes found straightforward venous transpositions to be most unsatisfactory. Eventually he settled for what almost amounted to the Lillehei procedure with the difference that, instead of direct anastomoses, he used aortic homografts between the inferior vena cava and the left atrium and between the right pulmonary veins and the right atrium. Because the amount of blood carried in these new channels was practically the same, the balance between the circulations was maintained. His first patient, a girl of three-and-a-half years, made a satisfactory recovery and began to walk for the first time in her life[12].

A year after his first report in 1956, Baffes had operated on 38 patients; 15 died in the immediate postoperative period and four others soon after leaving hospital. The remaining 19 – the youngest a baby of six weeks, the oldest aged 12 years – all had a most welcome alleviation of their symptoms. As his experience increased Baffes found that the grafts did not grow with the patients, but if operation could be delayed until the child was over six weeks old a sufficiently large graft could be used to make this of no importance. At this time he was also contemplating a second-stage operation to transplant the superior vena cava and left pulmonary veins and thus complete the correction. Although this was not done clinically – and would call for an extracorporeal circulation – animal experiments had shown it to be quite feasible[13].

The Baffes operation became popular and held the field for nearly 10 years. Yet even as it was making its debut, surgeons were moving inside the atria and taking the first tentative steps towards the technique that was to supersede it.

In 1956 Kay and Cross changed over from the arterial side to the venous and with an intricate remoulding procedure transposed the venous returns actually inside the atria. They operated on two patients with the help of an extracorporeal circulation. Both died, the first three hours and the second 25 hours afterwards. In both cases other defects were repaired[14].

On March 20, 1957, Alvin Merendino of the University of Washington School of Medicine removed the entire interatrial septum from a girl of six-and-a-half years and inserted a plastic prosthesis into the combined cavities. This was designed to direct the flow entering from the pulmonary veins (bringing oxygenated blood) into the right atrium, and the flow entering from the venae cavae and coronary sinus into the left atrium. The operation was carried out with an extracorporeal circulation and elective cardiac arrest; unfortunately, Merendino had to stop the heart twice because he failed to mould the prosthesis to 'compartmentalize' all the orifices of the pulmonary veins at the first attempt. The girl's heart went into irreversible ventricular fibrillation and she died. A second patient, a girl of six years, died from cerebral embolus[15].

The idea of remodelling the atrial chambers was, however, catching on, and in 1957 Senning reconstructed the chambers in such a way that flaps produced what he called venous and arterial atria; sometimes he used small prostheses to help in directing the flow. Of four cases reported on in 1959[10], one was a success and the function of that patient's atria seemed to be good.

John Kirklin of the Mayo Clinic took up Senning's technique and by 1961 had operated on 11 patients, using extracorporeal hypothermia at 12°C. Four survived, though one of these died two-and-a-half months afterwards owing to apparently unrelated pneumonia[16].

Success was hard to come by with any method so the next one should serve to alert us to the work of a surgeon in South Africa whose achievements were not then widely known to the world outside. At the Groote Schuur Hospital, Cape Town, on February 13, 1961, a 16-year-old Cape Coloured boy was operated on by Christiaan Barnard. The lad had always been cyanosed and dyspnoeic; his development was retarded and he could do very little. Using extracorporeal cooling at 15°C Barnard completely excised the atrial septum and, much as Merendino had done, inserted a plastic prosthesis into the cavity. This was so designed that the pulmonary venous return drained through it to the anatomical right (but functional left) ventricle, and the systemic venous return flowed around it to reach the anatomical left (but functional right) ventricle. A major problem was to ensure a normal flow during diastole, and Barnard had to do a lot of plastic surgery to get a good fit and avoid obstruction. Yet all went well and a year later the boy was doing excellently[17].

Four months after this operation a baby girl was born in Canada. She was far from well and became increasingly cyanosed. When she was 21 days old something had to be done: that something was a Blalock-Hanlon operation, as the creation of an atrial-septal defect in patients with transposition was now called. Her heart rate increased and her colour improved, but when she reached one-and-a-half years she began to go downhill again. So on May 16, 1963, Mustard operated a second time, using a pump-oxygenator. First he closed a small ventricular-septal defect, then he excised the entire atrial septum. This he replaced with a flaplike sheet or baffle of pericardium that almost completely divided the atria into two separate chambers – but functionally correct chambers. The perfusion lasted for 50 minutes and after operation the girl made an uneventful recovery to the point that she looked normal and walked and played normally[18].

Since pericardium had a poor reputation for surviving inside the heart, Mustard countered possible criticism by pointing out that pericardial grafts in low-pressure areas did not shrink and underwent minimal fibrosis. Nowhere, he said, was the pericardium a tunnel, and this was important as far as future growth was concerned. Nevertheless, experiments with piglets had suggested that the pericardial flap would grow with the patient[18].

In 1966 Mustard analysed the results in four patients. All showed full arterial oxygen saturation and had normal arterial blood pressures. Pressure tracings in the atria suggested that the pericardial baffle interfered not at all with function. So, Mustard concluded, it was possible to give normal cardiac function and systemic oxygenation[19].

27

VALVE REPLACEMENT

T he complete surgical replacement of heart valves destroyed by disease
was inevitable. We have already seen some of the opening moves of
the 1950s: Murray inserting cadaver aortic valves into the descending
aorta and into the mitral orifice[1], Hufnagel putting ball valves also in the
descending aorta[2], and Lillehei making good deficiencies of valve cusps with
plastic buttresses[3]. These operations had great significance because they
showed that both natural and prosthetic valves functioned inside the body and
that plastic materials were tolerated as part of the valve cusps. They also
indicated the division of opinion between the supporters of natural and
man-made materials – a division that is still far from being resolved. Yet even
when surgeons were able to move safely inside the heart for sufficiently long
periods, there was no wild rush to insert new valves; so much remained to be
learned, particularly about their behaviour and the likely long-term results, that
progress was cautious and backed up by a great deal of laboratory research.
Patients received new valves only when nothing else could be done for them.

The two valves we are most familiar with – the mitral and the aortic –
attracted practically all the attention since the problems posed by the other two
were different in nature or degree and could mostly be dealt with by standard
procedures. Right from the beginning work on natural and artificial
replacements ran in separate channels with the choice of the one seeming
often to be governed by the deficiencies of the other; eventually the results in
large series of patients produced a more positive approach – though not
necessarily a changing of sides.

The first successful attempt at experimental valve replacement with an artificial prosthesis was made by Rehmi Denton of Albany, New York, in 1949, using a closed technique. His polyethylene prosthesis for the mitral orifice had no moving parts and was shaped like a short, stubby, thick-walled tube with a rounded lower end. In one type the lumen went straight through; in two others it curved and came out at the side of the lower or ventricular end. Denton worked through the left atrium; by temporarily putting a metal cylinder with a rubber diaphragm into the incision, he was able to place the anchoring sutures without great loss of blood. Then, quickly removing the cylinder, he inserted the prosthesis into the valve orifice and tied the sutures which were already attached to the prosthesis. While this was being done the new 'valve' was held through its lumen with a metal clamp specially designed to allow the blood to continue flowing. Six of Denton's eight dogs survived and one (with a curved-lumen valve) was healthy and active a year later. The technique was, however, abandoned owing to difficulties in getting the prosthesis into the proper place and in fixing it securely[4].

The achievement of a firm union between prosthesis and surrounding tissues was indeed one of the major problems facing the early workers; another was the alarmingly high incidence of clot formation. So the hunt was on for suitable materials and designs. The versatility of plastics made them the obvious choice of material though a lot of hard work was needed to develop substances that met the surgeons' demands. The valve itself had to stand up to constant stress and strain without deterioration, and the fixation device had virtually to be incorporated into the body by in-growth of tissue. Metals also came into the picture when cages were required for ball-and-cage valves. The question of design produced two schools of thought: one that tried to imitate nature as closely as possible and the other which aimed to produce valves that functioned efficiently, even though the design was strange to the body.

By 1959, Charles Hufnagel had developed a replacement for a single cusp of the aortic valve to use in cases of aortic incompetence. The new cusp was made of Dacron cloth impregnated with silicone rubber under high pressure (to prevent tissue from growing into the material which would impair its flexibility) and molded into the correct anatomical shape. The edge of the cusp that was to be fixed to the aortic annulus, however, was not impregnated to allow it to heal firmly in place. Some of these cusps had small pins at this edge which were simply passed through the aortic wall and bent like staples without the need for stitching[5]. In 1961 Hufnagel said he had repaired more than 150 incompetent aortic valves under cardiopulmonary bypass with local cooling of the heart. The cusps had been inserted either singly or in groups of three united at the commissures. His experience, though, had led him to believe that most patients with severe aortic incompetence needed complete replacement, since the replacement of one cusp merely led to the breakdown of the remaining valve tissue during the next few months. He had, in fact, operated a second time on two patients for this very reason. Improvement in Hufnagel's patients was judged by the disappearance of angina pectoris and of evidence of congestive cardiac failure[6].

Dwight McGoon of the Mayo Clinic approached the problem of aortic incompetence rather differently, for he placed more stress on retaining those elements of the valve that were still able to function; if part of a cusp was destroyed but the remnant was flexible, he incorporated it into the replacement. His prosthesis started off as a tube of closely knitted Teflon which was cut and flattened to the approximate shape beforehand and the free leaflet edges stiffened slightly with polyurethane. When he saw precisely what the patient needed he trimmed the base of the prosthesis accordingly. In this way the length of original tubing could be transformed into a bicuspid or tricuspid valve that was stitched to the aortic annulus or to remnants of flexible cusps as appropriate. The anchoring was completed at the commissures with sutures of knitted Teflon tape. McGoon operated on seven patients in 1960 (the first on July 18); three died of apparently unrelated causes within the first 24 hours[7].

The mitral valve was technically more difficult than the aortic to replace, not only from the fixation and suturing points of view but also because of its chordae tendineae or 'guy ropes' which the aortic valve does not possess. Nina Braunwald and Andrew Morrow of the National Heart Institute, Bethesda, Maryland, pondered on the problems for some time and finally came down on the side of copying the normal anatomy. During their experiments on dogs (carried out with cardiopulmonary bypass) they continually modified and improved the design of the prosthesis. Eventually, four of the animals lived for eight to 40 hours; as the deaths were believed to be due to technical difficulties in suturing which would not be encountered in human patients and as the valves were covered only by a thin layer of fibrin but no clot they decided to move into the operating theatre[8].

The first complete excision and replacement of the mitral valve took place on March 10, 1960. A 16-year-old girl with severe mitral regurgitation was linked up to a heart-lung machine; her mitral valve was excised from its annulus and the papillary muscles and chordae were removed. In their place Morrow stitched the new valve which was made of polyurethane reinforced with Dacron fabric. Besides the leaflets, it had tails that were passed through the ventricular wall and sutured to act as imitation chordae. These tails were essential, as the leaflets were so flexible that they had to have something to keep them from flapping back into the atrium with each ventricular contraction. Unfortunately, they were inaccurately placed and the girl died 60 hours later[8].

But before the outcome was known, Morrow had operated again (on March 11), this time successfully; the 44-year-old woman patient made an uneventful, although slow, recovery and was alive and well two months after operation[8].

Perhaps influenced by the trouble with artificial chordae, Henry Ellis[9,10] of the Mayo Clinic experimented with a single, hinged plastic cusp for replacement of the whole mitral valve. His prosthesis was made of Mylar which, guided by Braunwald's experience, he sometimes coated with polyurethane. He inserted it in such a way that the suture line and knots at the annulus were covered leaving a smooth surface. Of 42 dogs, 33 survived; 12 lived for more than a month and one for 10 months. All the survivors were given an anticoagulant drug but this did not prevent the death of seven of the animals from the results of massive thrombosis. The commonest complication though was fracture of the valve hinge and this, in fact, caused all the later deaths. Nevertheless, Ellis drew some comfort from studies in three dogs which suggested that when there was firm healing between the ring of the prosthesis and the mitral annulus, a relatively normal haemodynamic state could be maintained – until the hinge broke.

But the days of the imitate-nature-with-plastics school were numbered (at least for the time being). Already the ball-and-cage proponents were beginning to make their presence felt. Hufnagel had succeeded for years with ball valves in the descending aorta so what could be more fitting than that surgeons should try to put them in the proper place once they had come to terms with the technical problems of surgery in the area. In May, 1960, Dwight Harken in Boston reported on the first patients in whom he had replaced the aortic valve with a prosthesis consisting of a Lucite ball in a stainless-steel cage with a Teflon-backed ring that was anchored by silk sutures. The operations were carried out with the help of extracorporeal cooling at about 26°C. All the patients were practically beyond help and five of the seven died, probably because of the poor state of their left ventricles[11]. He then decided to wait a year to see how the two survivors fared before inserting any more valves. At the end of the period they were both back at work and showed no evidence of damage to the blood cells or of peripheral emboli. As they had been cardiac invalids before operation, Harken was well satisfied[12].

In 1961 a most significant paper was published by Albert Starr and his engineer colleague, Lowell Edwards, of the University of Oregon Medical School, Portland[13]. They admitted that at the start they were prejudiced against the ball-and-cage valve which they called a 'repugnant' intracardiac appliance. However, at that time no survivals of mitral-valve replacement beyond three months had been reported so they felt justified in giving it a trial. Immense care went into the manufacture of the valve: the cage was cast in one-piece stainless steel which was shaped and given a mirror finish by buffing and electropolishing; the surface was then silicone-coated and inspected for flaws, however minute. (In their first two cases only, the cage was made of Lucite.) The fixation ring was made of knitted Teflon cloth and attached to the cage by

Teflon spreader rings and braided Teflon cloth. (In the first seven cases the spreader rings were of stainless steel, but these were discarded in favour of Teflon to avoid the possibility of electrolytic corrosion.) The ball was of medical grade, heat-cured silastic. In the laboratory, the valve had responded well to accelerated fatigue tests, but Starr and Edwards knew there could be a world of difference between satisfactory behaviour on the bench and prolonged efficient functioning in the human body. Indeed, their whole approach was one of great caution as they insisted that the patients must be otherwise hopeless cases and that if any other procedure might seem better when the diseased valve was inspected, it should be tried. Since the prosthesis could be inserted quickly in about 20-25 minutes, and as the patients were operated on with extracorporeal cooling at 32°C there was plenty of time to assess the situation adequately.

Starr went in through the left atrium and excised the mitral valve, leaving a margin which allowed sutures to be put in on the aortic side without danger of injury to the aortic valve through the party wall; around the remainder of the periphery this margin acted as a marker and tough anchoring tissue. The prosthesis was fixed into the annulus by 16 or 20 sutures with the cage hanging, upside down as it were, in the left ventricle. During diastole, when the blood flowed into the ventricle from the atrium, the ball fell into the cage, but during systole (ventricular contraction) it was forced back into the ring at the base of the cage. Starr's first patient was a woman of 33 who had previously had a roll of Ivalon sponge sutured to a valve leaflet in an attempt to relieve her regurgitation; she was operated on on August 25, 1960, but died of air embolism 10 hours later. It was thus most important, said Starr, to make sure that all air was removed from the heart before restarting the circulation. The next operation took place on September 21 and the 52-year-old man, who had suffered from both mitral incompetence and stenosis, was back at work at the time of the report. All the patients began taking anticoagulants by mouth on the seventh day after operation, though Starr was not convinced of the need for this, as some of his dogs had survived for a long time after valve replacement without the drugs.

So much then for replacement of single valves, but when the cause of the damage is rheumatic fever, as it so often is, more than one valve may be seriously affected. Would it prove possible to replace two or more valves at the same operation? After months of laboratory studies Robert Cartwright of Pittsburgh worked out a means of getting at the aortic valve through the left atrium[14] – remember Brock had had an unhappy experience with this route, but replacement of the mitral valve had not been part of his plans[15]. On November 1, 1961, Cartwright operated on a man of 35 who had rheumatic disease of both mitral and aortic valves and was in severe congestive cardiac failure despite intensive medical treatment. Through the left atrium Cartwright removed the major leaflet of the mitral valve to give himself access to the left ventricle and thus to the aortic valve which was excised and replaced with a Starr-Edwards ball-and-cage valve. He then removed the remainder of the mitral valve and inserted another Starr-Edwards prosthesis. The patient was on extracorporeal bypass for one hour and 55 minutes at 25°C and saline ice sludge was packed around the heart to produce hypothermic arrest. During the procedure the aorta was clamped to prevent risk of emboli and during closure of the left atrium the operation field was flooded with carbon dioxide to displace the air. This works because carbon dioxide is absorbed safely.

All went well and the man returned to full activity after three months, but four-and-a-half months after operation he died suddenly because two of the sutures holding the mitral prosthesis in place broke loose and caused a fatal leak.

Starr himself was not slow to see the possibilities of multiple valve replacement and in 1964 he reported on 13 patients who had had new aortic and mitral valves inserted; two had even had their tricuspid valves replaced as well[16]. The first operation took place on June 16, 1962, but he was unable to resuscitate the 45-year-old male patient. Starr's first success was with one of the triple replacements: on February 21, 1963, a man of 31 was on high-flow cardiopulmonary bypass at 30°C with intermittent coronary perfusion for five hours and eight minutes; for two hours and 31 minutes of this time his heart was in cold arrest. After a stormy convalescence he was much improved. For these multiple replacements Starr found he had no need to make any major modifications to the valve design; each insertion was carried out as if it was the only one, with the mitral prosthesis going in first, followed by the aortic and finally the tricuspid.

Eight of the patients survived and six left hospital in excellent condition and were restored to full activity. All but one were taking anticoagulants. Even if the mortality rate seems high, these were excellent results as Starr operated only on patients who could not be helped in any other way[16].

With the arrival of the ball-and-cage valve, other types of prosthetic valve replacements began to fade from the scene. Quite a number of different versions were subsequenly produced but the most popular and the best known remained the Starr-Edwards. Modifications were introduced to overcome some of their more immediate defects, yet it was time that revealed their more serious disadvantages. The same may, however, be said of valves derived from human and animal sources.

In many ways the development of valve transplantation was like an echo of prosthetic replacement a year or two later. First there was an attempt to do the job without interrupting the circulation; this was followed by a pause until surgeons felt competent to come to grips with the difficulties, and finally there was the choice to be made on material and design. This matter of choice is not so strange as may at first sight seem because the materials could come from a dead human body, an animal or, as time went on, from the patient himself, and for design the surgeon had the four valves of the heart to choose from. In fact only two are of practical value: the aortic, which proved the most popular, and the pulmonary, which was used when the patient's own valve was given a new home.

In previous chapters we have seen how a variety of tissues, such as pericardium, vein, tendon, and so forth, were used inside the heart in attempts to remedy valvular dysfunction but no one had tried replacing valve tissue with valve tissue until 1952 when Robert Litwak of Boston carried out experiments on dogs. This was before the days of the open heart so he designed an instrument that allowed him to operate under direct vision on one cusp only, of either the pulmonary or aortic valve. It was a clamp-like device with two blades, one flat with a rim, the other a ring that fitted inside the rim. The flat blade was introduced into the heart through an incision protected by a purse-string suture in the ventricular wall and passed up through the valvular orifice. The ring blade was clamped on the outside. When an incision was made in the tissue held by the ring, there was a valve cusp sitting on the flat blade and effectively isolated from the circulation. Litwak excised the cusp. For the replacement he used either a cusp from another dog (a homograft) or a piece of the animal's own pericardium stitched round a segment of aortic wall taken from another dog and cut to shape[17].

The composite replacements functioned well, and tests showed that they were physiologically competent. But the homografts all fibrosed and became useless due to shrinkage after varying periods of time – all, that is, except one, and Litwak admitted to being puzzled by its success[17]. The trouble was that practically nothing was known about the fate of tissue implanted in the heart. Autografts (taken from the animal's own body) had a pretty poor reputation for survival – possibly because they were asked to do jobs so utterly different to what nature had designed them for – yet they were looked on as angels compared with homografts. Hence Litwak's puzzlement at even one success.

The prospect for human-valve replacement was far from rosy until Murray took a hand. Admittedly he put the homograft aortic valve in the descending aorta, but it worked[1]. Other surgeons repeated Murray's experimental work along these lines but considerable confusion arose from the fact that the grafted valve only survived if the animal's own aortic valve was made incompetent. Arthur Beall, Denton Cooley and Michael De Bakey of Houston, Texas, performed the operation in 1961 on four patients with severe aortic regurgitation[18,19] and three years later three were doing well; the fourth had been killed in a car accident and the surgeons only heard about it when it was too late to carry out a postmortem to see how the transplanted valve had fared[19]. Nevertheless, people did not really sit up and take notice of homografts until they realized that Murray's first patient, operated on in 1955, was still living six-and-a-half years later[20].

The earliest attempts at actual replacement of the aortic and mitral valves with aortic homografts in human patients were carried out in Toronto by Murray's colleague, Raymond Heimbecker; their group had been working on the problems experimentally in dogs since 1959[21]. In 1961, using cardiac bypass and coronary perfusion, Heimbecker removed a patient's aortic valve and replaced it with one obtained aseptically from a cadaver and kept till needed in a saline-penicillin mixture at 4°C. The graft was sutured into the normal, or subcoronary, position by running stitches with reinforced mattress sutures at the commissures which were tied outside the aorta over small pads. The patient died after 24 hours from coronary thrombosis. Heimbecker's attention was then diverted to prosthetic valves and he did not repeat the performance with a homograft for three years by which time encouraging preliminary reports of their use from other centres made him decide to have another look at their possibilities[22].

His two operations on the mitral valve had scarcely better results. The first was on a man of 35 who had already had two mitral commissurotomies for rheumatic mitral stenosis. On March 23, 1962, Heimbecker went in again with the patient on cardiac bypass at 30°C. He excised the stenosed cusps and stitched the aortic valve homograft into the mitral annulus with much the same technique as he had used in the aortic area, although the valve obviously had to be upside down to allow the flow to be in the correct direction. The patient did well immediately after operation but he died a month later from a chest infection and electrolyte imbalance. Postmortem examination showed the donor valve to be apparently normal and working satisfactorily. Heimbecker's second patient survived for one day[21]. So, for replacement of the mitral valve as well as the aortic, he turned to the increasingly popular Starr-Edwards prosthesis.

At the Radcliffe Infirmary, Oxford, Alfred Gunning and the Spaniard, Carlos Duran, were confident that the use of natural valves in the aortic area should be pursued. After all, they said, homologous valves had been shown to work for at least six-and-a-half years in the descending aorta, and the subcoronary position had presented no barriers to prosthetic replacements. Why not combine the two observations and put a natural valve in a natural position? But first the technical details of preparation and insertion had to be worked out.

They removed the aortic valve from a cadaver with a cuff of tissue above and below. This was trimmed right down to the bare essentials of the three commissural struts and the cusps, the non-coronary cusp being marked for orientation purposes. The valve was anchored through the struts by three sutures tied on the outside over small pads of Teflon felt and by a running suture round the annulus. A valve transplanted in this manner worked efficiently on a piece of apparatus known as a pulse duplicator[23].

Meanwhile Donald Ross, a South African working at Guy's Hospital, had also been studying valve homotransplantation. By oversight a valve had been left in tap water for more than a week and had started to decompose, but it still functioned in the pulse duplicator and continued to do so efficiently for at least three months when tested for a short period every day[24]. This suggested that the important working parts had a very tough skeleton – by allowing the decomposition of soft tissues to continue, Ross had arrived at a Gunning-type preparation[24,25].

His first patient was a man of 43 with a severely calcified aortic valve who came to him with increasing symptoms and begging for surgical relief. On July 24, 1962, Ross operated; he started by doing a valvotomy but the valve disintegrated and had to be excised. This forced his hand. Although his work was still only in the experimental stage he inserted a freeze-dried homograft that had been prepared by the Gunning method. The operation was carried out with the patient on full-flow cardiac bypass at normal temperature; the coronary arteries were cannulated and perfused, also at normal temperature[25].

The man made an uncomplicated recovery and remained in the hospital for six weeks taking anticoagulants and cortisone to prevent thrombosis and rejection of the homograft – whenever tissue from another human being or animal is grafted into the body there is always the danger that the body will 'recognize' it as foreign and take steps to reject it. Exceptions occur when the graft is required to act as scaffolding for the body to build around as, for instance, in bone grafts. Fortunately as it turned out, valve tissue is composed of collagen, which is immunologically non-specific and avascular and gives rise to only a very mild reaction.

By 1964 Ross had operated on 11 more patients with aortic-valve disease, eight of whom survived. In all he tried débridement of the valve or some form of reconstruction with pericardial tissue before deciding that transplantation was the real answer. Despite some of the patients having grossly hypertrophied ventricles and being on the bypass for an average of one-and-a-half to two hours, he had no immediate operative deaths. After the first eight patients he stopped using cortisone, realizing that his fears of rejection were unfounded[24].

Owing to the limited supply of valves, one difficulty was finding the correct size; so when the available replacement was too big Ross decided it was better to make a comfortable fit by suspending the valve from a suitable place slightly higher up the aorta, rather than to cram it in and cause distortion. He obtained the valves as soon as possible (24-48 hours) after the death of the donor – this was usually satisfactory if the body had been kept in the mortuary refrigerator – and put them in sterile containers which were flooded with ethylene oxide. They were then freeze-dried and the sealed containers stored on a shelf at room temperature[24].

Now, once again, we see how the same bright idea occurs to different people when the time is ripe. Brian Barratt-Boyes at the Green Lane Hospital, Auckland, New Zealand, unaware of the work going on in England, on August 23, 1962, replaced the incompetent aortic valve of a 14-year-old girl with a homograft which, however, had somewhat more tissue left on it than the Gunning preparation. Sixteen months later the girl was doing well[26].

By that time Barratt-Boyes had operated on a total of 44 patients, 21 with aortic incompetence, 17 with calcific aortic stenosis, and six with multivalvular disease. Although 28 were in a very advanced state, 41 survived and had normally functioning valves. The operations were carried out with the help of cardiac bypass at 30°C with continuous perfusion of both coronary arteries. Most of Barratt-Boyes's valves were removed from the cadaver within 15 hours of death by a sterile technique and stored in a nutrient medium or by freeze-drying. An alternative was to have the pathologist collect the valve at the routine postmortem and sterilize it with beta-propiolactone, but he felt this was second best, even though sterile removal made more demands on the surgeon's valuable time[26].

Like other surgeons at this period Barratt-Boyes reserved valve transplantation for serious cases. He considered it the treatment of choice for gross aortic incompetence; for calcific aortic stenosis he would first try decalcification, but later his experience told him that this should be discarded entirely despite other reports indicating that it had a place. In 1967 he report-ed on 76 patients whose stenotic aortic valves had been treated by débride-ment valvotomy. Forty of these had been followed up for between 21 and 70 months; 38 had developed significant stenosis again which, in many, was sufficiently severe to warrant further surgery[27].

The difficulties of obtaining human valves in sufficient quantities and in suitable sizes to meet the growing demand made people think about using animal valves instead – an idea that was encouraged by the absence of an immune rejection response to homograft valves (a very mild cellular reaction would subside in about two weeks). In 1965 Duran and Gunning reported they had transplanted freeze-dried aortic valves of pigs into the descending aortas of 17 dogs. All the animals died within eight months but this was due to local problems in the aortic wall; the cusps of the transplanted valves were in good condition[28].

A little later the same year Duran, Jean-Paul Binet, and two other Parisian colleagues recorded the first successes with animal valves in human patients[29]. (*En passant* they mentioned an operation by Duran and Gunning in 1964 when a heterologous aortic valve had been inserted into a very ill patient who had died 24 hours afterwards from causes unrelated to the heterograft.) The French team used a pig's aortic valve in a 48-year-old woman with calcific aortic stenosis on September 23, 1965, and on September 30 they transplanted a calf's aortic valve into another woman of 56 with aortic incompetence. All five of their patients made uncomplicated recoveries and none received anticoagulant drugs. The valves in these cases were stored in a solution of mercurochrome antiseptic.

The technical problems of replacing the aortic valve with a transplant, whether of human or animal origin, were thus overcome, and the early results influenced John Kirklin of the Mayo Clinic. America was the home of the prosthetic valve, but Kirklin was dissatisfied because of the thrombo-embolic hazards and the need for keeping the patient on anticoagulant drugs. So he turned to homografts and between June, 1965, and June, 1966, treated 50 patients with aortic disease. There were three deaths after operation but these were not due to dysfunction of the transplanted valve. In their paper in 1967 Kirklin and his colleagues wrote in support of Barratt-Boyes that homograft replacement was the treatment of choice in these cases[30].

However, if all seemed to be going well with aortic replacement, the same could not be said for the mitral valve. The difficulties were due to the relative flimsiness of the valve ring which meant that the chordae tendineae and their papillary muscles were needed to keep the cusps at the correct tension to prevent their falling back into the atrium. Both Ross and Barratt-Boyes were working on replacement by the whole valve complex but, although a technique was evolved in experiments on dogs, the early clinical results in 1965-66 were not very encouraging as the chordae were prone to rupture. Could the chordae be dispensed with by using a valve other than the mitral? M Hubka and his colleagues in Bratislava, Czechoslovakia, thought they could.

Why not use an aortic valve, inserted upside down (to allow the valve to operate in the correct direction) in the atrium just above the mitral orifice. Among the advantages conferred by this position was a free outflow tract for the left ventricle – a ball-and-cage valve in the mitral position projects into the left ventricle and can interfere with the flow of blood being pumped into the aorta.

Their plan came to them quite early on, for their first dog was operated on in October, 1964, with the aid of extracorporeal circulation and moderate hypothermia. Hubka removed the valve cusps and a portion of aortic wall in the region of the commissures from the donor animal. Then, having excised the recipient's mitral valve, he stitched the aortic wall to the mitral annulus, and the ring of the new valve to the wall of the atrium a little higher up. In this way he achieved a fairly rigid valve seating and the funnelling effect into the mitral orifice was retained. Five of Hubka's eight dogs were alive and in good condition after at least a year when his report was published in 1967[31]. Yet before it appeared the principle had been applied in the operating theatre by Marian Ionescu and Geoffrey Wooler at Leeds General Infirmary.

Since these two surgeons had difficulty with adjusting the chordae of mitral heterografts, they changed to aortic-valve heterografts and put in a vast amount of experimental work to adapt the grafts in the best possible manner to their new task. They settled for heterografts (taken from animals) for the two main reasons of ease of supply and size – in mitral incompetence of a degree severe enough to merit this type of operation, the mitral ring is dilated and normal human valves are too small but aortic valves from pigs, one-and-a-half or two years old, fill the bill nicely. These valves were sterilized with beta-propiolactone and then instantly frozen and freeze-dried in the manner described by Barratt-Boyes.

Starting in February, 1967, Ionescu and Wooler operated on 13 patients with only two deaths; the early results were good but the follow-up period was short[32]. The cuff of the pig's valve was sutured to the mitral annulus, although the technique differed from Hubka's in that a semi-rigid Teflon ring was put in the atrium above the mitral annulus and the annulus of the donor aortic valve was sutured to it. In this way the atrial wall was brought to the valve and any possible distortion of the valve thereby prevented.

Early difficulties with graft replacements of the aortic valve had included regurgitation when the original valve was badly calcified and left little suitable tissue for attachment. This was largely overcome by Barratt-Boyes's technique of inserting a double row of sutures. Another problem was leakage around the edges of the transplant before new tissue had incorporated it into the body. This was avoided by destroying the surface of the area of implantation to achieve a quick and effective inflammatory union. But by 1966 the long-term fate of valve replacement with grafts was becoming known: the valves were prone to degenerate and become calcified. Because he believed in the benefits of graft valves – freedom from embolic complications and a normal flow through a central orifice with none of the turbulence produced by pros-theses – Ross wondered whether there could be any way round the late changes. The method of preparation of the graft came in for consideration and also the possibility of changing the 'material'. What about the patient's own pulmonary valve? In theory it should prove to be a better graft than any from an outside source; and as the stresses and strains in the pulmonary area were less than those in the aortic area, a donor valve could be inserted there with a better chance of long-term survival. In addition, if the donor valve in the pulmonary orifice did deteriorate, the effects would be less troublesome.

In 1967 Ross reported on 12 patients in whom he had used their own pulmonary valves. The excision of the valve entailed no great technical difficulty, but he had to take care not to damage the left main coronary artery during the dissection. Between the time of its removal and its insertion the valve was left lying in the blood of the left ventricle or aortic root. In two cases the pulmonary valve was used to replace a mitral valve by a technique similar to that of Ionescu and Wooler. These patients were alive and well two and

three months after operation. Two of those who had had aortic-valve replacements had died from unrelated causes; the others were progressing satisfactorily although the longest follow-up was then only five months[33]. However, at
the end of 1968 Ross told a meeting of the International College of Surgeons
in Tokyo that he had then carried out the operation on 33 patients with
satisfactory follow-up of up to 16 months[34].

The chief complication of the prosthetic valves is thrombosis with
subsequent embolism. In some early series this reached the alarmingly high
figure of 85-90 percent though when the practice of covering the metal parts
with velour cloth was introduced, the rate fell quite dramatically to about 15-20
percent. To help combat the danger of thrombosis patients have to take
anticoagulant drugs, and these are not without risk. The fact that ball-and-cage
valves sit in the blood flow causes turbulence and leads to destruction of the
blood cells and anaemia. In addition there is the possibility of mechanical
failure with degeneration or fracture of the ball, though sometimes it swells and
becomes impacted. Infection with bacteria (thrombosis predisposes to this) or
with fungi is also a danger.

By comparison, homografts would seem to be a better bet, and certainly
for the first three or four years after their insertion the majority function
satisfactorily. But, as we have seen, after that time their cusps are inclined to
thin and develop holes or become calcified. This calcification starts in the
aortic wall and spreads into the cusps to produce stenosis. In their favour, during the first few years, is the absence of clotting (thus the patient does not need
to take anticoagulants), their incorporation into the body tissues, their flexibility
and 'normality', and above all their ideal design which does not interfere with
the flow of blood.

These rather disappointing observations are necessary to put valve
replacement in perspective. But the patients who received new valves in the
early years were seriously ill with only a short time to live. Replacements
brought a fresh lease of life to a great many of them. Yet there still remained
some with serious multivalvular disorders whose disease was too far advanced
to be helped even by replacement. For these and others with irreparable heart
damage, the only hope lay in a new heart.

28

ARTIFICIAL HEARTS AND
SUPPORT OF THE CIRCULATION

When cardiac surgery spread its wings and began to fly the possibilities of using the pump-oxygenator as a treatment in its own right were explored. The first surgeon to employ the apparatus solely to help a failing heart was Clarence Dennis of New York who had been working on the problems of cardiac bypass since 1947[1] and in 1951 had almost been the first to operate successfully with a heart-lung machine. On November 1, 1954, he was confronted with a 54-year-old housewife whose circulation was rapidly failing due to rheumatic disease of three of her heart valves. He took her to the operating theatre and, with all sterile precautions, connected her to the apparatus by taking the blood from her left great saphenous vein and returning it through her left brachial artery. Perfusion continued for four hours and resulted in the disappearance of the signs of pulmonary oedema and hydrothorax and in a marked benefit to her difficult breathing. This improvement lasted for 10 days before her condition steadily deteriorated. Dennis speculated that by treating patients with severe (Class IV) mitral stenosis in this manner, it might be possible to improve their symptoms and convert them to Class III patients. The advantage of this in terms of operative mortality rate would have been a reduction from about 40 percent (in Class IV patients) to between 5 and 10 percent (in Class III patients)[1].

Dennis, however, next moved on to studying the possibilities of the machine as a life-saver in selected cases of myocardial infarction. The patients he chose were those in shock with signs of progressive and medically unmanageable deterioration and a systolic blood pressure below 80mm of mercury. The idea was to provide a 'crutch' for the heart until the surviving muscle was able to resume its job (assuming there was enough of it left). Under local anaesthesia he inserted a catheter through the saphenous vein in the thigh into the common iliac vein. The blood was pumped through a disc oxygenator with a bubble trap and returned to the body by a cannula in a brachial artery. A coil in a warm water bath was incorporated in the circuit to keep the blood at body temperature. On February 27, 1957, a man of 52 who had been in severe pain for 12 hours after a heart attack was admitted to Dennis's hospital. Twenty-four hours later he was put on the machine for three hours. Perfusion was then stopped as blood appeared in the urine (indicating damage to the red cells), but the patient slowly recovered and after six weeks was ready for discharge. Two other patients died despite perfusion; postmortem examination in one revealed such extensive occlusions of the coronary arteries that failure was inevitable[2].

In 1962 Dennis and Åke Senning reported on a modification of this technique by which they completely bypassed the left heart. They thought it might be of use in aortic- or mitral-valve disease or after open-heart surgery as well as in myocardial infarction. In their dogs they had passed a catheter down a jugular vein into the right atrium and *through* the septum into the left atrium. The blood withdrawn by the catheter was pumped into the machine and returned by another catheter inserted in a femoral artery. The damage to the heart proved to be of no clinical importance and the hole between the atria healed without trouble in three months[3].

The technique was tried on one patient whose ventricular septum had ruptured six days after an acute episode of coronary occlusion. Signs of shock disappeared after about three hours on the bypass and he was taken to the operating theatre for repair of his ventricular septum. Extracorporeal cooling was instituted, but when the surgeon put in a plastic patch the whole septum just disintegrated and nothing further could be done to save the man's life[3].

Because the pump-oxygenator had been primarily intended to take over the function of the heart and lungs during open-heart surgery it was unsuitable for prolonged support of the failing myocardium. When surgeons realized this they put their minds to designing something specially suited to the job.

From the early 1960s Michael De Bakey of Baylor University College of Medicine, Houston, Texas, had been interested in helping the heart mechanically. The ultimate objective was complete replacement but De Bakey considered this had too many problems and he therefore concentrated on bypassing or assisting the left ventricle with apparatus implanted inside the chest. In 1962 he and his colleagues, who included Denton Cooley and Arthur Beall, designed a bypass that went from the left atrium to the ascending aorta[4], but in the next year they described a variation that went instead to the descending aorta. This, they said, was an improvement as it was safer, easier to insert, and allowed a tube-type pump to be used. The blood flowed through a Silastic tube reinforced with Dacron and with ball-type valves at each end to ensure that the blood flowed in the correct direction; outside this tube was another with a single inlet connected to an external source of air. The volume of air pumped into the outside tube could be adjusted from zero to 60ml per stroke, and the pumping arrangement could be connected electronically to the electrocardiogram so that each stroke was triggered by the R wave. The air in the outside tube thus squeezed the blood smoothly along its way, in synchrony with the appropriate stage in the heart's cycle. This apparatus had been used to support the left ventricle in experimental animals for weeks or months without significant blood changes and in 1963 De Bakey reported its use in a patient[4].

On July 18 a 42-year-old man in severe congestive heart failure had his calcified stenotic aortic valve replaced with a Starr-Edwards prosthesis. The next morning his heart stopped beating. Immediately his chest was opened and cardiac massage started. Although this was successful, it was soon evident that his brain was seriously damaged and his lungs waterlogged. Because De Bakey believed the waterlogging was caused by left ventricular failure he thought this was an ideal opportunity to study the effects of assisting the circulation. On the evening of July 19 he inserted the air-driven bypass pump which did its job continuously and efficiently during the last four days of the patient's life[5].

The next occasion on which De Bakey implanted a pump, he used one that worked on a different principle – diastolic counterpulsation. This is a rather frightening term to describe something really quite simple. The pump sucks blood out of the aorta in time with the contraction of the heart, and pumps it back in again while the heart is relaxing. In this way the pump takes some of the burden off the left ventricle by lowering the resistance against which it has to work, and by returning the blood during diastole improves the flow into the coronary arteries thus increasing the oxygen supply to the heart.

The principle of diastolic counterpulsation had been worked on about 1961 by a number of surgeons including Dwight Harken and his group at Boston. In their case, the pump had been a somewhat large device outside the animal's body and the blood had been pulsed by means of a cannula passed into the aorta through the femoral, iliac, or left subclavian artery[6].

At any rate, in April, 1966, De Bakey replaced the rheumatic mitral valve of a 65-year-old miner with a Starr-Edwards prosthesis. At the end of the operation he was faced with the problem of getting the patient safely off the pump-oxygenator. The man's heart was in poor condition and the pressure in his pulmonary circuit was high. A form of temporary mechanical assistance was the only solution, so De Bakey inserted an air-driven counterpulsator type of pump. Although the tubes went into the aorta, the small pump itself sat outside on the chest wall. Unfortunately, although the apparatus kept a normal circulation going for a few days, it was not sufficient to save the man's life[7].

Later that year De Bakey returned to the squeezing type of tube pump which, by this time, had been improved by lining it with velour cloth to prevent clotting. On August 8, 37-year-old Mrs Esperanza del Valle Vasquez was critically ill with severe aortic and mitral valve disease and left ventricular failure. De Bakey replaced both valves, but as her ventricle just could not cope he inserted the bypass pump. For days it pumped away; on several occasions the ventricle showed signs of failing and each time the output of the pump was increased with dramatically good results. When, after 10 days, her heart was equal to its task unaided, the pump was removed, and 18 days later Mrs Vasquez was discharged from hospital. A year later she was free of symptoms and working as a beautician[8].

De Bakey and his team only used the device when the patient's heart muscle could not pump adequately at the end of the operation. In other words, if the patient was taken off the pump-oxygenator he would die – nevertheless, the heart muscle had to be in a potentially recoverable condition.

Among other surgeons hard at work on apparatus to assist the left ventricle was Adrian Kantrowitz at Maimonides Hospital, Brooklyn. His device was similar to De Bakey's tube-type pump in that it was composed of one tube inside another and driven by compressed air. It differed in the important respect that it was designed for permanent implantation and had no valves. Two Dacron tubes at the ends of the pump itself were inserted into the ascending and descending aorta and the intervening aorta was divided and the stumps sewn up. This meant that all the blood pumped out by the heart had to pass through the device. The external source of power to pump the air was synchronized with the R wave of the patient's electrocardiogram. Once in place the amount of assistance could be varied between none at all and taking over 80 percent of ventricular work[9].

The first person to have one of Kantrowitz's devices inserted was a man of 33 who had been admitted in heart failure; he died 20 hours after operation on February 4, 1966, from a combination of causes including previous liver disease. For the first 10 hours or so he had seemed to be doing well and had talked with his doctors. The second patient in whom Kantrowitz inserted his pump (on May 18, 1966) was a woman of 63 who was seriously ill with congestive heart failure, diabetes mellitus and impaired liver and kidney function. She lived for 12 days with intermittent support from the pump before dying of a stroke[9].

At this stage Kantrowitz realized that a bypass would not help many patients whose heart failed after an infarction but who had sufficient muscle left to make recovery possible if the initial catastrophe could be overcome. So he produced a more simple device which looked after both the coronary and the peripheral circulations[10]. A balloon at the end of a catheter was introduced through a femoral artery and passed up the aorta until it lay just distal to the origin of the left subclavian artery. The outside end of the catheter was connected to a pump. The pump was synchronized with a sensor in the tip of the tiny balloon, so that when the blood pressure in the aorta rose, a burst of helium gas expanded the balloon. This forced the blood forward into the peripheral circulation, thereby easing the work of the heart; and, in addition, it increased the pressure in the aorta on the heart side of the balloon during diastole and thus improved the coronary circulation. The pump could also be triggered by synchronizing it with the electrocardiogram.

At a meeting of the American Society for Artificial Organs in 1968, Kantrowitz reported that 15 patients had been intermittently assisted by the balloon for periods lasting one-and-a-half to 55 hours. One of the first two patients in 1967 was still alive at the time of the report. In all, six had recovered from their infarctions with the aid of the balloon and had been discharged from hospital. 'Our results', he said, 'indicate that intermittent balloon pumping effectively supports the circulation and can be continued for prolonged periods without deleterious effects to either the patient or the pumping apparatus.'[11]

Despite these successes, however, dissentient voices were heard. For instance, John H Kennedy of the Cleveland Metropolitan General Hospital had used various forms of circulatory assistance on 22 patients, 11 of whom recovered from their heart failure[12]. But his experiments on dogs made him wonder whether left-heart bypass really helped the heart as the animals developed biochemical upsets, low blood pressure and some even seemed to deteriorate during the procedure. Perhaps, he speculated, the body and the pump, each with its own special control systems, were in conflict[13].

Another to doubt the merits of the auxiliary pumps was Walton Lillehei[14, 15]. In his view these devices might well have a built-in defect since there were few clinical conditions in which only one side of the heart was in trouble; both usually were involved, and relieving the work of one side added to the burden on the other. The answer was *total* heart relief and to this end he had developed a portable, pumpless oxygenator constructed of perforated propylene plates interfolded with thin Silastic membrane. In his animal experiments, carried out at the University of Minnesota before he moved in 1967 to Cornell University Medical College, Lillehei had attached the oxygenator to the femoral artery and vein. The oxygenator was pumpless because, when oxygen was introduced under pulsatile pressure, it could support the animal's circulation. Two units, one attached to the axillary vessels, the other to the femoral vessels, would in theory be sufficient to support the entire circulation of an adult human being.

Other forms of assistance that came and went, mostly in the laboratory, rarely in the operating theatre, included two-layered squeezing devices slipped over both ventricles; they worked by rhythmic inflation with air. However, the friction they produced was liable to damage the outside of the heart.

And so we come to the dream of those who put their faith in the tremendous technological advances of that era – and it is a dream still unfulfilled. The idea of the complete replacement of the human heart by a machine within the chest is attractive and to some appeals more than heart transplantation, because the surgeon is not dependent on the death of a donor with a sound heart.

In 1937, Vladimir Demikhov of Moscow was working on cardiac resuscitation when he decided to try replacing the heart with a mechanical pump. The machine he constructed consisted of two membrane pumps side by side, and was the size of the normal heart. It was primed with a physiological solution[16].

Demikhov inserted the venous (input) cannulae of the apparatus through the atrial appendages and tied them in with thick ligatures. Next the arterial (output) cannulae were introduced into the aorta and pulmonary artery under cover of elastic clamps; ligatures were tied tightly around the bottom of both ventricles, the ventricles removed, and the pump switched on. This part of the operation had to be done quickly (in five or six minutes) as the circulation was interrupted from the moment of inserting the arterial cannulae. The machine was driven by an electric motor outside the body, which meant that the 'shaft' had to pass through the chest wall; the exit point was carefully sutured to make it airtight. Demikhov carried out three experiments in 1937 and five more in 1958. The longest survival was for five-and-a-half hours, during which time 'all signs of life were observed'. He regarded the apparatus as a unique method for storing the organs of a dead donor while awaiting a suitable recipient[16].

Kazuhiko Atsumi and his colleagues at the Tokyo University School of Medicine began their research in 1958, and constructed a variety of pumps. Their first was a hydraulically driven plastic heart which maintained a dog's circulation for five-and-a-half hours. Then, in January, 1960, they successfully substituted both sides of a dog's heart for 13 hours with two small roller-type pumps driven by a miniature motor. The operation was done with the help of Drew's method of deep hypothermia, the body temperature being lowered to 10°C. But, as might be expected, they ran into the problem of thrombosis; so, to try to avoid this, they built a small bellows type of pump of specially treated natural rubber. This they inserted into the chests of four dogs (using deep hypothermia) and kept one alive for seven hours[17]. In one experiment in 1967, the dog lived for 27 hours, and other dogs survived overnight after awakening from the anaesthetic[18]. The commonest causes of death among their animals were pulmonary oedema and brain damage[17].

The problems of achieving a physiological circulation are immense, and, as Atsumi has said, it seems that the primary job of the heart is to pump whatever blood appears at its inlet into whatever pressure level exists at its outlet. The heart itself should neither influence the venous return nor be influenced by the systemic arterial pressure. Therefore Atsumi worked hard at developing a control system for his hearts so that they responded to all manner of changes (hormonal, biochemical, pressure and so on) that affect the normal heart. A computer was fed with the relevant information so that it could order the necessary changes in pumping action and with a correct time delay[18].

In America, another team. headed by the Dutchman, Willem Kolff (who emigrated to the United States after the war), and including Tetsuzo Akutsu and later Yukihiko Nosé were also studying the problems. On June 26, 1959, Kolff removed a dog's heart and implanted in its place a pendulum type of artificial heart in which the ventricles emptied alternately. The animal breathed spontaneously for two hours after its chest was closed and retained its corneal, wink, and tendon reflexes. The pump kept the blood pressure above 80mm of mercury for five hours at which time the experiment was ended. At the postmortem there was no sign of pulmonary oedema[19].

Three days later Kolff repeated the experiment, but this time he implanted a simple roller type of artificial heart which had only one valve on each side (corresponding to the aortic and pulmonary valves). Again the ventricles emptied alternately. This experiment lasted only two hours[20].

In 1965 the same team from Cleveland, Ohio, reported that a calf had lived for 31 hours and 15 minutes after a one-piece, four-chambered heart had been implanted in its pericardial sac[21].

However, a compact power source suitable for implantation in the patient's body is one of the many stumbling blocks in producing a permanent artificial heart, and various suggestions, such as electrical energy transmitted through the chest wall and a tiny battery charged by muscular contraction, were suggested. Even nuclear energy was proposed, an idea pursued at the National Heart Institute, Bethesda, Maryland. The artificial heart in the chest would be driven by a small atomic steam engine implanted in the lower abdomen with a heat exchanger in the upper abdomen to cool things down. As one medical news magazine observed: 'Since the power system is self-contained, there will be no steam exhaust.'[22]

29

TRANSPLANTATION OF THE HEART
– THE BACKGROUND

'Transplantation of protoplasm is of the widest occurrence in Nature. The very existence of the higher plants and animals is proof of this, for it is through transplantation of protoplasm – fertilization, as it is called – that such organisms originate.'

These words opened the chapter on 'Transplantation of tissues' in Charles Guthrie's book *Blood-vessel surgery and its applications*[1]. They were written in 1912 when Guthrie was 32 and professor of physiology and pharmacology at the University of Pittsburgh. During the previous seven years he had experimentally transplanted a vast array of tissues and organs, much of the work being done with Alexis Carrel when they were together at the University of Chicago. Quite a number of other research workers at this time were exploring along the same lines, largely with kidneys, and the clue to this burst of enthusiasm is found in the title of Guthrie's book. Unless you can stitch blood vessels together effectively, you can't transplant organs, for organs must have an efficient blood supply.

The situation was deplorable at the start of the last century, and in 1902 only 21 'successful' arterial sutures had been reported in man. Surgeons were still influenced by the bad old days of the pre-antiseptic era when non-absorbable sutures and ligatures were left with long ends so that when the inevitable suppuration occurred they could be pulled out. This event was eagerly awaited, since it was thought to indicate that the body was doing its job and that, with luck, healing would continue. Then with the arrival of anti-sepsis and, later, asepsis and the progress in abdominal surgery, absorbable catgut could safely be left in the abdomen when intestines were stitched together. So when blood vessels required suturing small intestinal needles and thin gut were used, and the vessels stitched as though they were intestine – with conspicuous failure. The few apparent successes proved nothing as obstruction of an artery does not invariably have dire results, particularly if there is a good collateral circulation. Attempts to improve matters made little headway until about 1905 when Carrel and Guthrie perfected the technique: small tapered needles of polished steel, fine silk thread or human hair, and stitches taken through all coats of the vessel wall[2]. This simplicity and their painstaking attention to detail opened up a whole new surgical vista though it was many years before all the possibilities were exploited.

Between them Guthrie and Carrel (who had started his work on blood vessels in 1901-02 at the University of Lyons) transplanted kidneys, adrenals, thyroids, parathyroids, ovaries, legs, arms, loops of intestine, the lower half of the body, the head and neck, and the heart[3,4,5]. Some of these tissues and organs were transplanted into the necks of recipient animals to study their function (this was the prime purpose of the experiments), but the outstanding successes were achieved with ovaries and kidneys transplanted into their correct sites. Fowls and guinea-pigs gave birth after receiving new ovaries (in 1906 Robert Morris reported the birth of a child to a woman whose ovaries had been removed and replaced with those of another four years previously[6]), and cats and dogs lived for a few weeks after abdominal transplantation of both kidneys. One cat that had had its own kidneys removed and replaced was in good health two years later.

Their experiments on heart transplantation came almost as an anticlimax. As Guthrie remarked, the operation was complicated by the fact that the heart has a double blood supply: the nutritional supply through the coronary system, and the functional supply through the heart's chambers. Their heart transplants in 1905 were all into the necks of recipient animals. In one experiment with dogs, only the nutritional supply was kept going. This was achieved by join-ing the aortic stump of the donor heart to the central cut end of the recipient's common carotid artery (the pressure of blood in the artery filled the coronary arteries of the donor heart) and the stump of the donor superior vena cava to the central cut end of the recipient's external jugular vein (to drain off the blood entering the donor's right atrium from the coronary sinus). The donor heart's circulation was thus ensured; all the remaining cut vessels were tied off. In a second experiment the anastomoses in the neck were so arranged that the heart functioned. A donor pulmonary vein was joined to the peripheral end of the recipient's cut common carotid artery. The aorta was joined to the central end of the carotid artery. One of the venae cavae was joined to the peripher-al end of the recipient's cut jugular vein; and the pulmonary artery was joined to the peripheral end of the carotid artery or jugular vein on the other side of the recipient's neck. This arrangement thus allowed for each side of the donor heart to receive its correct sort of blood (arterial or venous) and to work against approximately normal pressures.

The circulation was re-established through the heart about an hour-and-a-quarter after removal from the donor; 20 minutes later blood was flowing through the coronary circulation. About an hour after the operation the ventricles began to beat effectively at a rate of 88 per minute, compared with the rate of the recipient's own heart of 130 per minute. After two hours the experiment was ended when the blood began to clot in the heart chambers[5].

Their final experiment was to transplant the lungs and heart of a week-old kitten into the neck of an adult cat. 'The aorta was anastomosed to the peripheral end of the carotid, and the vena cava to the peripheral end of the jugular vein,' wrote Carrel. 'The coronary circulation was immediately reestablished and the auricles began to beat. The lungs became red, and after a few minutes effective pulsations of the ventricles appeared. But the lungs soon became oedematous, and distention of the right part of the heart occurred. This accident seems difficult of prevention. A phlegmon [infection] of the neck terminated this observation two days later.'[5]

The big stumbling block in the transplantation of organs between animals was the fairly rapid destruction of the grafted tissue even though the blood supply was still intact. That it was not due to severance of the nervous supply, Carrel and Guthrie knew from their successes with autotransplants. In some way the host's blood was toxic to the graft: 'It would seem that with our present knowledge a consideration of the biolysins (or biotoxins) would be rational. From the same standpoint it is conceivable that perhaps by preliminary processes of immunization of the donor or recipient, or both, different results might be observed.'[5]

A consideration of biolysins did not, however, trouble Pien Ch'iao. In blissful ignorance of immunology, this honourable and cultured Chinese doctor of the third century BC, slipped a knockout potion into the drinks of a couple of soldiers. While they were sleeping he opened them up and swapped over a number of internal organs, including their hearts. Three days later the soldiers awoke, none the worse for their experience. Credit must, however, be given to Pien Ch'iao's colleague, a Chinese pixie who could see through the body and diagnose disease. It was he who suggested the transplantation, presumably to test his immunosuppressive agent. Unfortunately for posterity, the case report was not published.

Legend this may be, but it is significant in the history of transplantation, for it shows that the idea has been around for a good number of years. Another legendary transplantation was performed by the twin brothers Cosmas and Damian who, after their martyrdom in the third century AD, became the patron saints of surgery. In one version of the story the brothers, during their lifetime, removed the cancerous leg of a white man and replaced it with the leg of a recently deceased Moor. In another, the saints appeared to the sick man in a dream some three centuries after their death. One brother amputated the leg, while the other went to a local cemetery and removed the leg of the Moor who had been buried that day. The following morning, it seems, the patient had trouble convincing his friends, despite the different colours of his legs, so everyone trooped off to the cemetery and opened the Moor's grave – sure enough, the cancerous leg was there.

Legends, however, are one thing, indicating as they do some deep-rooted human desire such as the wish to be free of disease or to achieve eternal life – though eternal life has its drawbacks if the myth of Tithonus and the tales of the Flying Dutchman and the Wandering Jew are anything to go by. It is quite another matter when dreams show every sign of becoming fact, particularly in the case of heart transplantation which implies the death of one human being that another may have life.

Since December, 1967, it has been only too evident that heart transplantation is not simply a problem of surgical technique. Many, many other issues have become involved, and to understand why, we really have to explore the whole of mankind's history – his attitudes to life, his beliefs, and the reasons for them. Aristotle's statement that the heart is the seat of the soul, of the emotions, of the intellect – is indeed the very source of life – is of immense importance, for this outlook is still very close to the surface even in an educated and sophisticated society. The Greeks and Romans tried un-successfully to make the liver the home of the soul; had the idea caught on, or had someone decided instead on the kidneys, there would doubtless have been an outcry when these organs were first transplanted, and the heart would have escaped with scarcely a murmur. Admittedly the heart is an unpaired organ, but so is the liver. No, transplantation of the heart is extremely difficult to view dispassionately, for is it not also the shrine of romantic love?

Ezekiel did his best to overcome resistance to the idea of transplantation: 'Thus saith the Lord God....A new heart also will I give you, and a new spirit will I put within you: and I will take away the stony heart out of your flesh, and I will give you an heart of flesh.' (Chapter 36, verse 26). He would have made a good publicity agent too, for he had previously used almost the same words in Chapter 11, verse 19. The word stony was well chosen, when we remember that calcification of the coronary vessels and of the heart valves pro-duces some of the conditions for which transplantation is the only treatment. However, it must be accepted that Ezekiel was speaking only metaphorically.

Next, if we are to put heart transplantation into perspective, we have to know something about the history of surgery and how rarely operations appear as finished products. We need to realize that many procedures started life with high mortality and morbidity rates and that it often took years before they became acceptable – still with a degree of morbidity and mortality attached to them. For instance, at the start of the modern era of surgery for mitral stenosis, some people believed the whole thing to be impracticable on account of the nature of the disease and the large number of patients involved. But as time went by the problems were ironed out, the back-log of patients was dealt with and, as so often happens, an operation that at first demanded the attentions of a virtuoso became a routine procedure for many thoracic surgeons. And again, only by putting an operation to the test on human patients can the rough edges be trimmed from it, perhaps leading to some different technique or approach of far greater value.

More specifically, we must take a glimpse at the history of organ transplantation. This is a comparatively recent departure that entered clinical practice in the 1950s, although it did not really get off the ground until the discovery of the immunosuppressant drugs in the early 1960s. Nevertheless, grafting of tissues such as bone and cornea is much older, and we must not ignore the few abortive attempts to transplant animal kidneys into human patients (usually onto arm blood vessels) at the beginning of the last century. Many organs were transplanted in the middle years of that century, either experimentally or clinically, but most experience was gained with kidneys, and the early results were worse than those of heart transplantation. The stimulus for the operation, and consequently for much of the surge of interest in transplantation, came from the development of the artificial kidney machine. Before 1944 prospects were terribly dim, but in that year the world learned of the remarkable achievement of Willem Kolff. During the Nazi occupation of Holland he had built an artificial kidney and used it successfully at the Municipal Hospital, Kampen, despite the dialysing membrane's being composed of nothing more nor less than cellophane[7,8]. Once the technical imperfections of the machine had been overcome, surgeons began to think seriously of transplantation as gravely ill patients could be brought to a reasonably fit state to withstand operation. It also provided something they could fall back on if the kidney transplant was rejected or failed.

Another important event of 1944 was Peter Medawar's demonstration that the rejection of skin grafts was in fact due to an immunological reaction[9,10]. By the end of the 1950s the same mechanism was shown to be the cause of rejection of organs. Understanding the nature of a problem may not solve it, but it helps to direct the attack in a more fruitful direction. In this case, attempts were made to suppress the immune reaction of the body, at first with whole-body doses of radiation and then with special immunosuppressive drugs that came to the fore in the early 1960s. Because these methods also destroy the patients' resistance to infection, great care has to be taken with their nursing, though as soon as possible they have to be weaned back to a normal environment complete with all its bacteria, fungi and viruses.

In an attempt to damp down rejection, tissues and organs were 'typed' or matched before grafting, in much the same way as blood is grouped. So far as is known, a complete correspondence between all the many antigens is an impossibility (except between identical twins), but it is often possible to match the most important.

Much of the informed criticism of heart transplantation was not that it had happened, but that it had happened too soon. Much greater progress, these critics believed, should have been made in understanding and combating the immunological problems before the operation was carried out on human patients. Yet, as has been said many times before in other contexts, are we to wait for tomorrow's advances before helping those in need today?

Transplantation of the heart took many people, both medical and others, by surprise. This in itself is surprising, for its coming had been writ large. After Guthrie and Carrel, organ transplantation pursued a pretty desultory course, and after the mid-1920s most research workers had given up in despair. Nothing more was done about the heart until 1933, when Frank Mann of Rochester, Minnesota, inaugurated the modern era in the sense that his paper[11] was quoted by most investigators when the ball really started rolling some 20 years later. Mann's studies were sparked by one of the co-authors of the paper, Jacob Markowitz (of Washington, DC), who wanted a denervated heart for an experiment. All the transplants were between dogs, with the donor heart attached to vessels in the recipient's neck; the technique was basically much the same as Carrel's and Guthrie's. Mann, too, emphasized the importance of restoring the coronary circulation as quickly as possible, otherwise the heart muscle would lose its tone and the valves fail to work properly. He managed this part of the operation with a gap of only five minutes between cessation of the coronary circulation in the donor's body and its re-establishment in the recipient. He found, though, that if he joined the donor aorta to the *peripheral* end of the recipient's cut carotid artery (rather than the *central* end, as Carrel had done) the lower pressure was more acceptable to the donor heart, and did not lead to incompetence of the aortic valve. This was significant for them, as the most frequent cause of failure was distension of the heart with blood before it began to beat. However, only the right side of the heart was made functional by anastomosing the donor pulmonary artery to the recipient's jugular vein – the blood that the right ventricle pumped out came from the coronary-sinus return. In successful cases, beating started at once at a constant rate between 100-130 beats per minute; this increased with exercise or struggling by about 15 beats per minute. The longest survival Mann achieved was eight days, with an average of four.

He concluded that 'The general behavior of such a transplanted organ as regards function, period of survival and cytologic change is similar to that of other homotransplanted organs.'[11] So, important though his work was in confirming Carrel's and Guthrie's findings, it did not extend the frontiers of knowledge.

Now we come to the breathtaking work of Vladimir Demikhov, but because of language and other barriers this was unknown to the West until 1962, when the book he had published in Russian in 1960 was translated into English[12]; and by this time Western scientists had more or less caught up. Although Demikhov had repeated many of the transplantation procedures carried out by Carrel and Guthrie, this in no way dims the brilliance of his studies, for by sheer persistence and with the intention of paving the way for human operations he refined the techniques and rubbed off many of the rough edges.

Among the multitude of his experiments was the transplantation of puppies' heads and necks to the necks of adult dogs. These heads reacted normally to their surroundings and would lap up water when thirsty; when the donor preparation included the forelegs, these sometimes gave running movements. The longest survival was 29 days.

Besides kidneys, Demikhov transplanted the adrenals, the whole of the gastrointestinal tract and pancreas, and the liver. He also transplanted the lower half of the body which, he said, offered the opportunity of transplanting all the organs just mentioned at one operation. But most of his work concerned the heart.

His experiments began in 1940, at Moscow State University, with the transplantation of hearts into the inguinal region (or groin), using Carrel's technique of suturing blood vessels. Then came the war, and he was unable to continue until 1946, by which time he had decided to put the heart in the chest – not in place of the recipient's heart but along with it. His reason for doing this was to make the heart work as an auxiliary pump, which was not the case in other sites where it was not connected to the lungs. Between February 24, 1946, and July 31, 1958, Demikhov carried out 250 of these experiments in 24 different ways. All the time he was trying to work out which were the best vessels to join to which, how to get good filling of both sides of the heart and a mass of other technical details. Often an encouraging method had to be abandoned because it was too difficult and time-consuming. To make room for the new heart, he removed different parts of the recipient dog's lungs and sometimes he transplanted a lobe of the donor's lung with its heart to reduce the number of anastomoses required. The longest survival Demikhov achieved was 32 days in a dog named Borzoi who was given a second heart on October 4, 1956. Although an infarct developed in the posterior wall of the transplant in the early days after surgery, Borzoi did well and played with other dogs. Electrocardiograms taken at the times of expected rejection showed no alterations. The dog was sacrificed on the 32nd day when the transplant started fibrillating.

The commonest cause of death in this series was thrombosis and embolic phenomena, and infection in the transplanted lung. In the early stages every animal died on the operating table, but with experience and a careful analysis of his mistakes Demikhov reduced the operative mortality rate to nil – an incredible achievement when considering that these and all his other experiments were done without the help of a heart-lung machine or any other supportive technique. He attributed his success to his technique of anaesthesia, controllable respiration, and the maintenance of arterial pressure by temporary compression of the aorta and intra-arterial transfusion.

Shortly after the start of these experiments, Demikhov realized that the number of anastomoses required was enormously time-consuming and could lead to damage of the animal's brain from anoxia, so he decided to begin a second series of experiments in which the heart and lungs were transplanted as a complete unit. With the two animals lying side by side, he used rubber tubes as temporary anastomoses in such a way that the whole procedure could be carried out without interrupting the circulation in the recipient animal or the donor organs. The first encouraging result came on October 20, 1946, when the recipient lived for two hours supported by its new heart and lungs; the operation was, however, not completed owing to a technical error. Only by the 15th experiment was Demikhov able to remove a live animal from the table.

In all, 67 operations were done in this series with Damka, a bitch operated on on June 12, 1951, being the longest survivor at six days. Because the usual cause of death was infection of the transplanted lungs, Demikhov decided to have a try at transplanting the heart alone. For a long time he had believed this to be technically impossible in view of the large number of vessels to be joined (dogs have more pulmonary veins than human beings) and the consequent risk of thrombosis. But, never one to give up, he devised a technique whereby transplantation could be done without interrupting the circulation. To overcome the problem of the pulmonary veins he separated the left atrium from the right so as to leave the whole of the recipient's left atrium in its body. This was possible, but in the first experiment (on Christmas Day, 1951) the wall between the atria was perforated and the animal died.

Twenty-two operations were performed and all the deaths – mostly on the table – were due to technical imperfections. The last two animals reported had their operations in January, 1955, and they lived for 13 $\frac{1}{2}$ and 11 $\frac{1}{2}$ hours, respectively.

Demikhov was not the only Russian to be working on heart transplantation. NP Sinitsyn, between 1941 and 1957, experimented with frogs and managed in some incredible manner to change the heart over by working through the animals' mouths[13]. The frogs lived for a considerable time (at least three months) after their experience. Sinitsyn also transplanted the hearts of warm-blooded animals, using the same technique as Mann and getting the same sort of results.

In 1947, BV Ognev described his transplantation of the heart into the inguinal region[14]. He joined the high-pressure femoral artery to the pulmonary veins, which caused overfilling of the left side of the heart and failure in 50 minutes.

Back on the Western side of the Iron Curtain, Emanuel Marcus and his colleagues at the Chicago Medical School began the battle all over again, publishing the first of their papers in 1951. Like Mann, they transplanted hearts into the necks, groins, and lower abdomens of recipient animals; to avoid the danger of the donor heart suffering from anoxia they brought a third animal on to the scene which they used to perfuse the coronary arteries of the heart while it was awaiting transplantation. By this technique of 'interim parabiotic perfusion' an uninterrupted blood supply was assured during the whole procedure. In their first set of experiments only the right side of the donor heart was functioning and to prevent overdistension they sometimes created an interatrial septal defect. This was effective because it transferred the blood to the left side of the heart which was doing no work; the carotid anastomosis to the aorta provided the coronary system with its blood. Ten of the 22 operations were successfully completed, though no heart beat for longer than 48 hours[15].

Marcus realized that the greatest stumbling block was the biological problem of tissue specificity, but he speculated that one day a heart might be transplanted to a delimited region where it would act as an accessory pump and decrease the work load of an overburdened heart. It might also, he said, be used to replace a patient's diseased heart, although that 'must be considered, at present, a fantastic dream'[15].

By 1952, Marcus had introduced two new procedures and had also tried to reduce the risk of rejection by cross-matching the bloods of the donor and recipient animals. In the Marcus II operation, the anastomoses were arranged to give both sides of the heart a job to do, with the left ventricle providing the pressure for filling its own coronary arteries. The first 22 experiments were all successful, though again no donor heart beat for more than 48 hours, by which time an angry-looking inflammatory oedema had affected it and the surrounding tissues. With increasing experience and an improved technique they managed to achieve survivals of up to six-and-a-half days[16].

The Marcus III procedure was more ambitious as it involved the transplantation of donor heart and lungs into the lower abdomen; the donor trachea was led to the surface through a hole in the recipient's abdominal wall which allowed artificial respiration to be carried out. This remarkable arrangement was able to support the recipient's life when its own heart and lungs were excluded from the circulation. The maximum survival time in eight of these experiments was nine hours[16].

At this stage, Marcus was puzzling away at the cause of rejection. It could not be anoxia, because his interim parabiotic perfusion technique avoided that. It was not contact of the donor heart with the tissues of the recipient since wrapping the heart in non-irritant cellophane made no difference to the results.

Needless to say he did not find the explanation[17].

By 1952 methods for obtaining an open heart were helpful laboratory tools, even though they were not quite ready for clinical use. Brian Cookson, Wilford Neptune and Charles Bailey were getting on nicely with their research into hypothermia and had been able to stop an animal's circulation completely for 30 minutes without harm. One can almost sense their minds ticking over and wondering what use they could make of this time. Yes, transplantation of the heart and lungs – with the organs mobilized before the circulations of the two animals were stopped, they were able to do the actual substitution in less than 15 minutes[18].

They performed three experiments. The dogs were cooled in a beverage cooler to 21-25°C rectally. The aortas were anastomosed first; then the supeior venae cavae were temporarily united by sliding them over polyethylene tubing and partial circulation resumed. An endotracheal tube was inserted for artificial respiration, the inferior venae cavae were connected over polyethylene tubing and the complete circulation restored. When the new heart was beating satisfactorily, the surgeons joined up the tracheas, removed the tubing (which had been used simply to speed up the anastomoses) and stitched the great veins properly.

The third dog lived for six hours with the new heart maintaining its circulation. Its reflexes returned, it breathed spontaneously and its electrocardiogram was normal (for 24°C)[18,19]. Why it died was never fully explained though the Philadelphia team thought that shock might have been responsible[19]. Their remark that this was the first time a transplanted heart had fully supported a recipient's circulation rather irked Demikhov who apparently failed to understand why knowledge of his work had not travelled beyond Eastern Europe.

The next Western achievement came from Puerto Rico, where a group led by the head of Charles Bailey's research laboratory, Gumersindo Blanco, reported their experiments in 1958. Their technique, as might be expected, was similar to Cookson's except that they used a pump-oxygenator with elective arrest (produced by potassium citrate) of the donor heart during the period it was cut off from a blood supply. Shortly after the new heart was in place and arterial blood was perfusing its coronary circulation, it began to contract. The beats gradually became co-ordinated and gathered strength. Although Blanco attempted the operation eight times, only six experiments were completed; in these the new heart worked effectively for a half hour to four-and-a-half hours. Again, the cause of failure was a mystery, but Blanco wondered whether in some cases it might not have been prolonged extracorporeal circulation producing anoxia of the brain[20].

From that time on things really began to move. An ever increasing number of papers was published reporting on all aspects of cardiac transplantation. Although valuable information was gleaned that was applicable to the normal heart, the primary objective had become the study of the *transplanted* heart. It is most important to appreciate this. Besides work on the homotransplanted heart (between animals of the same species). a great deal was done on autotransplanted hearts (removal and replacement in the same animal). With autotransplants the effects of transplantation could be studied by themselves without the intrusion of the bothersome problem of rejection. The heart's metabolism, its response to drugs, the microscopic changes that took place in its cells, its physiology and response to exercise were all intensively investigated. In the early 1960s, however, some conflicting results appeared; early deaths and disturbances of heart rhythm in autotransplant survivors were attributed to cutting the heart off from its nerve supply or, perhaps, from its lymphatic connections[21]. But fortunately, animals in other series, particularly those of Norman Shumway at Stanford University, California, did not suffer from these effects. As time went on, his dogs with autotransplanted hearts continued to live for one, two, five years, giving every evidence of normal cardiac function and even of autonomic innervation[22]. Why there should have been the initial discrepancies has never been satisfactorily answered.

Technical details were constantly modified and improved; among the most important was the method of dealing with the venous return and the atria. Demikhov had already rebelled against suturing all the pulmonary veins separately and had left the recipient's left atrium in its body to reduce the number of anastomoses. In 1957, the same idea occurred to Mauricio Golberg and Edgar Berman in Baltimore, though the amount of atrium they retained was less. Like Blanco, they had two teams working simultaneously on the donor and the recipient, and they too used a pump-oxygenator with potassium-citrate arrest of the donor heart[23]. (Unlike Blanco, and Cookson before him, they only transplanted the heart.) However, ventricular fibrillation kept recurring and none of their dogs lived longer than two hours.

A further advance was made at Guy's Hospital, London, in 1959, by Russell Brock and Henry Cass, an Australian postgraduate, who left both atria behind to avoid individual suturing of the venae cavae as well as of the pulmonary veins. With technical aspects their sole concern they performed five autotransplants and one homotransplant on dogs using a pump-oxygenator and potassium arrest. Bleeding and tearing of sutures (always problems in canine hearts) were among the difficulties they encountered, and their longest survival was one hour. Nevertheless they wrote: 'At first sight an attempt to transplant the heart appears almost fantastic but more leisured thought indicates that is not necessarily so. The basically simple function of the heart as a pump. invites the possibility, either when the muscle itself is diseased or failing, or when the valve mechanisms are otherwise irreparable.'[24]

Back on the Western side of the Atlantic, Norman Shumway and Richard Lower were beginning the studies which, probably more than any other, influenced the progress of heart transplantation to the operating theatre. Independently of Brock and Cass, they arrived at the same technical solution: 'The [recipient's] heart is excised, and there is left only the common posterior atrial wall containing the ostia of the venae cavae, the pulmonary veins, and a ridge of atrial septum. The aorta and pulmonary artery are divided about a centimeter distal to the commissures.'[25] They were careful to preserve the so-called volume-receptor nerves to the posterior atrial wall, as these were important to future function. Shumway's name became associated with this technique; hard, maybe, on Brock and Cass and the others whose work paved the way, but nevertheless a deserved tribute to Shumway's persistence and markedly better results.

The Stanford surgeons paid no attention to breed in selecting their dogs, and they made no attempt to alter their immunological status. The donor's heart was removed in the same manner as the recipient's and immersed in normal saline solution at 4°C for about five minutes during which time the temperature of its muscle fell to 12-15°C. It was then implanted by joining the atrial walls, and the atrial septum to the posterior atrial wall, with a continuous suture. As soon as the heart was adequately warmed it was defibrillated, but Shumway did not take the animal off the pump-oxygenator until the transplant was fully capable of maintaining the circulation[25].

At first their animals lived only a matter of hours, yet this quickly became days and in 1960 one dog lived 21 days. Before they died, the dogs were normally active and had a normal tolerance for exercise, but when the end came it came rapidly, usually in 24 hours[26].

If the immunological mechanisms could be overcome, wrote Lower and Shumway in 1960, 'in all likelihood it [the heart] would continue to function adequately for the normal life span of the animal.'[25] And with the arrival of the immunosuppressive drugs attempts were soon under way to prolong the survival of transplants.

So far as hearts were concerned, Keith Reemtsma of Tulane University School of Medicine increased the maximum time a heart survived in the neck from 10 days in untreated, control animals to 27 days in animals treated with methotrexate[27] (seven to 10 days is the critical period when rejection first shows itself). Two years later, in 1964, he inserted the donor heart in the recipient's chest parallel with its own heart (which was not removed). The control animals still only lived for a maximum of 10 days, but others given azathioprine lived for as long as 32 days[28].

David Blumenstock of Cooperstown, New York, managed to have one animal survive for 42 days with the help of methotrexate after a complete transplant. His report in 1963 made no mention of controls and 42 of the 50 animals operated on died within 24 hours[29].

Adrian Kantrowitz and his colleagues at Maimonides Hospital, Brooklyn, were also doing great work, and in 1964 they achieved the longest survival to that date – as if to confuse the issue they did it without using immunosuppressive drugs[30]. How to explain this is extraordinarily difficult but it may have been due to their technique, to their use of three-month-old puppies (a weaker immune response than in full-grown animals), or to luck in picking compatible animals.

When Kantrowitz used a pump-oxygenator he obtained no long-term survivors, but when he turned to deep hypothermia without a pump-oxygenator at all, the picture changed. Twenty-four out of 40 puppies lived more than a day, one died after 57 days, and one was still living at the time of the report (published in 1965) – 112 days after operation. The animals were cooled by total immersion in ice-cold water; the recipient to 16-17°C and the donor to 27-29°C rectally. This allowed the recipient's circulation to be safely stopped for the 45 minutes or so that the transplantation required. The heart was massaged while the animal was rewarmed and at 27°C was defibrillated.

Chest complications were a nuisance but on the credit side was the fact that microscopic examination of the hearts in the long-term survivors showed no unequivocal evidence of rejection. Also the hearts steadily increased in size, keeping pace with the growth of the puppies, and showed signs of gradual reinnervation. Kantrowitz regarded this as encouraging for the eventual use of heart transplants in infants.

Although others adopted Kantrowitz's method, none achieved comparable results, and nearly all the attention was focused on immunosuppressive drugs. But despite the rather dismal immunological picture hearts were technically ready for transplantation. 'Furthermore,' wrote Shumway and Lower in 1964[31], 'with a definite increase in survival of renal homografts, it seems logical to conclude that cardiac homografts are just around the corner.' And they ended most perspicaciously: 'Perhaps the cardiac surgeon should pause while .society becomes accustomed to resurrection of the mythological chimera'.

This was not the writing on the wall; this was its interpretation.

30

TRANSPLANTATION OF THE HEART
– THE ACHIEVEMENT

The cardiac surgeon did not pause; it would have been unrealistic to imagine he could. Research at such an advanced stage could not be shut off like a tap. And society, if it thought about the matter at all, still regarded transplantation of the human heart as a 'fantastic dream'; its collective mind was not even ready to accept the possibility, let alone become accustomed to it.

Yet at the beginning of 1964, before Shumway's and Lower's advice was published, the first cardiac transplantation on a human patient had taken place at the University Hospital of the University of Mississippi Medical Center. The reason why this failed to create an upheaval in the outside world is simple and significant: the donor heart came from a chimpanzee, not from another human being. Mr Everyman could still sleep soundly, free of the irrational fear of his heart being cut from his body while he still had life.

James Hardy entered the arena well prepared and with his eyes wide open. Since 1956 he and his colleagues had performed more than 200 animal heart transplants. During the developmental phases they made countless mistakes and had great difficulty with oozing from raw surfaces which was responsible for the rapid demise of many of their dogs. At first they transplanted the heart and lungs together; six animals survived for 75 minutes to 22 hours, but in none of them could normal respiration be restored[1]. As Watts R Webb and Hector Howard (members of Hardy's team) said in 1957, they reckoned they had reached an impasse because of the failure of totally denervated lungs to function on their own[1]. (This is another example of the puzzles sent to try experimental workers, for others did not find the same problem and in 1961 Shumway and Lower transplanted hearts and lungs with the return of spontaneous respiration which sustained life until rejection occurred. Nevertheless, they admitted that the problem of long-term survival after pulmonary denervation remained unanswered[2].) Webb had the same trouble with autotransplanted hearts and lungs, but he found that when he transplanted one lung only with the heart, the lung seemed to function satisfactorily.

In 1958 these same two members of the Mississippi team were doing better and had 12 technical successes with the heart and right lung. They also left some of the left atrium behind, but for a different reason from the others who had the same idea: 'All vessels were left long and, to obtain additional length, the pulmonary veins may be divided with a cuff of atrium.'[3] The donor organs were refrigerated at 4°C before insertion and in 10 of the dogs the hearts maintained blood pressures for 30 minutes to seven-and-a-half hours.

By 1962 Hardy was ready to transplant heart or lungs in a human patient if all the circumstances – such as suitable donor and suitable recipient available at the same time – were favourable. As far as the heart was concerned, he had thrashed out all the moral and ethical issues with 'many thoughtful persons', both medical and lay. He had done mock operations on human cadavers and had the whole team completely prepared. But circumstances decreed that the lung should have priority, and on June 11, 1963, Hardy performed the first human lung transplantation, having done more than 400 experiments on dogs[4]. After operation the patient was given drugs and cobalt radiotherapy; the transplanted lung worked well right from the start, but on the 18th day the man died from pre-existing kidney disease. Postmortem examination revealed no evidence that the new lung was being rejected. This was decidedly encouraging not only for lungs but also for hearts. since Shumway's experiments in 1961 had shown that pathological changes in transplanted hearts were less severe than those in transplanted lungs[2].

Six months later on January 18, 1964, Hardy went into his operating theatre fully organized to transplant a heart. The intended recipient was a man of 36 who, after repair of a knife wound of his left ventricle carried out elsewhere in April, 1963, had had a succession of emboli from the heart that caused a right hemiplegia, mental impairment, double incontinence, the loss of both legs (amputated) and gangrene of his intestines. But removal of his heart proved unnecessary. This episode – which Hardy referred to as a 'dry run' because a donor was ready who died at the opportune moment – gave valuable experience, as it showed that the whole procedure could have gone smoothly[5].

There had also been another donor available. Hardy had recently visited New Orleans where he had been impressed with Keith Reemtsma's use of primate kidneys for renal heterotransplants[6]. The possibility of using a chimpanzee heart seemed remote, but if there had been no other solution to the problem Hardy was prepared to go ahead.

Within a few days conditions once again seemed favourable for a human transplant. A 68-year-old man was admitted to the hospital with hypertensive cardiovascular disease and severe coronary arteriosclerosis. His blood pressure was so low it could not be measured. In the recovery ward lay a young man almost dead from irrecoverable brain damage. On January 23 the older man was taken to theatre and put on cardiopulmonary bypass. His own heart failed. Hardy waited. But the younger man lingered on. A decision was imperative. Since the patient had given his permission for a chimpanzee heart to be used, Hardy believed the circumstances were now such that the operation would be well within ethical and moral boundaries. His decision made, Hardy acted.

The chimpanzee's heart was removed and the coronary sinus perfused with cold oxygenated blood until transplantation was completed. The new heart beat well but, regrettably, its previous owner weighed only 96 pounds (44 kg) – considerably less than the recipient – and it was too small to cope with the return of venous blood. In vain Hardy implanted pacemakers to boost its rate; it just could not do the work and the patient died after a few hours.

'By the time the operation was over,' Hardy wrote[5], 'almost 25 persons, many of them physicians, had gained entrance to the operating suite on one pretext or another, despite the fact that a doorkeeper had been placed at the only unlocked entrance.' He knew there would be excitement, because someone had tipped off the press about the previous dry run and the hospital had had difficulty in convincing reporters that no transplantation had taken place. Hardy was in the public eye. So on the occasion of the real transplantation, a press announcement was made. Unfortunately this did not state that a chimpanzee heart had been used, and when a report appeared in 'a distant city' of a human heart having been transplanted a revised statement was given out to check the rumour. This it did pretty effectively and the press soon lost interest.

'The clinical transplantation of a human heart might prompt controversy, and the clinical transplantation of the primate heart was even more likely to arouse controversy.' How wrong could Hardy be? Four years later everyone knew the answer when the name of Christiaan Barnard hit the world's headlines.

This son of a Dutch Reformed Church missionary graduated from Cape Town University in 1946. After a spell in general practice he began his surgical career and spent from 1954 to 1956 at Minneapolis working under Walton Lillehei. On his return to South Africa he became Director of Surgical Research at Cape Town Medical School. Much of his energy was directed at congenital anomalies of the heart, but the results of his work at Groote Schuur Hospital in all aspects of cardiac surgery bore favourable comparison with the best in the world[7]. He preceded a new operation with meticulous animal experiments and followed up his patients closely and in detail.

Since 1964 he and his brother Marius had been studying heart transplantation in dogs employing Shumway's technique, with the preservation of as much atria and atrial septum as possible in the recipient animal. The donor dog was immersed in an ice bath – until its temperature fell to 30-32°C – for five to 10 minutes before insertion of its heart into the recipient which had been cooled extracorporeally to 26-28°C. In 90 percent of the dogs the transplanted heart supported the circulation quite satisfactorily at the end of the operation. The investigations were, however, concerned only with the techniques of surgery[8].

Christiaan Barnard was, nevertheless, ready.

And so, on the night of December 2/3, 1967, was Louis Washkansky when a 24-year-old girl was admitted dying from head injuries. Washkansky was a 54-year-old diabetic who had had heart attacks in 1959, 1960 and 1965, which had irreparably damaged his heart. He was now in intractable heart failure, and had readily agreed to the hope offered by transplantation. The girl had compatible red-cell antigens and a similar leucocyte antigen pattern to Washkansky's. The stage was set.

In the early hours of the morning of the third, Washkansky was taken to the operating theatre, anaesthetized, and his chest opened. A direct examination of his heart proved that nothing other than transplantation could help him. Meanwhile the girl had been taken to an adjoining theatre after a neurosurgeon had stated that her brain injuries were beyond treatment. When she was certified as dead she was attached to a pump-oxygenator and cooled to 26°C. Then her aorta was clamped so that only her heart was cooled; this continued until its temperature had fallen to 16°C. In two minutes it was removed and put in a bowl of physiological solution at 10°C and taken to the other theatre where, after an gap of only four minutes, it was again being perfused with blood.

By this time Washkansky was on a Lillehei-DeWall pump-oxygenator; extra-corporeal cooling was started, and when his mid-oesophageal temperature had reached 30°C, his heart was excised. Following Shumway's technique, Barnard divided the atrial septum as close to the ventricles as possible and left cuffs of atria around the entering veins. He trimmed the donor heart to make it a good fit and began sewing it into its new home. First he joined the left atria, then the right atria and the pulmonary arteries. At this point, perfusion of the donor heart was stopped and the aortas anastomosed. Rewarming now began, and when Washkansky's mid-oesophageal temperature reached 36°C the first shock from a defibrillator restored a good ventricular contraction at a rate of 120 beats per minute. Rewarming continued for another 15 minutes. The bypass – by this time only partial – was discontinued at the third attempt when the heart was able to maintain a satisfactory blood pressure unaided[9].

The donor heart had arrived in the theatre at 3.01 am. At 6.13 am the oper-ation was concluded. Afterwards, sitting down with a cup of tea, someone asked: 'What shall we do now?'

A silence, then Barnard said: 'Let's tell the medical superintendent.'

And in one short phone call the news was told. 'Sir, we have just transplanted a heart and the patient is well.'

Surgically the operation was a success; but now began the most testing part of the whole procedure – postoperative care. Fluids and electrolytes were kept in balance and drugs were given to ensure adequate cardiac function. The danger of rejection was anticipated by giving Washkansky corticosteroid drugs and azathioprine from the first day, with local cobalt irradiation to the heart on the fifth, seventh and ninth days. (Because of this treatment, Washkansky's resistance to infection was lowered and he was nursed in isolation; this was effective so far as the hospital staff was concerned, but Barnard had trouble keeping reporters out.) The response was remarkable. The signs of heart failure disappeared almost miraculously, and the patient lost quantities of retained fluid; his waterlogged legs returned to their normal shape, and by the third day his grossly enlarged liver was also a normal size. His diabetes became much easier to control.

The implications, said Barnard, were clear: the heart was a pump and it was possible to replace this function with a transplant. The new heart could recognize when more work was required of it, for example when infection occurred, and could respond by an increase in rate and output. How this happened, Barnard did not know, although he wondered whether it might be due to some built-in mechanism or to humoral control.

Thirteen days after operation Washkansky showed signs of a lung infection which did not respond to treatment, and on December 21 he died. The transplanted heart had, nevertheless, maintained a good circulation until the end.

Because there was some confusion over whether the heart showed signs of rejection or not, the summary of the article in the *British Medical Journal* by James Thomson, the professor of pathology at Cape Town who carried out the postmortem, is quoted in full:

'Necropsy on the first heart transplantation in man confirmed that death was due to extensive bilateral pneumonia and not to rejection of the heart. Signs of rejection, however, were demonstrated histologically, but were of a low order compared with those seen in the transplanted dog heart. How far the mildness of the rejection signs is to be ascribed to species differences, immuno-suppressive drugs and procedures, postoperative rest, and nursing and medical care, or to the good matching of leucocyte antigens cannot at the moment be assessed.'[10]

While Washkansky was still alive, the second human heart homo-transplantation was performed. The surgeon was Adrian Kantrowitz, and the recipient a two-and-a-half-week-old boy who had a lethal congenital cardiac anomaly. The donor heart came from an infant born with a grossly deficient brain, but it beat for only six-and-a-half hours in its new body[11].

Then on January 2, 1968, came Barnard's second transplantation which, as time progressed, confounded his critics and surprised and even puzzled his most ardent supporters. The recipient, Philip Blaiberg, lived for 593 days, successfully overcoming a number of rejection crises and giving every indication of thoroughly enjoying his extra life, despite – or perhaps because of – being virtually a human pillbox. In June, 1969, Blaiberg's health suddenly deteriorated, and he died two months later, on August 17. This 58-year-old Cape Town dentist had received the heart of a Cape Coloured man of 24 who died suddenly from a brain haemorrhage; it transformed him from a breathless cardiac cripple into a man able to look after himself, drive a car, and bathe in the sea[12].

By the time of Blaiberg's operation, however, publicity was becoming a headache for the Groote Schuur team; despite their endeavours, it was not to be avoided. For instance, before Blaiberg had been operated on, someone, in an unguarded moment, said that the next patient would be a dentist who was so ill he could no longer practise. A journalist thereupon telephoned every dentist in Cape Town and so identified Blaiberg.

Indeed, the publicity that enveloped all credible and incredible aspects of heart transplantation exceeded anything ever before given to a medical subject and jammed the surgeons well and truly into a cleft stick. These operations were news; the public was avid for information and the press was going to see that it got what it wanted, names, family details, and all. The surgeons found themselves forced into giving press conferences. It was no longer possible to announce their work in reasoned articles in medical journals.

The world had at last woken up to the reality of heart transplantation and was going to have its say, belatedly maybe, on the moral, social, ethical, religious and economic issues involved. Comment by doctors and laymen alike was by no means entirely favourable and at times the criticism looked remarkably like hysteria born of fear – fear deeply rooted in the beliefs of mankind; fear that the heart would be used for transplantation before the body was dead.

But despite this atmosphere, in the 20 months after the first human heart homotransplantation, 143 operations were performed in countries all over the world. Twenty-nine of the 141 recipients (two patients had the operation twice) were still alive, and one of them had survived for more than six months. More than half the transplantations (84) took place in the United States of America. Encouragingly, many of the teams who jumped on the transplantation bandwagon inadequately prepared realized what they were up against and withdrew from the fray: the 143 heart-transplant operations were performed by 56 teams, but only about 10 were still carrying on after those 20 months. Almost at random, we will have a look at one or two representative cases.

On January 6, 1968, Norman Shumway put into effect his years of experimental preparation when he transplanted the heart of a 43-year-old woman into Michael Kasperak who was dying from chronic viral myocarditis. Misfortune dogged the way from the start. The diseased heart was so enlarged that after its removal the cavity was almost three times the size of the donor heart. This produced technical problems and five hours after operation the 54-year-old patient had to be taken back to the theatre where his chest was reopened and fluid removed from the pericardial space. Then two days later his kidneys and liver began to fail (they were in poor condition before operation owing to his long-standing heart condition) and he bled from his gastrointestinal tract – a manifestation of liver failure. The kidney failure was treated by peritoneal dialysis and the bleeding by really massive transfusion. On the eighth day another liver crisis resulted in the surgical removal of his gall bladder under local anaesthesia. On January 21, he died[13].

The cost of Kasperak's last 16 days was $28 845 which included $7200 for 288 pints (163 litres) of blood[14]. This large sum, not at all exceptional for the early transplants, generated a lot of criticism, much of it concerned with how better the money would have been spent on preventive medicine. No one denies the importance of prevention of heart disease, but we come back to the old argument of helping the sick we have with us now. Also, these high costs of the first operations should be regarded as developmental costs and spread over the years that followed. Thus by the end of 1968, Denton Cooley at St Luke's Hospital, Houston, had reduced the expense of his operations quite considerably to about $200 or $300 per day[15].

Cooley had graduated from Johns Hopkins University School of Medicine where, in due course, he became surgical resident to Alfred Blalock. Yet, with all his previous vast experience of cardiac surgery he admitted: 'Dr Barnard showed that a heart transplant patient could survive. Otherwise I would have hesitated.'[16] At the beginning of May, 1968, his team had been on 24-hour alert for three months. Then by a remarkable coincidence he obtained three donors and three suitable recipients within a four-day period. The first patient, a man of 47, received on May 3 the heart of a 15-year-old girl who had shot herself in the head. The second, another man of 47, was operated on on May 5; his heart came from a 15-year-old boy. And the third, a man of 62, received his new heart on May 7[17]. In an addendum to the report of these cases, Cooley mentioned that one patient had received the heart of a sheep: he died. By the beginning of October, 1968, Cooley had performed 10 human heart transplants with seven survivors at that time. Some of the patients had returned to work.

Denton Cooley was renowned for his swiftness in operating, with not one unnecessary movement. 'Remember,' he said, 'that in surgery the longer you take, the sicker the patient gets.'[16] But he was not stressing speed for speed's sake. By sheer skill and organization he reduced the length of operation from about four-and-a-half hours to one hour and 45 minutes, skin to skin. In certain respects his transplantation technique differed from that of others such as Barnard and Shumway. For instance, he neither cooled nor perfused the donor heart; at first this was a controversial point, but it was eventually endorsed by a number of other cardiac surgeons. Cooley also modified the details concerning those parts of the recipient's heart that should be left behind. He placed great emphasis on preserving the intrinsic nerve conduction pathway from the sinus node to the atrio-ventricular node as failures in other transplants could be traced to interference with this pathway. In Blaiberg's case and in his own surviving patients the pathway had been kept intact.

Another cause for technical failure, in Cooley's opinion, was thrombosis – with subsequent embolism – starting in the atrial appendages of the remnants of the recipient heart. For this reason he always removed them.

Cooley was the first surgeon to add antilymphocytic globulin to the patient's postoperative drug treatment, and indeed he recommended that transplants should not be carried out unless the surgeon had a supply of this rare commodity. Because lower doses of other immunosuppressive drugs could then be given, the risk of infection was reduced and Cooley removed his patients from strict bacteriological isolation soon after operation. He also allowed his patients out of bed in 48 hours provided they had not been too disabled before surgery.

The first time a heart and lungs were transplanted as a unit in a human patient was on September 15, 1968, at St Luke's Hospital. A two-month-old girl had been born with a severe congenital heart anomaly which had affected her lungs. Because of this Cooley felt that surgery on her heart alone could not succeed, so he transplanted the heart and lungs from a dead anencephalic infant. The heart worked well, but gradually the lungs ceased functioning and the baby girl died after 14 hours[18].

On the same day (May 3, 1968) that Cooley carried out his first heart transplant, the first British operation was performed by Donald Ross at the National Heart Hospital in London. The recipient was a 45-year-old man who for three years had had a chronic heart condition and was now in severe con- gestive failure. Ross had been looking for a suitable donor for some time and during the previous week had been searching hard. Then on May 2, a man of 26 sustained serious head injuries in a fall on a building site. He was operated on at King's College Hospital but could not be saved. The following afternoon, Ross knew he had a donor, and all preparations were made while the body was rushed across London in an ambulance with the circulation maintained by external cardiac massage[19]. The recipient, Frederick West, lived for 45 days.

With the arrival of heart transplantation, one might be tempted to think that Stephen Paget's words of more than a century ago were at last justified: 'Surgery of the heart has probably reached the limits set by Nature to all surgery.'[20] One day, perhaps, rheumatic fever might be preventable, so even might coronary artery disease and congenital abnormalities. But that is not yet. Today, tomorrow, for many, many years to come, the surgeon's scalpel will still be called upon to treat disease of the human heart.

SOURCES

CHAPTER 1: PROLOGUE

1 For an account of the development of modern surgery from the discovery of anaesthesia to the 1950s, see: Richardson RG. (1958). *The surgeon's tale*. London; Allen and Unwin.

2 Bigelow HJ. (1846). 'Insensibility during surgical operations produced by inhalation.' *Boston Medical and Surgical Journal*, **35**, 309-17; 379-82.

3 Lister J. (1867). 'On a new method of treating compound fracture, abscess, etc. with observations on the conditions of suppuration.' *Lancet*, **1**, 326-9; 357-9; 387-9; 507-9; **2**, 95-96.

4 Lister J. (1867). 'On the antiseptic principle in the practice of surgery.' *British Medical Journal*, **2**, 246-8.

5 Pasteur L. (1862). 'Mémoire sur les corpuscles organisés qui existent dans l'atmosphère, examen de la doctrine des générations spontanées.' *Annales de Chimie et de Physique*, **64**, 5-110.

6 Schimmelbusch C. (1892). *Anleitung zur Aseptischen Wundbehandlung*. Mit einem Vorwort des Herrn Geh.-Rath Professor Dr. E. von Bergmann. Berlin; Hirschwald.

7 Schimmelbusch C. (1894). *The aseptic treatment of wounds*. With a preface by Prof. Bergmann. Translated by A.T. Rake from the second German edition. London; Lewis.

8 Koch R. (1878). *Untersuchungen über die Aetiologie der Wundinfections-krankheiten*. Leipzig; Vogel.

CHAPTER 2: THE CIRCULATION

1 *Leonardo da Vinci Quaderni Anatomie*. Vol IV, folio 11v. Edited by Vangensten OCL, Fohahn H, Hopstock H. (1911). Oslo; Cristiana University.

2 Vesalius A. (1543). *De humani corporis fabrica*. Basel; Oporinus.

3 Columbus R. (1559). *De re anatomica*. Venetiis; Nicolai Benilacquae.

4 Servetus M. (1553). *Christianismi restitutio*. Vienne. Translation in: O'Malley CD. (1953). *Michael Servetus*. Philadelphia; American Philosophical Society.

5 Fabricius H. (1603). *De venarum ostiolis*. Patavii; Laurentij Pasquati. Facsimile edition with introduction, translation, and notes: Franklin KJ. (1933). *De venarum ostiolis 1603 of Hieronymus Fabricius of Aquapendente (1533?-1619)*. Springfield, Ill. and Baltimore; Thomas.

6 Harvey W. (1628). *Exercitatio anatomica de motu cordis ex sanguinis in animalibus*. Francofurti; Guilielmi Fitzeri.

7 Malpighi M. (1686). 'De pulmonibus.' In: *Opera omnia*. Londini; Roberto Scott. [Two letters written to Borelli in 1661.]
[For a different approach to the events in this chapter, *see* Richardson R. (1999). *Medicine through the ages with Dr Baldassare*, chapters 14, 15. London; Quiller.]

CHAPTER 3: WOUNDS OF THE HEART

1 Sprengell CJ. (1708). *The aphorisms of Hippocrates and the sentences of Celsus*. Sect. 6, Aph. 18, p.159. London; (no publisher cited).

2   Galen. Translated into French by Daremberg C. (1856). *Oeuvres anatomiques, phys-iologiques et médicales de Galien.* Vol. II, X *Des lieux affectés,* livre 5, Ch. 2, p.628. Paris; Baillière.

3   Houllier J. (1644). *In aphorismos Hippocratis. Commenterij septem,* pp.343-6. Geneva; Chouët.

4   Cabrol B. (1604). *Alphabeton anatomikon.* Obs. 26, pp.104-5. Geneva; Chouët.

5   Zacchias P. (1651). *Quaestiones medico-legales,* 3rd ed. Lib. V, Tit. II, Quaest. II, sec 21, p.300. Amstelaedami; Joannis Blaeu.

6   Harvey W. Cited by Foy G. (1893). Letter to the editors. 'Some effects of wounds of the heart.' *Lancet,* **1**, 59.

7   Wolf I. (1704). *Observationum chirurgico-medicarum libri duo; cum scholiis et vari-is interspersis historiis medicis, editi a Joanne Chr. Wolfio.* Obs 21. Quedlimburgi; TP Calvisi. Cited by Fischer G. (1868). 'Die Wunden des Herzens und des Herzbeutels.' *Archiv für Klinische Chirurgie,* **9**, 571-910 (see p.852).

8   Bonet T. (1679). *Sepulchretum, sive anatomia practica ex cadaveribus morbo denatis.* Geneva; Chouët.

9   Bonet T. (1700). *Sepulchretum, sive anatomia practica, ex cadaveribus morbo denatis.* Revised edition with new commentaries by J.J. Mangetus. Vol.III, Book IV, Sect. III, Obs. XXIII, p.354; and new Obs. III and IV, pp.376, 378. Lugduni; Cramer and Perachon.

10 Morgagni GB. (1761). *De sedibus et causis morborum per anatomen indagatis libri quinque.* Venetiis; Remondiniana.

11 Morgagni GB. (1769) *.The seats and causes of diseases investigated by anatomy.* Translated from the Latin by B. Alexander. Book II, Letter 26, Article 18. Book IV, Letter 53, Articles 1-41. Book V, Letter 69, Article 5. London; Millar, Cadell, and Johnson and Payne.

12 Rose E. (1884). '"Herztamponade." (Ein Beitrag zur Herzchirurgie.).' *Deutsche Zeitschrift für Chirurgie,* **20**, 329-410.

13 Fischer G. (1868). 'Die Wunden des Herzens und des Herzbeutels.' *Archiv für Klinische Chirurgie,* **9**, 571-910.

14 Balch GB. (1861). 'Case of gunshot wound, in which a leaden bullet remained twen-ty years in the walls of the heart.' *American Journal of Medical Science,* **42**, 293-4.

15 Callender GW. (1873). 'Removal of a needle from the heart. Recovery of the patient.' *Medico-Chirurgical Transactions, London,* **56**, 203-12.

16 Schechter D, Gilbert L. (1966). Reported in *World Medicine,* January 17, 1967, p.99.

17 Block (1882). In discussion following paper by Gluck in Eilfter Congress der Deutschen Gesellschaft für Chirurgie. *Verhandlungen der Deutschen Gesellschaft für Chirurgie,* **11**, 108-9.

18 Bülau G. (1891). 'Für die Heber-Drainage bei Behandlung des Empyems.' *Zeitschrift für Klinische Medizin,* **18**, 31-45.

19 Billroth T. (1864). In: *Handbuch der Allgemeinen und Speciellen Chirurgie.* Ed. v. Pitha and Billroth. Band 3. Abth. 2. A. Abschnitt VI, p.163. Stuttgart; Enke.

20 Origin and dating of Billroth's remark on heart suture given by: Nissen R. (1963). Letter to the Editor: 'Billroth and cardiac surgery', *Lancet,* **2**, 250-1.

21 Billroth T, Winiwarter v. A. (1884). *General surgical pathology and therapeutics.* Translated from the 4th edition and revised from the 10th by C.E. Hackney. London; Lewis.

22 Del Vecchio S. (1895). 'Sutura del cuore.' *Riforma Medica,* **2**, 38-40, 50-3.

23 Dalton HC. (1895). 'Report of a case of stab-wound of the pericardium, terminating in recovery after resection of a rib and suture of the pericardium.' *Annals of Surgery,*

21, 147-52.

24 Cappelen A. (1896). 'Valvus cordis; sutur of hjertet.' *Norsk Magazin for Laegevidenskaben*, **57**, 285-8.

25 Farina (1896). Cited by Durante in discussion. XI. Kongress der Italienischen chirurgischen Gesellschaft, gehalten in Rom vom 26-29. Oktober 1896. *Zentralblatt für Chirurgie*, **23**, 1224.

26 Farina G. (1896-7). 'Sutura del ventricolo destro.' *Bullettino di Accademia Medica di Roma*, **23**, 248.

27 Farina G. (1896). Letter quoted in: Bland-Sutton J. (1910). 'A clinical lecture on the treatment of injuries of the heart.' *British Medical Journal*, **1**, 1273-6.

28 Rehn (1896). 'Fall von penetrirender Stichverletzung des rechten Ventrikel's Herznaht.' Versammlung der Gesellschaft deutscher Naturforscher und Ärzte in Frankfurt a/M. vom 21. Bis 26. September 1896. *Zentralblatt für Chirurgie*, **23**, 1048-9.

29 Rehn (1897). 'The successful treatment of a wound of the heart.' Report of The Congress of the German Surgical Association. *Lancet*, **1**, 1306.

30 Pott P. (1775). *Chirurgical observations relative to the cataract, the polypus of the nose, the cancer of the scrotum, the different kinds of rupture and the modification of the toes and feet.* London; Hawes.

31 Collected data on repair of heart wounds: Peck CH. (1909). 'The operative treatment of heart wounds.' *Annals of Surgery*, **50**, 101-34.

32 Paget S. (1896). *The surgery of the chest.* Bristol; Wright. London; Simpkin, Marshall, Hamilton, Kent.

33 Stelzner (1887). 'Mittheilung einer Operation behufs Entfernung einer Nähnadel aus dem rechten Herzventrikel.' Report in: *Verhandlungen der Gesellschaft für Chirurgie*, **16**, 58-61.

34 Tuffier T. (1897). *Chirurgie du poumon en particulier dans les cavernes tuberculeuses et la gangrène pulmonaire*, p.31. Paris; Masson.

35 Tuffier T. (1889). *Etudes éxperimentales sur la chirurgie du rein; néphrectomie, néphrorrhapie, urétérotomie.* Paris; Steinheil.

36 Röntgen WC. (1895). 'Ueber eine neue Art von Strahlen.' *Sitzungsberichte der Physikalisch-Medizinischen Gesellschaft*, **29**,132-41.

37 Jones R, Lodge O. (1896). 'The discovery of a bullet lost in the wrist by means of the Roentgen rays.' *Lancet*, **1**, 476-7.

38 Tuffier T. (1903). 'Extraction d'une balle implantée dans la paroi de l'oreillette gauche du coeur.' *Bulletin et Mémoires de la Société de Chirurgie de Paris*, **29**, 957-65.

CHAPTER 4: THE PERICARDIUM

1 Riolan J. (1649) *Encheiridium anatomicum et pathologicum.* Lib. III, Cap. IV, p.206. Lugduni Batavorum; Adriani Wyngaerden.

2 Senac (1749). *Traité de la structure du coeur, de son action, et de ses maladies.* Vol. II, Lib.IV, Chap. V, VII, p.365. Paris; Vincent.

3 Romero F. (1814-15). 'Extrait d'un mémoire de M. le docteur F. Romero, médecin de Catalogne, sur l'hydrothorax et l'hydropéricarde; et du rapport qui en a été fait par MM. Husson et Mérat.' *Bulletins de la Faculté de Médecine de Paris*, **4**, 373-6.

4 Skielderup M. (1818). 'De trepanatione ossis sterni et aperture pericardii.' *Acta Regiae Societatis Medicae Hayniensis*, **5**, 130-41.

5 For a biography of Baron D J Larrey, see: Richardson R. (2000). *Larrey: Surgeon-in-Chief to Napoleon's Imperial Guard.* London; Quiller Press.

6 Larrey DJ. (1812-17). *Mémoires de chirurgie militaire, et campagnes.* 4 vols. **1**, 151-2. Paris; Smith.

7 Soubiran A. (1966). *Le Baron Larrey. Chirurgien de Napoléon*, pp.96-97. Paris; Fayard.

8 Larrey DJ. (1812-17) *Mémoires de chirurgie militaire, et campagnes.* 4 vols. **4**, 74-6. Paris; Smith.

9 Larrey DJ. (1810). 'Sur une blessure du péricarde, suivie d'hydro-péricardie.' *Bulletin des Sciences Médicales*, **6**, 255-73.

10 Larrey DJ. (1829-36). *Clinique chirurgicale, exercée particulièrement dans les camps et les hôpitaux militaires, depuis 1792 jusqu'en 1829.* 5 vols. **2**, 284-303; 303-37. Paris; Gabon (1829 – also vol. **3**). (Vols **4** and **5**, Paris; Baillière, 1832 and 1836, respectively.)

11 Botallo L. (1660). 'De curandis vulneribus sclopetorum.' In: *Opera omnia*, pp.599-801. Lugduni Batavorum; Danielis and Abrahami. [Originally published in 1560 in Lyons.]

12 Desault PJ. (1803). *Cours théorique et pratique de clinique externe.* 'Des maladies par solution de continuité,' **2**,147 et seq. Paris; Delaplace.

13 Hilsmann FA. (1875). 'Ueber die paracentese des perikardiums.' *Schriften der Universität zu Kiel*, **22**, No. 7.

14 Langenbeck B von (1888). *Vorlesungen über Akiurgie*, pp.449-50. Berlin; Hirschwald.

15 Rosenstein S. (1881). 'Ein Fall von Incision des Pericardium.' *Berliner Klinische Wochenschrift*, **18**, 61-3.

16 West S. (1883). 'Purulent pericarditis treated by tapping.' (In a report of a meeting of the Pathological Society of London.) *British Medical Journal*, **2**, 1129.

17 Roberts JB. (1881). 'The surgery of the pericardium.' *Annals of Anatomy and Surgery*, **4**, 247-52.

18 Dieulafoy G. (1873). *A treatise on the pneumatic aspiration of morbid fluids*, pp.219-44. London; Smith, Elder.

19 Delorme E, Mignon. (1895). 'Sur la ponction et l'incision du péricarde.' *Revue de Chirurgie*, **15**, 797-838; 987-1022.

20 Balance C. (1920). 'The Bradshaw Lecture on: The surgery of the heart.' *Lancet*, **1**, 1-5; 73-9; 134-9.

21 Weill E. (1895). *Traité clinique des maladies du coeur chez les enfants*, pp.128-9. Paris; Octave Doin.

22 Delorme (1898). 'Sur un traitement chirurgical de la symphyse cardo-péricardique.' *Bulletin et Mémoires de la Société de Chirurgie de Paris*, **24**, 918-22.

23 Hallopeau MP. (1921). 'Un cas de cardiolyse.' *Bulletin et Mémoires de la Société de Chirurgie de Paris*, **47**, 1120-1.

24 Rehn L. (1913). 'Die Chirurgie des Herzens und des Herzbeutels.' *Berliner Klinische Wochenschrift*, **50**, 241-6.

25 Sauerbruch F, O'Shaughnessy L. (1937). *Thoracic surgery.* London; Arnold.

26 Brauer (1902). 'Ueber chronische adhäsive Mediastino-Perikarditis und deren Behandlung.' *Münchener Medizinische Wochenschrift*, **49**, 1072.

27 Brauer (1902). In discussion: 'Die Erfolge der Kardiolysis.' *Münchener Medizinische Wochenschrift*, **49**, 1732.

28 Brauer L. (1909). 'Lungenkollapstherapie unter anwendung einer extrapleuralen thorakoplastik.' Report in: *Münchener Medizinische Wochenschrift*, **56**, 1866.

29 Mackenzie W. (1906). 'Pericarditis in children considered surgically.' *Intercolonial Medical Journal of Australia*, **11**, 492-6.

30 Morison A. (1908). 'On thoracostomy in heart disease.' *Lancet*, **2**, 7-12.

CHAPTER 5: CARDIAC ARREST

1   Dana RH. (Editor) (1848). 'A history of the ether discovery.' *Littell's Living Age*, **16**, 529-71; 575. [Richard Henry Dana (1815-1882) worked his passage round Cape Horn to California and back, writing of his experiences in *Two years before the mast* (1840) – a best-seller in its day.]
2   Morton WTG. (1847). *Circular. Morton's Letheon*, 5th ed. Boston; Dutton and Wentworth. [First edition, 1846.]
3   Morton WTG. (1847). *Remarks on the proper mode of administering sulphuric ether by inhalation.* Boston; Dutton and Wentworth.
4   Simpson JY. (1847). 'On a new anaesthetic agent, more efficient than sulphuric ether.' *Lancet*, **2**, 549-50.
5   Report of Inquest (1848). 'Fatal application of chloroform.' *Lancet*, **1**, 161-2.
6   Simpson JY. (1848). 'Remarks on the alleged case of death from the action of chloroform.' *Lancet*, **1**, 175-6.
7   Morton WTG. (1850). *On the physiological effects of sulphuric ether, and its superiority to chloroform.* Boston; David Clapp.
8   Snow J. (1858). *On chloroform and other anaesthetics: their action and administration.* Edited, with a memoir of the author, by Benjamin W Richardson, MD. London; Churchill.
9   Report of the Second Hyderabad Chloroform Commission (1890). *Lancet*, **1**, 149-59; 421-9; 486-510; 1140-2; 1369-88.
10 Lawrie E. (1891). 'The Hyderabad Chloroform Commission.' *Lancet*, **1**, 591.
11 Levy AG. (1911). 'Sudden death under light chloroform anaesthesia.' *Journal of Physiology*, **42**, iii-vii; **43**, xviii-xix.
12 Vesalius A. (1543). *De humani corporis fabrica*, Lib. VII, cap. 19, p.658. Basel; Oporinus.
13 Bleeck C. (1850). Letter to the Editor: 'Alarming results of chloroform.' *Lancet*, **1**, 283.
14 Ricord P. (1850). 'New method of remedying the accidents caused by chloroform.' *Lancet*, **1**, 208-9.
15 Metcalf JT. (1857). 'On the priority and use of chloroform.' *Transactions of the New York Academy of Medicine*, **1**, 139-58.
16 A Mirror of the Practice of Medicine and Surgery in the Hospitals of London (1850). 'Guy's Hospital. Neuralgia after amputation of a finger; inhalation of chloroform; sudden death. (Under the care of Mr. Cock.)' *Lancet*, **2**, 21.
17 Silvester HR. (1858). 'A new method of resuscitating still-born children, and of restoring persons apparently drowned or dead.' *British Medical Journal*, **volume for 1858**, 576-9.
18 Hake TG. (1874). 'Studies on ether and chloroform, from Prof. Schiff's physiological laboratory.' *Practitioner*, **12**, 241-50.
19 Schiff M. (1894-6). 'Ether et chloroform. De la différence entre l'anesthésie par l'éther et par le chloroform.' Zusätze, 1895. *Gesammelte Beiträge zur Physiologie.* Vol III, p.11. Lausanne; Benda.
20 Block (1882). In discussion following paper by Gluck in Eilfter Congress der Deutschen Gesellschaft für Chirurgie. *Verhandlung der Deutschen Gesellschaft für Chirurgie*, **11**, 108-9.
21 Zesas DG. (1903). 'Über Massage des freigelegten Herzens beim Chloroformkollaps.' *Zentralblatt für Chirurgie*, **30**, 588-90.

22 Watson BA. (1887). 'An experimental study of the effects of puncture of the heart in cases of chloroform narcosis.' *Transactions of the American Surgical Assosciation*, **5**, 275-302. (Discussion, 303-9.)

23 Paget S. (1896). *The surgery of the chest*. Chapter 24. Bristol; Wright. London; Simpkin, Marshall, Hamilton, Kent.

24 Tuffier, Hallion (1898). 'De la compression rythmée du coeur dans la syncope cardiaque par embolie.' *Bulletin de la Société de Chirurgie de Paris*, **24**, 937-9.

25 Igelsrud K. (1904). 'Abdominal hysterectomy; chloroform collapse; massage of the heart; recovery.' Personal communication to WW Keen, published in: Keen WW. (1904). 'A case of total laryngectomy (unsuccessful) and case of abdominal hysterectomy (successful), in both of which massage of the heart for chlorform collapse was employed, with notes of 25 other cases of cardiac massage.' *Therapeutic Gazette*, **28**, 217-30 (see p.220).

26 Starling EA, Lane WA. (1902). 'Reflex inhibition of the heart during administration of ether in which manual compression of the heart was successful in restoring the circulation.' *Lancet*, **2**, 1397.

27 Crile G. Cited in: Keen WW. (1904). See 25, above.

28 Crile GW. (1904). 'Some observations on the surgical physiology of the vascular system.' *Therapeutic Gazette*, **28**, 230-3.

29 Boehm R. (1878). 'V. Arbeiten aus dem pharmakologischen Institute der Universität Dorpat: 13. Ueber Wiederbelebung nach Vergiftungen und Asphyxie.' *Archiv für Experimentelle Pathologie und Pharmakologie*, **8**, 68-101. [External cardiac massage on cats, with some good results.]

30 Koenig F. (1883). *Lehrbuch der Allgemeinen Chirurgie*, pp.60-1. Berlin; Hirschwald.

31 Maas (1892). 'Die Methode der Wiederbelebung bei Herztod nach Chloroformeinathmung.' *Berliner Klinische Wochenschrift*, **29**, 265-8.

32 McKendry JBR. (1962). Letter to the Editor: 'Closed chest cardiac massage: an early case report.' *Canadian Medical Association Journal*, **87**, 305-6.

33 Stout HA. (1957). 'Cardiac arrest: massage without incision.' *Journal of the Oklahoma State Medical Association*, **50**, 112-4.

34 Krogh A. (1938). 'Extracellular and intracellular fluid.' *Acta Medica Scandinavica*, suppl. 90, 9-18.

35 Rainer EH, Bullough J. (1957). 'Respiratory and cardiac arrest during anaesthesia in children.' *British Medical Journal*, **2**, 1024-8.

36 Rainer EH. (1960). Letter to the Editor: 'External cardiac massage.' *British Medical Journal*, **2**, 1880.

37 Jude JR, Kouwenhoven WB, Knickerbocker GG. (1964). 'External cardiac resuscitation.' *Monographs in the Surgical Sciences*, **1**, 59-117.

38 Kouwenhoven WB, Jude JR, Knickerbocker GG. (1960). 'Closed-chest cardiac massage.' *Journal of the American Medical Association*, **173**, 1064-7.

39 Jude JR, Kouwenhoven WB, Knickerbocker GG. (1961) 'A new approach to cardiac resuscitation.' *Annals of Surgery*, **154**, 311-9.

40 Nixon PGF. (1961). 'The arterial pulse in successful closed-chest cardiac massage.' *Lancet*, **2**, 844-6.

41 Tossach W. (1771). 'A man dead in appearance recovered by distending the lungs with air.' *Medical essays and observations*, 5th ed., vol. V, Part II, pp.108-112. Published by a Society in Edinburgh.

42 Hawes W. (Editor) (1774-84). *Transactions of the Royal Humane Society from 1774-1784: with an appendix of miscellaneous observations on suspended animation, to the year 1794*. Printed by Ino. Nichols and sold for the Society by Rivingtons, Dilly,

Johnson and Hookham.

43 Keith A. (1909). 'Three Hunterian Lectures on the mechanism underlying the various methods of artificial respiration practised since the foundation of the Royal Humane Society in 1774.' *Lancet*, **1**, 745-9, 825-8, 895-9.

44 Larrey DJ. (1814). *Memoirs of military surgery, and campaigns of the French armies.* Translated by RW Hall. Vol. I, pp.38-9. Baltimore; Cushing.

45 Beck CS, Pritchard WH, Feil HS. (1947). 'Ventricular fibrillation of long duration abolished by electric shock.' *Journal of the American Medical Association,* **135**, 985-6.

46 Brockman SK, Webb RC, Bahnson HT. (1958). 'Monopolar ventricular stimulation for the control of acute surgically produced heart block.' *Surgery*, **44**, 910-8.

47 Weirich WL, Gott VL, Lillehei CW. (1957). 'The treatment of complete heart block by the combined use of a myocardial electrode and an artificial pacemaker.' *Surgical Forum*, **8**, 360-3.

48 Clark RM, Ross DN, Taylor DG, George RE. (1959). 'Complete heart-block. Successful use of an electronic pacemaker after closure of ventricular septal defect.' *Lancet*, **1**, 392-4. [The surgeon in this case was Russell Brock.]

49 Druss RG, Kornfeld DS. (1967). 'The survivors of cardiac arrest. A psychiatric study.' *Journal of the American Medical Association*, **201**, 291-6.

CHAPTER 6: PULMONARY EMBOLISM

1 Trendelenburg F. (1908). 'Ueber die operative Behandlung der Embolie der Lungenarterie.' *Archiv für Klinische Chirurgie*, **86**, 686-700.

2 Trendelenburg F. (1908). 'Operative interference in embolism of the pulmonary artery.' *Annals of Surgery*, **48**, 772-4.

3 Krüger (1909). 'Ein nach Trendelenburg operierter Fall von Embolie der Lungenarterie.' *Zentralblatt für Chirurgie*, **36**, 757-62.

4 Schumacher (1914). Cited by: Nystrom G. (1930). Experiences with the Trendelenburg operation for pulmonary embolism.' *Annals of Surgery*, **92**, 498-532.

5 Kirschner M. (1924). 'Ein durch die Trendelenburgsche Operation geheilter Fall von Embolie der Art. pulmonalis.' *Archiv für Klinische Chirurgie*, **133**, 312-59.

6 Kirschner M. (1910). 'Die praktischen Ergebnisse der Fascien-Transplantation.' *Archiv für Klinische Chirurgie*, **92**, 888-912.

7 Kirschner M. (1920). 'Ein neues Verfahren der Oesophagoplastik.' *Archiv für Klinische Chirurgie*, **114**, 606-63.

8 Ohsawa T. (1930). 'Über die freie ventro-arco-diaphragmale Thorakolaparotomie bzw. Laparothorakotomie.' *Zentralblatt für Chirurgie*, **57**, 2467-72.

9 Ohsawa T. (1933). 'The surgery of the oesophagus.' *Archiv für Japanische Chirurgie*, **10**, 605-95.

10 Meyer W. (1930). In discussion of: Nyström G. (1930). 'Experiences with the Trendelenburg operation for pulmonary embolism.' *Annals of Surgery*, **92**, 498-532. [On pp.531-2, Meyer records Trendelenburg's gift of instruments to Kirschner.]

11 Obituary (1925). Of Professor Trendelenburg. *British Medical Journal*, **1**, 389-90.

12 Obituary (1925). 'Death of Prof. Trendelenburg.' *Lancet*, **1**, 47-8.

13 Meyer AW. (1930). 'The operative treatment of embolism of the lungs.' *Surgery, Gynecology and Obstetrics*, **50**, 891-8.

14 Meyer AW. (1931). 'Eine weitere (meine vierte) erfolgreiche Lungenembolieoperation. (Neues zur technik.)' *Deutsche Zeitschrift für Chirurgie*, **231**, 586-92.

15 Crafoord C. (1929). 'Two cases of obstructive pulmonary embolism successfully

operated upon.' *Acta Chirurgica Scandinavica*, **64**, 172-86.

16 Nyström G. (1930). 'Experiences with the Trendelenburg operation for pulmonary embolism.' *Annals of Surgery*, **92**, 498-532.

17 Sauerbruch EF. His many unsuccessful attempts at pulmonary embolectomy cited in: Meyer AW. (1930). 'The operative treatment of embolism of the lungs.' *Surgery, Gynecology and Obstetrics*, **50**, 891-8.

18 Crafoord C. Cited in: Benichoux R. (1951). 'The surgical treatment of massive pulmonary embolism. Report of 22 cases of Trendelenburg's operation.' *Journal International de Chirurgie*, **11**, 464-91.

19 Valdoni P. (1936). 'Un caso di embolia dell' arteria polmonare guarito con l'embolectomia.' *Policlinico, Sezione Pratica*, **43**, 911-8.

20 Lewis I. (1939). Trendelenburg's operation for pulmonary embolism. A successful case.' *Lancet*, **1**, 1037-41.

21 Marion P. (1953). 'Coeur pulmonaire aigu. Artériotomie pulmonaire gauche. Embolectomie rétrograde partielle. Guérison.' *Mémoires de l'Académie de Chirurgie*, **79**, 239-42.

22 Ochsner A. (1944). In discussion of: Neuhof H. (1944). 'The problem of embolism of the pulmonary artery. Report of a transcardiac operation.' *Annals of Surgery*, **120**, 488-93. (See p.493.)

23 Steenburg RW, Warren R, Wilson RE, Rudolf LE. (1958). 'A new look at pulmonary embolectomy.' *Surgery, Gynecology and Obstetrics*, **107**, 214-20.

24 Allison PR, Dunnill MS, Marshall R. (1960). 'Pulmonary embolism.' *Thorax*, **15**, 273-83.

25 Cooley DA, Beall SC Jr, Alexander JK. (1961). 'Acute massive pulmonary embolism: successful surgical treatment using temporary cardiopulmonary bypass.' *Journal of the American Medical Association*, **177**, 283-6.

CHAPTER 7: EARLY EXPERIMENTS AND ARGUMENTS

1 Becker O. (1872). 'Ueber die sichtbaren Erscheinungen der lutbewegung in der menschlichen Netzhaut.' *Archiv für Ophthalmologie*, **18**, pt I, 206-96 (see p.279).

2 Klebs E. (1876). 'Ueber Operative Verletzungen der Herzklappen und deren Folgen.' *Prager Medizinische Wochenschrift*, **1**, 29-52.

3 Cohnheim J. (1877). *Vorlesungen über Allgemeine Pathologie*, **I**, p.38. Berlin; Hirschwald.

4 Cohnheim J. (1889). *Lectures on general pathology*, **I**, pp.48-54. Translated from the second German edition by AB McKee. London; The New Sydenham Society.

5 Rosenbach O. (1878). 'Ueber Artificielle Herzklappenfehler.' *Archiv für Experimentelle Pathologie und Pharmakologie*, **9**, 1-30.

6 Milton H. (1897). 'Mediastinal surgery.' *Lancet*, **1**, 872-5.

7 Samways DW. (1898). 'Mitral stenosis: A statistical inquiry.' *British Medical Journal*, **1**, 364-5.

8 Samways DW. (1898). 'Cardiac peristalsis: its nature and effects.' *Lancet*, **1**, 927.

9 Brunton TL. (1867). 'On the use of nitrite of amyl in angina pectoris.' *Lancet*, **2**, 978.

10 Brunton L. (1902). 'Preliminary note on the possibility of treating mitral stenosis by surgical methods.' *Lancet*, **1**, 352.

11 Leading article (1902). 'Surgical operation for mitral stenosis.' *Lancet*, **1**, 461-2.

12 Brunton L. (1902). Letter to the Editor: 'Surgical operation for mitral stenosis.' *Lancet*, **1**, 547.

13 Samways DW. (1902). Letter to the Editor: 'Surgical operation for mitral stenosis.' *Lancet*, **1**, 548.

14 Lane WA. (1902). Letter to the Editor: 'Surgical operation for mitral stenosis.' *Lancet*, **1**, 547.

15 Shaw LE. (1902). Letter to the Editor: 'Surgical operation for mitral stenosis.' *Lancet*, **1**, 619.

16 Fisher T. (1902). Letter to the Editor: 'Surgical operation for mitral stenosis.' *Lancet*, **1**, 547-8.

17 Mackenzie J. (1908). *Diseases of the heart*, pp.220 *et seq.* London; Oxford University Press.

18 Mackenzie J. (1925). *Diseases of the heart*, 4th ed. London; Oxford University Press.

19 Munro JC. (1907). 'Ligation of the ductus arteriosus.' *Annals of Surgery*, **46**, 335-8.

20 Cushing HW. (1905). 'The special field of neurological surgery.' *Bulletin of the Johns Hopkins Hospital*, **16**, 77-87.

21 MacCallum WG. (1906). 'On the teaching of pathological physiology.' *Bulletin of the Johns Hopkins Hospital*, **17**, 251-4.

22 Cushing H, Branch JRB. (1907-08). 'Experimental and clinical notes on chronic valvular lesions in the dog and their possible relation to a future surgery of the cardiac valves.' *Journal of Medical Research*, **17**, 471-85.

23 Bernheim BM. (1909). 'Experimental surgery of the mitral valve.' *Bulletin of the Johns Hopkins Hospital*, **20**, 107-10.

24 Carrel A. (1902). 'La technique opératoire des anastomoses vasculaires et la transplantation des viscères.' *Lyon Médicale*, **98**, 859-64.

25 Carrel A, Guthrie CC. (1906). 'Anastomoses des vaisseaux sanguins.' *XV Congrès International de Médecine* (Lisbon, April 1906). Section de Chirurgie, 238-49.

26 Carrel A, Guthrie CC. (1906). 'Uniterminal and biterminal venous transplantations.' *Surgery, Gynecology and Obstetrics*, **2**, 266-86.

27 Carrel A. (1908). 'Results of the transplantation of blood vessels, organs and limbs.' *Journal of the American Medical Association*, **51**, 1662-7.

28 Dakin HD. (1915). 'On the use of certain antiseptic substances in the treatment of infected wounds.' *British Medical Journal*, **2**, 318-20.

29 Carrel A. (1916). 'Carrel-Dakin solution.' *Journal of the American Medical Association*, **67**, 1777-8.

30 Carrel A. (1910). 'On the experimental surgery of the thoracic aorta and the heart.' *Transactions of the American Surgical Association*, **28**, 243-54.

31 Tuffier T, Carrel A. (1914). 'Patching and section of the pulmonary orifice of the heart.' *Journal of Experimental Medicine*, **20**, 3-8.

32 Carrel A. (1914). 'Experimental operations on the sigmoid valve of the pulmonary artery.' *Journal of Experimental Medicine*, **20**, 9-18.

33 Jeger E. (1913). *Die Chirurgie der Blutgefässe und des Herzens*, pp.325-7. Berlin; Hirschwald.

CHAPTER 8: THE PROBLEM OF THE OPEN THORAX

1 Van Slyke DD. (1917). 'Studies in acidosis. II. A method for the determination of carbon dioxide in solution.' *Journal of Biological Chemistry*, **30**, 347-68.

2 Beecher HK, Murphy AJ. (1950). 'Acidosis during thoracic surgery.' *Journal of Thoracic Surgery*, **19**, 50-70

3 Vesalius A. (1543). *De humani corporis fabrica*, Lib.I, p.200. Basel; Oporinus.

4 Trendelenburg (1871). 'Beitrage zu den Operationen an den Luftwegen.' *Archiv für Klinische Chirurgie*, **12**, 112-33.

5 Macewen W. (1886). 'On the radical cure of oblique inguinal hernia by internal abdominal peritoneal pad, and the restoration of the valved form of the inguinal

canal.' *Annals of Surgery,* **4**, 89-119.

6   Macewen W. (1893). *Pyogenic infective diseases of the brain and spinal cord.* Glasgow; Maclehose.

7   McEwen [*sic*] (1880). 'Transplantation of bone.' Report of a meeting of the Glasgow Pathological and Clinical Society. *British Medical Journal,* **1**, 364.

8   Macewen W. (1906). 'On some points in the surgery of the lung.' *British Medical Journal,* **2**, 1-7. [The 'left pneumonectomy' for tuberculosis took place on April 24, 1895. The patient was still alive in 1940.]

9   Macewen W. (1880). 'Clinical observations on the introduction of tracheal tubes by the mouth instead of performing tracheotomy or laryngotomy.' *British Medical Journal,* **2**, 122-4; 163-5.

10 O'Dwyer J. (1885). 'Intubation of the larynx.' *New York Medical Journal,* **42**, 145-7.

11 O'Dwyer J. (1887). 'Fifty cases of croup in private practice treated by intubation of the larynx, with a description of the method and of the dangers incident thereto.' *Medical Record,* **32**, 557-61.

12 Fell GE. (1887). 'Forced respiration in opium poisoning – its possibilities, and the apparatus best adapted to produce it.' *Buffalo Medical and Surgical Journal,* **27**, 145-57.

13 Matas R. (1900). 'Intralaryngeal insufflation. For the relief of acute surgical pneumothorax. Its history and methods with a description of the latest devices for this purpose.' *Journal of the American Medical Association,* **34**, 1371-5; 1468-73.

14 Kirstein A. (1895). 'Autoskopie des Larynx und der Trachea (Laryngoscopia directa, Euthyskopie, Besichtigung ohne Spiegel).' *Archiv für Laryngologie und Rhinologie,* **3**, 156-64.

15 Killian G. (1898). 'Ueber directe Bronchoskopie.' *Münchener Medizinische Wochenschrift,* **45**, 844-7.

16 Kuhn F. (1902). 'Die pernasale Tubage.' *Münchener Medizinische Wochenschrift,* **49**, 1456-7.

17 Mikulicz-Radecki J von (1886). 'Ein Fall von Resection des carcinomatösen Oesophagus mit plastischem Ersatz des excidirten Stückes.' *Prager Medizinische Wochenschrift,* **11**, 93-4.

18 Sauerbruch (1904). 'Zur Pathologie des offenen Pneumothorax und die Grundlagen meines Verfahrens seiner Ausschaltung.' *Mitteilungen aus den Grenzebietender Medizin und Chirurgie,* **13**, 399-482.

19 Sauerbruch F. (1904). 'Über die Ausschaltung der schädlichen Wirkung des Pneumothorax bei intrathorakalen Operationen.' *Zentralblatt für Chirurgie,* **31**, 146-9.

20 Sauerbruch (1904). 'Ueber die physiologischen und physikalischen Grundlagen bei intrathorakalen Eingriffen in meiner pneumatischen Operationskammer.' *Verhandlungen der Deutschen Gesellschaft für Chirurgie,* **33**, pt II, 105-15.

21 Mikulicz von (1904). 'Chirurgische Erfahrungen über die Sauerbruch'sche Kammer bei Unter- und Ueberdruck.' *Verhandlungen der Deutschen Gesellschaft für Chirurgie,* **33**, pt I, 34-41.

22 Brauer L. (1904). 'Die Ausschaltung der Pneumothoraxfolgen mit Hilfe des Ueberdruckverfahrens.' *Mitteilungen aus den Grenzgebieten der Medizin und Chirurgie,* **13**, 483-500.

23 Brauer L. (1903-04). 'Untersuchungen über die Leber.' *Zeitschrift für Physiologische Chemie,* **40**, 182-214.

24 Brauer (1904). 'Eine Modification des Sauerbruch'schen Verfahrens zur Verhütung der Pneumothoraxfolgen.' *Verhandlungen der Deutschen Gesellschaft für Chirurgie,*

33, pt I, 41-8.

25 Petersen W. (1904). 'Ueber Operationen in der Brusthöhle.' *Verhandlungen der Deutschen Gesellschaft für Chirurgie*, **33**, pt I, 48-52.

26 Sauerbruch, Petersen, Brauer (1904). Discussion. *Verhandlungen der Deutschen Gesellschaft für Chirurgie*, **33**, pt I, 52-4.

27 Sauerbruch EF. (1908). 'Present status of surgery of the thorax and the value of the Sauerbruch negative pressure procedure in the prevention of pneumothorax.' *Journal of the American Medical Association*, **51**, 808-15.

28 Tuffier T. (1897). *Chirurgie du poumon en particulier dans les cavernes tuberculeuses et la gangrène pulmonaire*, p.31. Paris; Masson.

29 Tuffier, Hallion (1896). 'Opérations intrathoraciques avec respiration artificielle par insufflation.' *Comptes Rendus des Séances de la Société de Biologie et de ses Filiales*, **10s**, **3**, 951-3.

30 Quénu, Longuet (1896). 'Note sur quelques recherches expérimentales concernant la chirurgie thoracique.' *Comptes Rendus des Séances de la Société de Biologie et de ses Filiales*, **10s**, **3**, 1007-8.

31 Barthélemy, Dufour (1907). 'L'anesthésie dans la chirurgie de la face.' *Presse Médicale*, **15**, 475-6.

32 Volhard F. (1908). 'Ueber künstliche Atmung durch Ventilation der Trachea und eine einfache Vorrichtung zur rhytmischen künstlichen Atmung.' *Münchener Medizinische Wochenschrift*, **55**, 209-11.

33 Meltzer SJ, Auer J. (1909). 'Continuous respiration without respiratory movements.' *Journal of Experimental Medicine*, **11**, 622-5.

34 Elsberg CA. (1910). 'The value of continuous intratracheal insufflation of air (Meltzer) in thoracic surgery: with description of an apparatus.' *Medical Record*, **77**, 493-5.

35 Tuffier T. (1913). 'Etat actuel de la chirurgie intrathoracique.' *Transactions of the XVII International Medical Congress, London*. Section 7, surgery, pp.247-327.

36 Rowbotham ES, Magill IW. (1921). 'Anaesthetics in the plastic surgery of the face and jaws.' *Proceedings of the Royal Society of Medicine*, **14**, 17-27.

37 Magill IW. (1936). 'Anaesthesia in thoracic surgery, with special reference to lobectomy.' *Proceedings of the Royal Society of Medicine*, **29**, 643-53.

38 Jackson DE. (1915). 'A new method for the production of general analgesia and anaesthesia with a description of the apparatus used.' *Journal of Laboratory and Clinical Medicine*, **1**, 1-12.

39 Waters RM. (1924). 'Clinical scope and utility of carbon dioxid [*sic*] filtration in inhalational anesthesia.' *Anesthesia and Analgesia; Current Researches*, **3**, 20-22, 26.

40 Crafoord C. (1938). 'On the technique of pneumonectomy in man. A critical survey of the experimental and clinical development and a report of the author's material and technique.' *Acta Chirurgica Scandinavica*, **81**, suppl. 54, p.142.

41 Nosworthy MD. (1941). 'Anaesthesia in chest surgery, with special reference to controlled respiration and cyclopropane.' *Proceedings of the Royal Society of Medicine*, **34**, 479-505.

42 Griffith HR, Johnson GE. (1942). 'The use of curare in general anesthesia.' *Anesthesiology*, **3**, 418-20.

43 Bernard C. (1849). 'Action physiologique des venins.' *Comptes Rendus des Séances et Mémoires de la Société de Biologie*, **1**, 90.

44 Pelouze, Bernard C. (1850). 'Reserches sur le curare.' *Comptes Rendus Hebdomadaires des Séances de l'Académie des Sciences*, **31**, 533-7.

CHAPTER 9: THE CURTAIN RISES

1 Tuffier T. (1913). 'Etat actuel de la chirurgie intrathoracique.' *Transactions of the XVII International Medical Congress, London.* Section 7, surgery, pp.247-327 (see p.317).

2 Tuffier (1914). 'Etude expérimentale sur la chirurgie des valvules du coeur.' *Bulletin de l'Académie de Médecine, 3me series,* **71**, 293-5.

3 Tuffier (1921). 'La chirurgie du coeur.' *Cinquième Congrès de la Société International de Chirurgie, Paris, 19-23 Juillet, 1920,* pp.5-75. Bruxelles; Hayez.

4 Doyen E. (1895). *Traitment chirurgical des affections de l'estomac et du duodénum,* p.221. Paris; Rueff.

5 Doyen (1913). Reported in: Association Française de Chirurgie XXVIᵉ Congrès (Paris 6-11 Octobre 1913). *Presse Médicale,* **21**, 860.

6 Doyen (1914). Reported in: XXVI Französischer Chirurgenkongress. Paris, 6.-11. Oktober 1913. *Zentralblatt für Chirurgie,* **41**, 1290.

7 Allen DS, Graham EA. (1922). 'Intracardiac surgery – a new method. Preliminary report.' *Journal of the American Medical Association,* **79**, 1028-30.

8 Allen DS. In discussion following: Cutler EC. (1926). 'The surgical aspect of mitral stenosis.' *Archives of Surgery,* **12**, 212-29.

9 Rhea I, Walker IC. Cited by: Cutler EC. (1948). 'The surgery of the heart and pericardium.' In: *Practice of surgery,* ed. Dean Lewis. Vol. IV, chap. 13, p.38. Hagerstown; Prior. [From internal evidence, Cutler wrote this chapter in 1926.]

10 Cutler EC, Levine SA. (1923). 'Cardiotomy and valvulotomy for mitral stenosis. Experimental observations and clinical notes concerning an operated case with recovery.' *Boston Medical and Surgical Journal,* **188**, 1023-7.

11 Cutler EC, Beck CS. (1929). 'The present status of the surgical procedures in chronic valvular disease of the heart. Final report of all surgical cases.' *Archives of Surgery,* **18**, 403-16.

12 Beck CS, Cutler EC. (1924). 'A cardiovalvulotome.' *Journal of Experimental Medicine,* **40**, 375-9.

13 Cutler EC. (1926). 'The surgical aspect of mitral stenosis.' *Archives of Surgery,* **12**, 212-29.

14 Goodall JS, Rogers L. (1924). 'Some surgical problems of cardiology. Technic of mitralotomy.' *American Journal of Surgery,* **38**, 108-12.

15 Goodall JC, Rogers L. (1924). 'The surgical treatment of mitral obstruction.' *New Zealand Medical Journal,* **23**, 242-6.

16 Obituary (1934). 'J. Strickland Goodall, M.B., F.R.C.S.Ed., M.R.C.P.' *British Medical Journal,* **2**, 1020-1. [Lambert Rogers's note is on p.1021.]

17 Souttar HS. (1925). 'The surgical treatment of mitral stenosis.' *British Medical Journal,* **2**, 603-6.

18 Ellis RH. (1965-6). 'The first trans-auricular valvotomy.' *The London Hospital Gazette,* **68**, Clin. Suppl. pp.x-xiv. [Details of Lilian Hines's history from the clinical notes in The London Hospital Records Department.]

19 Leading article (1923). 'Operative treatment of mitral stenosis.' *British Medical Journal,* **2**, 530-1.

20 Goodall JS, Rogers LC. (1925). Letter to the Editor: 'Surgical treatment of mitral stenosis.' *British Medical Journal,* **2**, 722.

21 Samways DM. (1925). Letter to the Editor: 'The surgical treatment of mitral stenosis.' *British Medical Journal,* **2**, 818.

22 Raven MO. (1925). Letter to the Editor: 'Surgical treatment of mitral stenosis.' *British Medical Journal,* **2**, 722.

23 Sainsbury H. (1925). Letter to the Editor: 'The surgical treatment of mitral stenosis.'

British Medical Journal, **2**, 818.

24 Pribram BO. (1926). 'Die operative Behandlung der Mitralstenose.' *Archiv für Klinische Chirurgie*, **142**, 458-65.

25 Wilson WC. (1930) 'Studies in experimental mitral obstruction in relation to the surgical treatment of mitral stenosis.' *British Journal of Surgery*, **18**, 259-74.

26 Graybiel A, Strieder JW, Boyer NH. (1938). 'An attempt to obliterate the patent ductus arteriosus in a patient with subacute bacterial endocarditis.' *American Heart Journal*, **15**, 621-4.

27 Gross RE, Hubbard JP. (1939). 'Surgical ligation of a patent ductus arteriosus: report of first successful case.' *Journal of the American Medical Association*, **112**, 729-31.

CHAPTER 10: CARDIAC CATHETERIZATION

1 *The Edwin Smith surgical papyrus* (1930). Translated by JH Breasted. Chicago; University of Chicago Press.

2 Morgagni GB. (1761). *De sedibus et causis morborum per anatomen indagatis libri quinque*. Venetiis; Remondiniana.

3 Auenbrugger L. (1761). *Inventum novum ex percussione thoracis humani ut signo abstrusos interni pectoris morbus detegendi*. Vindobonae; Trattner.

4 Corvisart JN. (1808). *Nouvelle méthode pour reconnaître les maladies internes de la poitrine par la percussion de cette cavité, par Auenbrugger*. Translated from the Latin with commentary in *Oeuvres de Corvisart*, vol II. Paris; Méquignon-Marvis.

5 Laennec RTH. (1819). *De l'auscultation médiate ou traité du diagnostic des maladies des poumons et du coeur, fondé principalement sur ce nouveau moyen d'exploration*. Paris; Brosson et Chaudé. [Second edition, 1826.]

6 Waller AD. (1887). 'A demonstration on man of electromotive changes accompanying the heart's beat.' *Journal of Physiology*, **8**, 229-34.

7 Einthoven W. (1903). 'Die galvanometrische Registrirung des menschlichen Elektrokardiogramms, zugleich eine Beurtheilung der Anwendung des Capillar-Elektrometers in der Physiologie.' *Archiv für Gesammte Physiologie* (Pflüger's), **99**, 472-80.

8 Chauveau A, Marey (1863). 'Appareils et expériences cardiographiques démonstration nouvelle du méchanisme des mouvements du coeur par l'emploi des instruments enregistreurs a indications continues.' *Mémoires de l'Académie Impériale de Médecine*, **26**, 268-319.

9 Bernard C. (1879). *Leçons de physiologie opératoire*, pp.277-86. Paris; Baillière.

10 Ehrlich P. (1911). 'Ueber Salvarsan.' *Münchener Medizinische Wochenschrift*, **58**, 2481-6.

11 Bleichröder F. (1912). 'Intraarterielle Therapie.' *Berliner Klinische Wochenschrift*, **49**, 1503-4.

12 Unger E. (1912). 'Bemerkungen zur intraarteriellen Therapie.' *Berliner Klinische Wochenschrift*, **49**, 1504.

13 Löb W. (1912). 'Bemerkungen zur intraarteriellen Therapie.' *Berliner Klinische Wochenschrift*, **49**, 1504-5.

14 Forssmann W. (1929). 'Die Sondierung des Rechten Herzens.' *Klinische Wochenschrift*, **8**, 2085-7; 2287.

15 Forssmann W. (1931). 'Ueber Kontrastdarstellung der Höhlen des lebenden rechten Herzens und der Lungenschlagader.' *Münchener Medizinische Wochenschrift*, **78**, 489-92.

16 Röntgen WC. (1895). 'Ueber eine neue Art von Strahlen.' *Sitzungsberichte der Physikalisch-Medizinischen Gesellschaft*, **29**, 132-41.

17 Moniz E. (1927). 'L'encéphalographie artérielle, son importance dans la localisation des tumeurs cérébrales.' *Revue Neurologique*, **2**, 72-90.

18 Robb GP, Steinberg I. (1938). 'A practical method of visualization of the chambers of the heart, the pulmonary circulation, and the great blood vessels in man.' *Journal of Clinical Investigation*, **17**, 507.

19 Robb GP, Steinberg I. (1939). 'Visualization of the chambers of the heart, the pulmonary circulation, and the great blood vessels in man. A practical method.' *American Journal of Roentgenology*, **41**, 1-17.

20 Cournand A, Ranges HA. (1941). 'Catheterization of the right auricle in man.' *Proceedings of the Society for Experimental Biology and Medicine*, **46**, 462-6.

21 Reboul H, Racine M. (1933). 'La ventriculographie cardiaque expérimentale.' *Presse Médicale*, **41**, 763-7.

22 Ponsdomenech ER, Núñez VB. (1951). 'Heart puncture in man for Diodrast visualization of the ventricular chambers and great arteries. I. Its experimental and anatomophysiological bases and technique.' *American Heart Journal*, **41**, 643-50.

23 Fariñas PL. (1946). 'Retrograde abdominal aortography. A contribution to the study of the abdominal aorta and iliac arteries.' *Radiology*, **47**, 344-8.

24 Seldinger SI. (1953). 'Catheter replacement of the needle in percutaneous arteriography. A new technique.' *Acta Radiologica*, **39**, 368-76.

25 Rousthöi P. (1933). 'Über angiokardiographie.' *Acta Radiologica*, **14**, 419-23.

26 Radner S. (1945). 'An attempt at the roentgenologic visualization of the coronary blood vessels in man.' *Acta Radiologica*, **26**, 497-502.

27 Hoyos JM, del Campo CG. (1948). 'Angiography of the thoracic aorta and coronary vessels.' *Radiology*, **50**, 211-3.

28 di Guglielmo L, Guttadauro M. (1952). 'A roentgenologic study of the coronary arteries in the living.' *Acta Radiologica*, suppl. 97.

29 Nordenström B. (1960). 'Contrast examination of the cardiovascular system during increased intrabronchial pressure.' *Acta Radiologica*, suppl. 200 (see p.97).

30 Arnulf G, Chacornac R. (1958). 'L'artériographie méthodique des artères coronaires grâce à l'utilisation de l'acétylcholine. Données expérimentales et cliniques.' *Lyon Chirurgicale*, **54**, 212-22.

31 Frische LH, Dotter CT. (1959). 'An improved method of coronary arteriography.' *Diseases of the Chest*, **35**, 546-53.

32 Sones FM, Shirey EK. (1962). 'Cine coronary arteriography.' *Modern Concepts of Cardiovascular Disease*, **31**, 735-8.

CHAPTER 11: ANGINA PECTORIS

1 Heberden W. (1806). *Commentaries on the history and cure of diseases*, p.364. 3rd edition. London; Payne. [His description of angina first appeared in 1768 in the *Medical Transactions of the College of Physicians*, **2**, 59-67.]

2 Fothergill J. (1776). 'Case of angina pectoris, with remarks.' *Medical Observations and Inquiries*, **5**, 233-51. Reprinted in: *A complete collection of the medical and philosophical works of John Fothergill...by John Elliot* (1781), pp.508-28. London;Walker.

3 Fothergill J. (1776). 'Farther account of the angina pectoris.' *Medical Observations and Inquiries*, **5**, 252-8. Reprinted in: *A complete collection of the medical and philosophical works of John Fothergill...by John Elliot* (1781), pp. 529-36.

4 Duchenne G-B. (1861). *De l'électrisation localisée et de son application a la pathologie et a la thérapeutique*, pp.961-72. 2nd edition. [First edition 1855.] Paris; Baillière. [Records the different ideas about the origin of angina.]

Sources

5   Hammer A. (1878). 'Ein Fall von thrombotischem Verschlusse einer der Kranzarterien des Herzens.' *Wiener Medizinische Wochenschrift*, **28**, 97-102.

6   Herrick JB. (1912). 'Clinical features of sudden obstruction of the coronary arteries.' *Journal of the American Medical Association*, **59**, 2015-20.

7   Brunton TL. (1867). 'On the use of nitrite of amyl in angina pectoris.' *Lancet*, **2**, 97-8.

8   François-Franck (1899). 'Signification physiologique de la résection du sympathique dans la maladie de Basedow, l'epilepsie, l'idiotie et le glaucome.' *Bulletin de l'Académie de Médicine*, **41**, 565-94.

9   Jonnesco T. (1920). 'Angine de poitrine guérie par la résection du sympathique cervico-thoracique.' *Bulletin de l'Académie de Médecine*, **84**, 93-102.

10 Mayo CH. In discussion following: Lilienthal H. (1925). 'Cervical sympathectomy in angina pectoris. A report of three cases.' *Archives of Surgery*, **10**, 531-43 (see p.541).

11 Earle G, Goodall JS, Handley WS. (1913). Cited by Goodall JS, Rogers L. (1924). Some surgical problems of cardiology. Technic of mitralotomy.' *American Journal of Surgery*, **38**, 108-12.

12 Daniélopolu D. (1923). 'Recherches sur la sensibilité viscérale. Possibilité d'améliorer l'angine de poitrine par la résection des racines postérieurs ou des nerfs spinaux correspondants.' *Bulletins et Mémoires de la Société Médicale des Hôpitaux de Paris*, 3s, **47**, 778-90.

13 Daniélopolu D. (1924). 'The pathology and surgical treatment of angina pectoris.' *British Medical Journal*, **2**, 553-7.

14 Daniélopolu D. (1926). 'The surgical treatment of angina pectoris.' *British Medical Journal*, **1**, 180-3.

15 Cutler EC. (1948). 'The surgery of the heart and pericardium.' In: *Practice of surgery*, ed. Dean Lewis, vol. IV, chap. 13, p.57. Hagerstown; Prior.

16 White JC. (1957). 'Cardiac pain. Anatomic pathways and physiologic mechanisms.' *Circulation*, **16**, 644-55.

17 Levine SA, Cutler EC, Eppinger EC. (1933). 'Thyroidectomy in the treatment of advanced congestive heart failure and angina pectoris.' *New England Journal of Medicine*, **209**, 667-79.

18 Blumgart HL, Levine SA, Berlin DD. (1933). 'Congestive heart failure and angina pectoris. The therapeutic effect of thyroidectomy on patients without clinical or pathologic evidence of thyroid toxicity.' *Archives of Internal Medicine*, **51**, 866-77.

19 Blumgart HL, Freedberg AS, Buka R. (1948). 'Treatment of euthyroid cardiac patients by producing myxedema with radioactive iodine.' *Proceedings of the Society for Experimental Biology and Medicine*, **67**, 190-1.

20 Blumgart HL, Freedberg AS. (1952). 'The heart and the thyroid: with particular reference to I[131] treatment of heart disease.' *Circulation*, **6**, 222-37.

CHAPTER 12: MYOCARDIAL REVASCULARIZATION

1   Beck CS. (1935). The development of a new blood supply to the heart by operation.' *Annals of Surgery*, **102**, 801-13.

2   Thorel C. (1903). 'Pathologie der Kreislauforgane.' *Ergebnisse der Allgemeinen Pathologie und Pathologischen Anatomie*. **9**, 559-1116.

3   O'Shaughnessy L. (1936). 'An experimental method of providing a collateral circulation to the heart.' *British Journal of Surgery*, **23**, 665-70.

4   O'Shaughnessy L. (1937). Report of a meeting of the West London Medico-Chirurgical Society. *Lancet*, **2**, 1378.

5   O'Shaughnessy L. (1937). 'Surgical treatment of cardiac ischaemia.' *Lancet*, **1**,

185-94.

6   Davies DT, Mansell HE, O'Shaughnessy L. (1938). 'Surgical treatment of angina pectoris and allied conditions.' *Lancet*, **1**, 1-10; 76-82.

7   Lezius A (1937). 'Die künstliche Blutversorgung des Herzmuskels.' *Archiv für Klinische Chirurgie*, **189**, 342-6.

8   Thompson SA, Raisbeck MJ. (1942). 'Cardio-pericardiopexy; the surgical treatment of coronary arterial disease by the establishment of adhesive pericarditis.' *Annals of Internal Medicine*, **16**, 495-520.

9   Thompson SA. (1957). 'The surgical treatment of coronary heart disease.' *American Practitioner and Digest of Treatment*, **8**, 406-8.

10 Harken DE, Black H, Dickson JF, Wilson HE. (1955). 'De-epicardialization: A simple, effective treatment for angina pectoris.' *Circulation*, **12**, 955-62.

11 Beck CS, Leighninger DS. (1954). 'Operations for coronary artery disease.' *Journal of the American Medical Association*, **156**, 1226-33.

12 Gross L, Blum L, Silverman G. (1937). 'Experimental attempts to increase the blood supply to the dog's heart by means of coronary sinus occlusion.' *Journal of Experimental Medicine*, **65**, 91-108.

13 Fauteux M. (1946). 'Surgical treatment of angina pectoris. Experiences with ligation of the great cardiac vein and pericoronary neurectomy.' *Annals of Surgery*, **124**, 1041-6.

14 Pratt FH. (1898). 'The nutrition of the heart through the vessels of Thebesius and the coronary veins.' *American Journal of Physiology*, **1**, 86-103

15 Roberts JT. (1943). 'Experimental studies on the nourishment of the left ventricle by the lumenal (Thebesial) vessels.' *Federation Proceedings*, **2**, 90.

16 Roberts JT, Browne RS, Roberts G. (1943). 'Nourishment of the myocardium by way of the coronary sinus.' *Federation Proceedings* **2**, 90.

17 Roberts JT, Spencer FD Jr, Browne RS. (1943). 'Drainage of the myocardium by cardial lumenal (Thebesian) vessels of the left ventricle.' *Federation Proceedings*, **2**, 90-1.

18 Beck CS, Stanton E, Batiuchok W, Leiter E. (1948). 'Revascularization of heart by graft of systemic artery into coronary sinus.' *Journal of the American Medical Association*, **137**, 436-42.

19 Battezzati M, Tagliaferro A, De Marchi G. (1955). 'La legatura della due arterie mammarie interne nei disturbi di vascolarizzazione del miocardio.' *Minerva Medica*, **46ii**, pt 2, 1178-88.

20 Zoja, Cesa-Bianchi. Cited by Battezzati *et al.* (Ref. 19 above).

21 Fieschi D. Cited by Battezzati *et al.* (Ref. 19 above).

22 De Marchi G, Battezzati M, Tagliaferro A. (1956). 'Influenze della legatura delle arterie mammarie interne sulla insufficienza miocardica.' *Minerva Medica*, **47ii**, pt 1, 1184-95.

23 Goldman A, Greenstone SM, Preuss FS, Strauss SH, Chang E. (1956). 'Experimental methods for producing a collateral circulation to the heart directly from the left ventricle.' *Journal of Thoracic Surgery*, **31**, 364-74.

24 Massino C, Boffi L. (1957). 'Myocardial revascularization by a new method of carrying blood directly from the left ventricular cavity into the coronary circulation.' *Journal of Thoracic Surgery*, **34**, 257-64.

25 Day SB, Lillehei CW. (1959). 'Experimental basis for a new operation for coronary artery disease: A left atrial-pulmonary artery shunt to encourage the development of interarterial intercoronary anastomoses.' *Surgery*, **45**, 487-95

26 Beck CS. (1957). 'Coronary artery disease – physiologic concepts – surgical opera-

tion.' *Annals of Surgery*, **145**, 439-60.

27 Vineberg AM. (1946). 'Development of an anastomosis between the coronary vessels and a transplanted internal mammary artery.' *Canadian Medical Association Journal*, **55**, 117-9.

28 Vineberg AM. (1954). 'Internal mammary artery implant in the treatment of angina pectoris: A three year follow up.' *Canadian Medical Association Journal*, **70**, 367-78.

29 Vineberg A, Munro DD, Cohen H, Buller W. (1955). 'Four years' clinical experience with internal mammary artery implantation in treatment of human coronary artery insufficiency including additional experimental studies.' *Journal of Thoracic Surgery*, **29**, 1-36.

30 Vineberg A, Pifarre R, Mercier C. (1962). 'An operation designed to promote the growth of new coronary arteries, using a detached omental graft: A preliminary report.' *Canadian Medical Association Journal*, **86**, 1116-8.

31 Smith S, Beasley M, Hodes R, Hall H, Biel E, Huth EW. (1957). 'Auxiliary myocardial vascularization by prosthetic graft implantation.' *Surgery, Gynecology and Obstetrics*, **104**, 263-8.

32 Vineberg A, Walker J. (1964). 'The surgical treatment of coronary artery heart disease by internal mammary artery implantation: report of 140 cases followed up to 13 years.' *Diseases of the Chest*, **45**, 190-206.

33 Sones FM, Shirey EK. (1962). 'Cine coronary arteriography.' *Modern Concepts of Cardiovascular Disease*, **31**, 735-8.

CHAPTER 13: CORONARY OCCLUSION

1 Carrel A. (1910). 'On the experimental surgery of the thoracic aorta and the heart.' *Transactions of the American Surgical Association*, **28**, 243-54.

2 Blumgart HL, Schlesinger MJ, Davis D. (1940). 'Studies on the relation of the clinical manifestations of angina pectoris, coronary thrombosis, and myocardial infarction to the pathologic findings.' *American Heart Journal*, **19**, 1-91.

3 Schlesinger MJ, Zoll PM. (1941). 'Incidence and localization of coronary artery occlusions.' *Archives of Pathology*, **32**, 178-88.

4 Gross RE. (1945). 'Surgical correction for coarctation of the aorta.' *Surgery*, **18**, 673-8.

5 Crafoord C, Nylin G. (1945). 'Congenital coarctation of the aorta and its surgical treatment.' *Journal of Thoracic Surgery*, **14**, 347-61.

6 Gross RE, Bill AH, Peirce EC. (1949). 'Methods for preservation and transplantation of arterial grafts. Observations on arterial grafts in dogs. Report of transplantation of preserved grafts in 9 human cases.' *Surgery, Gynecology and Obstetrics*, **88**, 689-701.

7 Murray G. (1953). 'Resection of atheromatous segments of coronary arteries and graft replacement.' Read before the *Congress of the International Society of Angiology*. Lisbon, September, 1953. [Not published in the proceedings.]

8 Murray G, Porcheron R, Hilario J, Roschlau W. (1954). 'Anastomosis of a systemic artery to the coronary.' *Canadian Medical Association Journal*, **71**, 594-7.

9 Demikhov VP. (1962). *Experimental transplantation of vital organs*, ch. 6, p.220-7. Translated by B Haigh. New York; Consultants Bureau.

10 Absolon KB, Aust JB, Varco RL, Lillehei CW. (1956). 'Surgical treatment of occlusive coronary artery disease by endarterectomy or anastomotic replacement.' *Surgery, Gynecology and Obstetrics*, **103**, 180-5.

11 May AM. (1957). 'Coronary endarterectomy. Curettement of coronary arteries in dogs.' *American Journal of Surgery*, **93**, 969-73.

12 Bailey CP, May A. (1957). 'Survival after coronary endarterectomy in man'. *Journal of the American Medical Association,* **164**, 641-6.

13 May AM, Bailey CP. (1958). 'Coronary endarterectomy.' *Journal of the International Journal of Surgeons,* **29**, 160-3.

14 Bailey CP, Musser BG, Lemmon WM. (1958). 'Appraisal of current surgical procedures for coronary heart disease.' *Progress in Cardiovascular Diseases,* **1**, 219-36.

15 Thal AP, Richards LS, Greenspan R, Murray MJ. (1958). 'Arteriographic studies of the coronary arteries in ischemic heart disease.' *Journal of the American Medical Association,* **168**, 2104-9.

16 Sones FM, Shirey EK. (1962) 'Cine coronary arteriography.' *Modern Concepts of Cardiovascular Disease,* **31**, 735-8.

17 Senning Å. (1961). 'Strip grafting in coronary arteries. Report of a case.' *Journal of Thoracic and Cardiovascular Surgery,* **41**, 542-9.

18 Sawyer PN, Kaplitt MJ, Sobel S, Di Maio D. (1967). 'Application of gas endarterectomy to atherosclerotic peripheral vessels and coronary arteries: Clinical and experimental results.' *Circulation,* (suppl. 1), **35**, **36**, 163-8.

19 Nardi GL, Shaw RS. (1963). 'Emergency coronary endarterectomy.' *Diseases of the Chest,* **44**, 193-6.

20 Favaloro R. (1970). *The surgical treatment of arteriosclerosis,* ch. 5, pp.39-66. Baltimore; Williams and Wilkins (see p.47).

21 Grüntzig A. (1978) Letter to the Editor: 'Transluminal dilatation of coronary-artery stenosis.' *Lancet,* **1**, 263.

CHAPTER 14: CARDIAC ANEURYSM

1 Sauerbruch F. (1931). 'Erfolgreiche operative Beseitigung eines Aneurysma der rechten Herzkammer.' *Archiv für Klinische Chirurgie,* **167**, 586-8.

2 Sauerbruch F. (1937). Report of a meeting of the West London Medico-Chirurgical Society. *Lancet,* **2**, 1377-8.

3 Beck CS. (1944). 'Operation for aneurysm of the heart.' *Annals of Surgery,* **120**, 34-40.

4 Beck CS. (1929). 'The effect of surgical solution of chlorinated soda (Dakin's solution) in the pericardial cavity.' *Archives of Surgery,* **18**, 1659-71.

5 Niedner FF. (1955). 'Die chirurgische Behandlung des Herzaneurysmas.' *Thorax-chirurgie,* **3**, 93-111.

6 D'Allaines F de G, Mouquin M, Hatt P-Y, Sauvan R, Fanjoux J, Latscha B-I. (1956). 'Opération plastique d'un anévrysme du coeur. Étude électrocardiographique péropératoire.' *Archives des Maladies du Coeur et des Vaisseaux,* **49**, 193-200.

7 Murray G. (1947). 'The pathophysiology of the cause of death from coronary thrombosis.' *Annals of Surgery,* **126**, 523-34.

8 Heimbecker RO, Chen C, Hamilton N, Murray DWG. (1967). 'Surgery for massive myocardial infarction. An experimental study of emergency infarctectomy.' *Surgery,* **61**, 51-8.

9 Likoff W, Bailey CP. (1955). 'Ventriculoplasty: excision of myocardial aneurysm.' *Journal of the American Medical Association,* **158**, 915-20.

10 Bailey CP, Bolton HE, Nichols H, Gilman RA. (1958). 'Ventriculoplasty for cardiac aneurysm.' *Journal of Thoracic Surgery,* **35**, 37-64.

11 Cooley DA, Collins HA, Morris GC Jr, Chapman DW. (1958). 'Ventricular aneurysm after myocardial infarction. Surgical excision with use of temporary cardiopulmonary bypass.' *Journal of the American Medical Association,* **167**, 557-60.

12 Lillehei CW, Levy MJ, DeWall RA, Warden HE. (1962). 'Resection of myocardial

aneurysms after infarction during temporary cardiopulmonary bypass.' *Circulation*, **26**, 206-17.

CHAPTER 15: FIELDS OF BATTLE
1   Bland-Sutton J. (1919). 'Missiles as emboli.' *Lancet*,**1**, 773-5.
2   Makins GH. (1922). 'Injuries to the pericardium and heart.' In: *History of the Great War medical services. Surgery of the war*, ed. Macpherson WG, Bowlby AA, Wallace C, English C. Vol. 1, ch. 16, pp.431-75. London; HMSO.
3   Yates JL. (1927). 'Wounds of the chest.' In: *The Medical Department of the United States Army in the World War.* Vol. XI Surgery. Part 1, p.393. Washington; Government Printing Office.
4   Ballance C. (1920). 'The Bradshaw Lecture on: The surgery of the heart.' *Lancet*, **1**, 1-5; 73-9; 134-9.
5   Hartmann H. Cited by: Ballance C. (1920). (Ref. 4 above.)
6   Deneke. Cited by: Ballance C. (1920). (Ref. 4 above.)
7   Duval P, Barnsby H. (1918). 'Balle de fusil mobile dans le segment péricardique de la veine cave inférieure. Extraction par péricardotomie et incision de la veine cave.' *Bulletin et Mémoires de la Société de Chirurgie*, **44**, 1138-42.
8   Fraser J. (1917). 'A case of suture of a perforating wound of the heart.' *Edinburgh Medical Journal*, **18**, 47-8.
9   Sampson HH. Cited in: Makins GH. (1922). (Ref. 2 above, pp.470-1.)
10 Moynihan B. (1919-1920). 'The surgery of the chest in relation to retained projectiles.' *British Journal of Surgery*, **7**, 444-86.
11 Head JR. In discussion following: Harken DE. (1947). (Ref. 19 below.)
12 Singleton AO. (1933). 'Wounds of the heart and a discussion of the causes of death.' *American Journal of Surgery*, **20**, 515-41.
13 Bigger IA. (1939). 'Heart wounds. A report of seventeen patients operated upon in the Medical College of Virginia Hospitals and a discussion of the treatment and prognosis.' *Journal of Thoracic Surgery*, **8**, 239-53.
14 Strieder JW. (1939). 'Stab wound of the heart. Report of a case treated conservatively.' *Journal of Thoracic Surgery*, **8**, 576-7.
15 United States Department of the Army (1942). *Technical manual TM 8-210: Guides to therapy for medical officers*, p.185. Washington; Government Printing Office. Cited by: Blalock A, Ravitch MM. (1943). (Ref. 16 below.)
16 Blalock A, Ravitch MM. (1943). 'A consideration of the nonoperative treatment of cardiac tamponade resulting from wounds of the heart.' *Surgery*, **14**, 157-62.
17 Brock RC. (1953). In: *History of the Second World War. Surgery*, ed. Cope Z, ch. 13, 'Thoracic surgery', pp.545-58. London; HMSO (see p.558).
18 Samson PC. (1948). 'Battle wounds and injuries of the heart and pericardium. Experience in forward hospitals.' *Annals of Surgery*, **127**, 1127-49.
19 Harken DE. (1947). 'The removal of foreign bodies from the pericardium and heart. A moving picture demonstration.' *Journal of Thoracic Surgery*, **16**, 701-4.
20 Duval P. (1919). 'L'extraction des projectiles cardio-pulmonaires.' *Bulletin et Mémoires de la Société de Chirurgie*, **45**, 863-7. [Deals mainly with radiological localization.]
21 Makins GH. (1922). See ref. 2 above, pp.472-3.
22 Miscall L. In discussion following: Harken DE. (1947). (Ref. 19 above.)

CHAPTER 16: BLUE BABIES AND SOME OTHERS
1   Crafoord C, Nylin G. (1945). 'Congenital coarctation of the aorta and its surgical

treatment. *Journal of Thoracic Surgery*, **14**, 347-61.

2   Gross RE, Hufnagel CA. (1945). 'Coarctation of the aorta. Experimental studies regarding its surgical correction.' *New England Journal of Medicine*, **233**, 287-93.

3   Gross RE. (1945). 'Surgical correction for coarctation of the aorta.' *Surgery*, **18**, 673-8.

4   Blalock A, Park EA. (1944). 'The surgical treatment of experimental coarctation (atresia) of the aorta.' *Annals of Surgery*, **119**, 445-56.

5   Clagett OT. (1947). 'Coarctation of the aorta: surgical aspects.' *Proceedings of the Staff Meetings of the Mayo Clinic*, **22**, 131-5.

6   Murray G. (1950). 'Vascular surgery.' In: *British surgical practice*, ed. Carling ER, Ross JP. Vol. 8, pp.489-528. London; Butterworth.

7   Gross RE. (1950). 'Coarctation of the aorta. Surgical treatment of one hundred cases.' *Circulation*, **1**, 41-55.

8   Blalock A, Taussig HB. (1945). 'The surgical treatment of malformations of the heart in which there is pulmonary stenosis or pulmonary atresia.' *Journal of the American Medical Association*, **128**, 189-202.

9   Fallot ELA. (1888). 'Contribution à l'anatomie pathologique de la maladie bleue (cyanose cardiaque). *Marseille-Médicale*, **25**, 77-93; 138-58; 207-23; 270-86; 341-54; 403-20.

10 Potts WJ, Smith S, Gibson S. (1946). 'Anastomosis of the aorta to a pulmonary artery.' *Journal of the American Medical Association*, **132**, 627-31.

11 Sellors TH. (1967). 'The genesis of heart surgery.' *British Medical Journal*, **1**, 385-93.

12 Lillehei CW, Cohen M, Warden HE, Read RC, Aust JB, De Wall RA, Varco RL. (1955). 'Direct vision intracardiac surgical correction of the tetralogy of Fallot, pentalogy of Fallot, and pulmonary atresia defects. Report of first ten cases.' *Annals of Surgery*, **142**, 418-45.

13 Kirklin JW, Ellis FH, McGoon DC, DuShane JW, Swan HJC. (1959). 'Surgical treatment for the tetralogy of Fallot by open intracardiac repair.' *Journal of Thoracic Surgery*, **37**, 22-51.

14 Lillehei CW. In discussion following: Kirklin JW, Ellis FH, McGoon DC, DuShane JW, Swan HJC. (1959). (Ref. 13 above.)

15 Rasmussen RA. In discussion following: Kirklin JW, Ellis FH, McGoon DC, DuShane JW, Swan HJC. (1959). (Ref. 13 above.)

16 Brock RC. (1948). 'Pulmonary valvotomy for the relief of congenital pulmonary stenosis. Report of three cases.' *British Medical Journal*, **1**, 1121-6.

17 Sellors TH. (1948). 'Surgery of pulmonary stenosis. A case in which the pulmonary valve was successfully divided.' *Lancet*,**1**, 988-9.

18 Campbell M. (1958). 'Late results of operation for Fallot's tetralogy.' *British Medical Journal*, **2**, 1175-84..

19 Brock RC. (1949). 'The surgery of pulmonary stenosis.' *British Medical Journal*, **2**, 399-406.

20 Tuffier T, Carrel A. (1914). 'Patching and section of the pulmonary orifice of the heart.' *Journal of Experimental Medicine*, **20**, 3-8.

21 Hufnagel CA. (1950). 'A method for the correction of pulmonary stenosis.' *Surgical Forum*, **1**, 246-50.

22 Kirklin JW, Openshaw CR, Tompkins RG. (1953). 'Surgical treatment of infundibular stenosis with intact ventricular septum. Report of a case.' *Annals of Surgery*, **137**, 228-31.

23 Temesvári A. (1958). 'A method of treating infundibular pulmonary stenosis.' *Thorax*, **13**, 165-8.

24 Gross RE. Cited by: Ross JK. (1961). 'The fate of autogenous tissue grafts in the heart.' *Annals of the Royal College of Surgeons of England*, **29**, 275-99.

CHAPTER 17: HOLES IN THE HEART

1 Murray G. (1948). 'Closure of defects in cardiac septa.' *Annals of Surgery*, **128**, 843-53.

2 Blakemore A. In discussion of: Murray G. (1948). (Ref. 1 above.)

3 Cohn R. (1947). 'An experimental method for the closure of inter-auricular septal defects in dogs.' *American Heart Journal*, **33**, 453-7.

4 Swan H. (1953). 'Surgical closure of interauricular septal defects.' *Journal of the American Medical Association*, **151**, 792-4.

5 Swan H, Stewart BD. (1953). 'A modified button technique for the closure of experimental interauricular septal defects.' *Journal of Thoracic Surgery*, **25**, 397-401.

6 Bailey CP, Downing DF, Geckeler GD, Likoff W, Goldberg H, Scott JC, Janton O, Redondo-Ramirez HP. (1952). 'Congenital interatrial communications: clinical and surgical considerations with a description of a new surgical technic: atrio-septo-pexy.' *Annals of Internal Medicine*, **37**, 888-920.

7 Shumacker HB. (1953). 'Surgical repair of atrial septal defects.' *Annals of Surgery*, **138**, 404-14.

8 Gross RE, Pomeranz AA, Watkins E, Goldsmith EI. (1952). 'Surgical closure of defects of the interauricular septum by use of an atrial well.' *New England Journal of Medicine*, **247**, 455-60.

9 Hufnagel CA, Gillespie JF. (1951). 'Closure of interauricular septal defects.' *Bulletin of the Georgetown University Medical Center*, **4**, 137.

10 Søndergaard T. (1954). 'Closure of atrial septal defects. Report of three cases.' *Acta Chirurgica Scandinavica*, **107**, 492-8.

11 Lewis FJ, Taufic M. (1953). 'Closure of atrial septal defects with the aid of hypothermia; experimental accomplishments and report of one successful case.' *Surgery*, **33**, 52-9.

12 Bailey CP, Lacy MH, Neptune WB, Weller R, Arvanitis CS, Karasic J. (1952). 'Experimental and clinical attempts at correction of interventricular septal defects.' *Annals of Surgery*, **136**, 919-36.

CHAPTER 18: MITRAL STENOSIS

1 Beck CS. (1954). 'The technique of opening the stenotic mitral valve.' *Journal of the American Medical Association*, **156**, 1400-1.

2 Cutler EC, Beck CS. (1929). 'The present status of the surgical procedures in chronic valvular disease of the heart. Final report of all surgical cases.' *Archives of Surgery*, **18**, 403-16.

3 Wilson WC. (1930). 'Studies in experimental mitral obstruction in relation to the surgical treatment of mitral stenosis.' *British Journal of Surgery*, **18**, 259-74.

4 Murray G, Wilkinson FR, MacKenzie R. (1938). 'Reconstruction of the valves of the heart.' *Canadian Medical Association Journal*, **38**, 317-9.

5 Murray G. (1950). 'Treatment of mitral stenosis by resection and replacement of valve under direct vision.' *Archives of Surgery*, **61**, 903-12.

6 Smithy HG. (1948). 'The control of arrhythmias occurring during operation upon the valves of the heart: experimental and clinical observations.' *Southern Surgeon*, **14**, 611-8.

7 Smithy HG, Boone JA, Stallworth JM. (1950). 'Surgical treatment of constrictive valvular disease of the heart.' *Surgery, Gynecology and Obstetrics*, **90**, 175-92.

Sources

8 Bailey CP. (1955). *Surgery of the heart*, p.487. London; Kimpton. [Follow-up of Smithy's patients.]

9 Deaths (1948). 'Horace Gilbert Smithy Jr.' *Journal of the American Medical Association*, **138**, 1250.

10 Bailey CP. (1949). 'Surgical treatment of mitral stenosis. Mitral commissurotomy.' *Diseases of the Chest*, **15**, 377-97.

11 Harken DE, Glidden EM. (1943). 'Experiments in intracardiac surgery. II. Intracardiac visualization.' *Journal of Thoracic Surgery*, **12**, 566-72.

12 Harken DE, Ellis LB, Ware PE, Norman LR. (1948). 'The surgical treatment of mitral stenosis. I. Valvuloplasty.' *New England Journal of Medicine*, **239**, 801-9.

13 Harken DE, Ellis LB, Norman LR. (1950). 'The surgical treatment of mitral stenosis. II. Progress in developing a controlled valvuloplastic technique.' *Journal of Thoracic Surgery*, **19**, 1-15.

14 Baker C, Brock RC, Campbell M. (1950) 'Valvulotomy for mitral stenosis. Report of six successful cases.' *British Medical Journal*, **1**, 1283-93.

15 Lutembacher R. (1916). 'De la sténose mitrale avec communication interauriculaire.' *Archives des Maladies du Coeur des Vaisseaux et du Sang*, **9**, 237-60.

16 Jarotzky A. (1926). 'Zur Frage der Operation im Innern des Herzens bei Stenosis mitralis.' *Zentralblatt für Chirurgie*, **53**, 140-2

17 Blalock A, Hanlon CR. (1948). 'Interatrial septal defect – its experimental production under direct vision without interruption of the circulation.' *Surgery, Gynecology and Obstetrics*, **87**, 183-7.

18 Bailey CP, Glover RP, O'Neill TJE. (1950). 'The surgery of mitral stenosis.' *Journal of Thoracic Surgery*, **19**, 16-49.

19 Cases from the Medical Grand Rounds Massachusetts General Hospital (1947-48). 'Case 53. A venous shunt for marked mitral stenosis.' *American Practitioner and Digest of Treatment*, **2**, 756-61. [Sweet and Bland's patient, Mrs Olivia CB.]

20 Sweet RH, Bland EF. (1949). 'The surgical relief of congestion in the pulmonary circulation in cases of severe mitral stenosis. Preliminary report of six cases treated by means of anastomosis between the pulmonary and systemic venous systems.' *Annals of Surgery*, **130**, 384-97.

21 D'Allaines, Lenègre J, Dubost C, Mathivat A, Scebat L. (1949). 'L'anastomose veine pulmonaire–veine azygos dans le rétrécissement mitral à propos d'un cas opéré avec succès.' *Archives des Maladies du Coeur et des Vaisseaux*, **42**, 456-61.

22 Blalock A. In discussion of: Sweet RH, Bland EF. (1949). (Ref. 20 above.)

23 Carrel A. (1910). 'On the experimental surgery of the thoracic aorta and the heart.' *Transactions of the American Surgical Association*, **28**, 243-54.

24 Jeger E. (1913). *Die Chirurgie der Blutgefässe und des Herzens*, pp.325-7. Berlin; Hirschwald.

25 Goodall JC, Rogers L. (1924). 'The surgical treatment of mitral obstruction.' *New Zealand Medical Journal*, **23**, 242-6.

26 Lowther CP, Turner RWD. (1962). 'Deterioration after mitral valvotomy.' *British Medical Journal*, **1**, 1027-36; 1102-7.

27 Bailey CP, Morse DP. (1959). 'Recurrent mitral stenosis: an increasingly common occurrence due to inadequate mobilization of the valve.' *Journal of the International College of Surgeons*, **31**, 8-23.

28 Dubost MC. (1954). 'Présentation d'un nouvel instrument dilateur pour commissurotomie mitrale.' *Presse Médicale*, **62**, 253. [In a report of a meeting of the Société Française de Cardiologie.]

29 Logan A, Turner R. (1959). 'Surgical treatment of mitral stenosis with particular ref-

erence to the transventricular approach with a mechanical dilator.' *Lancet*, **2**, 874-80.

CHAPTER 19: MITRAL INCOMPETENCE

1   Cutler EC. (1948). 'The surgery of the heart and pericardium., In: *Practice of surgery*, ed. Dean Lewis. Vol. IV, ch. 13, p.33. Hagerstown; Prior. [As noted in the references to Chapter 9, internal evidence would suggest that Cutler wrote the chapter in 1926.]
2   Murray G. (1950). 'Treatment of mitral valve stenosis by resection and replacement of valve under direct vision.' *Archives of Surgery*, **61**, 903-12.
3   Templeton JY, Gibbon JH. (1949) 'Experimental reconstruction of cardiac valves by venous and pericardial grafts.' *Annals of Surgery*, **129**, 161-76.
4   Bailey CP, O'Neill TJE, Glover RP, Jamison WL, Ramirez HPR. (1951). 'Surgical repair of mitral insufficiency. (A preliminary report.)' *Diseases of the Chest*, **19**, 125-37.
5   Logan A, Turner R. (1952). 'The diagnosis of mitral incompetence accompanying mitral stenosis. Review of eleven cases treated surgically.' *Lancet*, **2**, 593-8.
6   Bailey CP, Jamison WL, Bakst AE, Bolton HE, Nichols HT, Gemeinhardt W. (1954). 'The surgical correction of mitral insufficiency by the use of pericardial grafts.' *Journal of Thoracic Surgery*, **28**, 551-603.
7   Harken DE, Black H, Ellis LB, Dexter L. (1954). 'The surgical correction of mitral insufficiency.' *Journal of Thoracic Surgery*, **28**, 604-27.
8   Kay EB, Cross FS. (1955). 'Surgical treatment of mitral insufficiency.' *Journal of Thoracic Surgery*, **29**, 618-20.
9   Kay EB, Cross FS. (1955). 'Surgical treatment of mitral insufficiency.' *Surgery*, **37**, 697-706.
10 Davila JC, Mattson WW Jr, O'Neill THE, Glover RP. (1954). 'A method for the surgical correction of mitral insufficiency. I. Preliminary communication.' *Surgery, Gynecology and Obstetrics*, **98**, 407-12.
11 Glover RP, Davila JC. (1957). 'The treatment of mitral insufficiency by the purse-string technique. Initial clinical application.' *Journal of Thoracic Surgery* **33**, 75-101.
12 Nichols HT. (1957). 'Mitral insufficiency: treatment by polar cross-fusion of the mitral annulus fibrosus.' *Journal of Thoracic Surgery*, **33**, 102-22.
13 Nichols HT, Uricchio JF. (1958). 'Further experiences with the surgical correction of rheumatic mitral regurgitation by cross polar plication.' *Circulation*, **18**, 763. [Abstract of paper to 31st Scientific Sessions.]
14 De Wall RA, Warden HE, Lillehei CW, Varco RL. (1956). 'A prosthesis for the palliation of mitral insufficiency.' *Diseases of the Chest*, **30**, 133-40.
15 Lillehei CW, Gott VL, De Wall RA, Varco RL. (1958). 'The surgical treatment of stenotic or regurgitant lesions of the mitral and aortic valves by direct vision utilizing a pump-oxygenator.' *Journal of Thoracic Surgery*, **35**, 154-91.
16 Murray G. (1956). 'Homologous aortic-valve-segment transplants as surgical treatment for aortic and mitral insufficiency.' *Angiology*, **7**, 466-71.

CHAPTER 20: AORTIC STENOSIS

1   Tuffier T. (1913). 'Etat actuel de la chirurgie intrathoracique.' *Transactions of the XVII International Medical Congress, London*. Section 7, surgery, pp.247-327 (see p.317).
2   Brock RC. (1950). 'The arterial route to the aortic and pulmonary valves. The mitral route to the aortic valve.' *Guy's Hospital Reports*, **99**, 236-46.
3   Souttar HS. (1925). 'The surgical treatment of mitral stenosis.' *British Medical Journal*, **2**, 603-6.
4   Brock RC. (1957). 'Surgical treatment of aortic stenosis.' *British Medical Journal*, **1**,

1019-28.

5   Smithy HG, Parker EF. (1947). 'Experimental aortic valvotomy. A preliminary report.' *Surgery, Gynecology and Obstetrics*, **84**, 625-8.

6   Bailey CP. (1955). *Surgery of the heart*, ch. 21. London; Kimpton (see pp.738-45).

7   Bailey CP, Glover RP, O'Neill TJE, Ramirez HPR. (1950). 'Experiences with the experimental surgical relief of aortic stenosis. A preliminary report.' *Journal of Thoracic Surgery*, **20**, 516-41.

8   Bailey CP, Ramirez HPR, Larzelere HB. (1952). 'Surgical treatment of aortic stenosis.' *Journal of the American Medical Association*, **150**, 1647-52.

9   Bailey CP, Bolton HE, Jamison WL, Larzelere HB. (1953). 'Commissurotomy for aortic stenosis.' *Journal of the International College of Surgeons*, **20**, 393-408.

10 Harken DE, Black H, Taylor WJ, Thrower WB, Soroff HS. (1958). 'The surgical correction of calcific aortic stenosis in adults. Results in the first 100 consecutive transaortic valvuloplasties.' *Journal of Thoracic Surgery*, **36**, 759-76.

11 Clowes GHA, Neville WE. (1954). 'Experimental exposure of the aortic valve. Laboratory studies and a clinical trial.' *Surgical Forum*, **5**, 39-45.

12 Swan H, Kortz AB. (1956). 'Direct vision trans-aortic approach to the aortic valve during hypothermia. Experimental observations and report of successful clinical case.' *Annals of Surgery*, **144**, 205-14.

13 Lillehei CW, DeWall RA, Gott VL, Varco RL. (1956). 'The direct vision correction of calcific aortic stenosis by means of a pump-oxygenator and retrograde coronary sinus perfusion.' *Diseases of the Chest*, **30**, 123-32.

14 Sarnoff SJ, Case RB. (1955). 'Experimental by-pass of the aortic valve by valvular anastomosis between apex of the left ventricle and thoracic aorta.' *Cardiovascular Surgery; Proceedings of the Symposium held at Henry Ford Hospital.* Ed. Lam CR, pp.304-15. Philadelphia and London; Saunders.

CHAPTER 21: AORTIC INCOMPETENCE

1   Hufnagel CA, Harvey WP, Rabil PJ, McDermott TF. (1954). 'Surgical treatment of aortic insufficiency.' *Surgery*, **35**, 673-83.

2   Hufnagel CA, Vilkgas PD, Nahas H. (1958). 'Experiences with new types of aortic valvular prostheses.' *Annals of Surgery*, **147**, 636-45.

3   Bailey CP. (1955). *Surgery of the heart*, pp.819-20. London; Kimpton.

4   Bailey CP. (Ref. 3 above, p.824).

5   Murray G. (1956). 'Homologous aortic-valve-segment transplants as surgical treatment for aortic and mitral insufficiency.' *Angiology*, **7**, 466-71.

6   Kerwin AJ, Lenkei SC, Wilson DR. (1962). 'Aortic-valve homograft in the treatment of aortic insufficiency. Report of nine cases, with one followed for six years.' *New England Journal of Medicine*, **266**, 852-7. [The six-year follow-up was of Murray's patient.]

7   Murray G. (1960). 'Aortic valve transplants.' *Angiology*, **11**, 99-102.

8   Lillehei CW, Gott VL, DeWall RA, Varco RL. (1958). 'The surgical treatment of stenotic or regurgitant lesions of the mitral and aortic valves by direct vision utilizing a pump-oxygenator.' *Journal of Thoracic Surgery*, **35**, 154-91.

9   Lillehei CW, Gott VL, DeWall RA, Varco RL. (Ref. 8 above. See footnote on p.170.)

10 Scott W. In discussion of: Hufnagel CA, Vilkgas PD, Nahas H. (Ref. 2 above.)

CHAPTER 22: TUMOURS OF THE HEART

1   Morison A. (1907). 'An address on the nature and management of hypertrophy of the heart.' *Lancet*, **2**, 505-8.

2   Beck CS. (1942). 'An intrapericardial teratoma and a tumor of the heart: both removed operatively.' *Annals of Surgery*, **116**, 161-74.

3   Goldberg HP, Glenn F, Dotter CT, Steinberg I. (1952). 'Myxoma of the left atrium. Diagnosis made during life with operative and post-mortem findings.' *Circulation*, **6**, 762-7.

4   Crafoord C. (1955). In discussion of: Glover RP. 'The technique of mitral commissurotomy.' *Cardiovascular Surgery: Proceedings of the Symposium held at Henry · Ford Hospital*. Ed. Lam CR, pp.202-3. Philadelphia and London; Saunders.

5   Bahnson HT, Spencer FC, Andrus EC. (1957). 'Diagnosis and treatment of intracavitary myxomas of the heart.' *Annals of Surgery*, **145**, 915-26.

6   Bigelow WG, Dolan FG, Campbell FW. (1955). 'The effect of hypotyhermia upon the risk of surgery.' *XVI Congrès de la Société Internationale de Chirurgie*, pp. 631-44.' Brussels.

7   Scannell JG, Brewster WR, Bland EF. (1956). 'Successful removal of a myxoma from the left atrium.' *New England Journal of Medicine*, **254**, 601-4.

8   Scannell JG, Grillo HC. (1958). 'Primary tumors of the heart: a surgical problem.' *Journal of Thoracic Surgery*, **35**, 23-36.

9   Fatti L, Reid FP. (1958). 'Excision of atrial myxoma.' *British Medical Journal*, **2**, 531-4.

10 Chin EF, Ross DN. (1957). 'Myxoma of the left atrium. Successful surgical removal under hypothermia.' *British Medical Journal*, **1**, 1447-8.

11 Krčilková M, Musil J, Navrátil J, Olejník O. (1958). 'The successful removal of a tumour from the right atrium under hypothermia.' *Thorax*, **134**, 173-6.

CHAPTER 23: HYPOTHERMIA

1   Haecker R. (1907). 'Experimentelle Studien zur Pathologie des Herzens.' *Archiv für Klinische Chirurgie*, **84**, 1035-98.

2   Sauerbruch F. (1907). 'Die Verwendbarkeit des Unterdruck-verfahrens in der Herzchirurgie.' *Archiv für Klinische Chirurgie*, **83**, 537-45.

3   Rehn L. (1907). 'Zur Chirurgie des Herzens und des Herzbeutels.' *Archiv für Klinische Chirurgie*, **83**, 723-78.

4   Carrel A. (1914). 'Experimental operations on the sigmoid valves of the pulmonary artery.' *Journal of Experimental Medicine*, **20**, 9-18.

5   Lovatt Evans C. (1945). *Principles of human physiology* (Originally written by Prof. EH Starling, M.D., F.R.C.P., C.M.G., F.R.S.), ninth edition, ch. 32, pp.544-6. London; Churchill.

6   Heymans J-F. (1919). 'Iso-hyper-et hypothermisation des mammifères par calorification et frigorification du sang de la circulation carotido-jugulaire anastomosée.' *Archives Internationales de Pharmacodynamie et de Thérapie*, **25**, 1-215.

7   Swan H. In discussion of: Fisher B, Russ C, Fedor E, Wilde R, Engstrom P, Happel J, Prendergast P. (1955). 'Experimental evaluation of prolonged hypothermia.' *Archives of Surgery*, **71**, 431-48.

8   Fay T, Henny GC. (1938). 'Correlation of body segmental temperature and its relation to the location of carcinomatous metastasis. Clinical observations and response to methods of refrigeration.' *Surgery, Gynecology and Obstetrics*, **66**, 512-24.

9   Smith LW, Fay T. (1940). 'Observations on human beings with cancer maintained at reduced temperature of 23°C to 33°C.' *American Journal of Clinical Pathology*, **10**, 1-11.

10 McQuiston WO. (1949). 'Anesthetic problems in cardiac surgery in children.' *Anesthesiology*, **10**, 590-600.

11 McQuiston WO. (1950). 'Anesthesia in cardiac surgery. Observations on three hundred and sixty-two cases.' *Archives of Surgery*, **61**, 892-9.

12 Bigelow WG, Lindsey WK, Greenwood WF. (1950). 'Hypothermia. Its possible role in cardiac surgery: an investigation of factors governing survival in dogs at low body temperatures.' *Annals of Surgery*, **132**, 849-66.

13 Cookson BA, Neptune WB, Bailey CP. (1952). 'Hypothermia as a means of performing intracardiac surgery under direct vision.' *Diseases of the Chest*, **22**, 245-60.

14 Cookson BA, Neptune W, Bailey CP. (1952). 'Intracardiac surgery with hypothermia.' *Journal of the International College of Surgeons*, **18**, 685-94.

15 Lewis FJ, Taufic M. (1953). 'Closure of atrial septal defects with the aid of hypothermia; experimental accomplishments and report of one successful case.' *Surgery* **33**, 52-9.

16 Swan H, Zeavin I, Blount SG, Virtue RW. (1953). 'Surgery by direct vision in the open heart during hypothermia.' *Journal of the American Medical Association*, **153**, 1081-5.

17 Boerema I, Wildschut A, Schmidt WJH, Broekhuysen L. (1951). 'Experimental researches into hypothermia as an aid in the surgery of the heart.' *Archivum Chirurgicum Neerlandicum*, **3**, 25-34.

18 Delorme EJ. (1952). 'Experimental cooling of the blood stream. Preliminary communication.' *Lancet* **2**, 914.

19 Ross DN. (1954). 'Venous cooling. A new method of cooling the blood-stream.' *Lancet*, **1**, 1108-9.

20 Ross DN, Brock RC. (1955). 'Hypothermia. Part III. The clinical application of hypothermic techniques.' *Guy's Hospital Reports*, **104**, 99-113.

CHAPTER 24: EXTRACORPOREAL CIRCULATION

1 Jacobj C. (1890). 'Apparat zur Durchblutung isoliter überlebender Organs.' *Archiv für Experimentelle Pathologie und Pharmakologie*, **26**, 388-400.

2 Embley EH, Martin CJ. (1905). 'The action of anaesthetic quantities of chloroform upon the blood vessels of the bowel and kidney; with an account of an artificial circulation apparatus.' *Journal of Physiology*, **32**, 147-58.

3 Dale HH, Schuster EHJ. (1927-28). 'A double perfusion pump.' *Journal of Physiology*, **64**, 356-64.

4 Wesolowski SA, Sauvage LR, Pinc RD. (1955). 'Extracorporeal circulation: the role of the pulse in maintenance of the systemic circulation during heart-lung by-pass.' *Surgery*, **37**, 633-82.

5 Melrose D. (1960). 'Extracorporeal circulation in the surgery of the heart and great vessels.' In: *Modern trends in cardiac surgery*, ed. Harley HRS, ch. 20, p.259. London; Butterworths.

6 Schröder Wv. (1882). 'Ueber die Bildungsstätte des Harnstoffs.' *Archiv für Experimentelle Pathologie und Pharmakologie*, **15**, 364-402.

7 Frey Mv, Gruber M. (1885). 'Untersuchungen über den Stoffwechsel isoliter Organe. I. Ein Respirationsapparat für isolirte Organe.' *Archiv für Anatomie und Physiologie. Physiologische Abteilung*, **9**, 519-32.

8 Brukhonenko S. (1929). 'Circulation artificielle du sang dans l'organisme entier d'un chien avec coeur exclu.' *Journal de Physiologie et de Pathologie Générale*, **27**, 257-72.

9 Terebinskii NN. Cited by: Demikhov VP. (1962). *Experimental transplantation of vital organs*, ch. 3, p.50. Translated by B Haigh. New York; Consultants Bureau.

10 Gibbon JH. (1937). 'Artificial maintenance of the circulation during experimental

occlusion of the pulmonary artery.' *Archives of Surgery*, **34**, 1105-31.

11 Gibbon JH. (1954). 'Application of a mechanical heart and lung apparatus to cardiac surgery.' *Minnesota Medicine*, **37**, 171-80.

12 Dodrill FD. In discussion of Gibbon JH. (1954). (Ref. 11 above.)

13 Dennis C, Spreng DS, Nelson GE, Karlson KE, Nelson RM, Thomas JV, Elder WP, Varco RL. (1951). 'Development of a pump-oxygenator to replace the heart and lungs; an apparatus applicable to human patients, and application to one case.' *Annals of Surgery*, **134**, 709-21.

14 Kirklin JW, Donald DE, Harshbarger HG, Hetzel PS, Patrick RT, Swan HJC, Wood EH. (1956). 'Studies in extracorporeal circulation. I. Applicability of Gibbon-type pump-oxygenator to human intracardiac surgery. 40 cases.' *Annals of Surgery*, **144**, 2-8.

15 Björk VO. (1948). 'Brain perfusions in dogs with artificially oxygenated blood.' *Acta Chirurgica Scandinavica*, **96**, suppl. 137.

16 Björk VO. (1948). 'An artificial heart or cardiopulmonary machine: performance in animals.' *Lancet*, **2**, 491-3.

17 Aird I, Melrose DG, Cleland WP, Lynn RB. (1954). 'Assisted circulation by pump-oxygenator during operative dilatation of the aortic valve in man.' *British Medical Journal*, **1**, 1284-7.

18 Juvenelle AA, Lind J, Wegelius C. (1954). 'A new method of extracorporeal circulation. Deep hypothermia combined with artificial circulation.' *American Heart Journal*, **47**, 692-736.

19 Gerbode F, Osborn JJ, Melrose DG, Perkins HA, Norman A, Baer DM. (1958). 'Extracorporeal circulation in intracardiac surgery: a comparison between two heart-lung machines.' *Lancet*, **2**, 284-6.

20 Clark LC, Gollan F, Gupta VB. (1950). 'The oxygenation of blood by gas dispersion.' *Science*, **111**, 85-7.

21 Dogliotti AM, Costantini A. (1951). 'Primo caso di applicazione all'uomo di un apparecchio di circolazione sanguina extracorporea.' *Minerva Chirurgica*, **6**, 657-9.

22 De Wall RA, Warden HE, Read RC, Gott VL, Ziegler NR, Varco RL, Lillehei CW. (1956). 'A simple, expendable, artificial oxygenator for open heart surgery.' *Surgical Clinics of North America*, **36**, 1025-34.

23 Long DM Jr, Sanchez L, Varco RL, Lillehei CW. (1961). 'The use of low molecular weight dextran and serum albumin as plasma expanders in extracorporeal circulation.' *Surgery*, **50**, 12-28.

24 Zuhdi N, Carey J, Cutter J, Rader L, Greer A. (1963). 'Intentional hemodilution.' *Archives of Surgery*, **87**, 554-9.

25 Cooley DA, Beall AC, Grondin P. (1962). 'Open-heart operations with disposable oxygenators, 5 per cent dextrose prime, and normothermia.' *Surgery*, **52**, 713-9.

26 Melrose DG, Bramson ML, Osborn JJ, Gerbode F. (1958). 'The membrane oxygenator. Some aspects of oxygen and carbon dioxide transport across polyethylene film.' *Lancet*, **1**, 1050-1.

27 Melrose D. (1960). (Ref. 5 above, p.262.)

28 Boehm R. (1878). 'V. Arbeiten aus dem pharmakologischen Institute der Universität Dorpat: 13. Ueber Wiederbelebung nach Vergiftungen und Asphyxie.' *Archiv für Experimentelle Pathologie und Pharmakologie*, **8**, 68-101.

29 Ringer S. (1883). 'A further contribution regarding the influence of the different constituents of the blood on the contraction of the heart.' *Journal of Physiology*, **4**, 29-42.

30 Martin EG. (1904). 'The inhibitory influence of potassium chloride on the heart, and

the effect of variations of temperature upon this inhibition and upon vagus inhibition.' *American Journal of Physiology*, **11**, 370-93.

31 Melrose DG, Dreyer B, Bentall HH, Baker JBE. (1955). 'Elective cardiac arrest. Preliminary communication.' *Lancet*, **2**, 21-2.

32 Melrose DG. Personal communication. [Melrose did not publish an account of the first clinical elective cardiac arrest.]

33 Sergeant CK, Geoghegan T, Lam CR. (1956). 'Further studies in induced cardiac arrest using the agent acetylcholine.' *Surgical Forum*, **7**, 254-7.

34 Pratt FH. (1898). 'The nutrition of the heart through the vessels of Thebesius and the coronary veins.' *American Journal of Physiology*, **1**, 86-103.

35 Roberts JT. (1943). 'Experimental studies on the nourishment of the left ventricle by the lumenal (Thebesial) vessels.' *Federation Proceedings*, **2**, 90.

36 Lillehei CW, DeWall RA, Gott VL, Varco RL. (1956). 'The direct vision correction of calcific aortic stenosis by means of a pump-oxygenator and retrograde coronary sinus perfusion.' *Diseases of the Chest*, **30**, 123-32.

37 Mustard WT, Chute AL. (1951). 'Experimental intracardiac surgery with extracorporeal circulation.' *Surgery*, **30**, 684-8.

38 Mustard WT, Chute AL, Simmons EH. (1952). 'Further observations on experimental extracorporeal circulation.' *Surgery*, **32**, 803-10.

39 Mustard WT, Chute AL, Keith JD, Sirek A, Rowe RD, Vlad P. (1954). 'A surgical approach to transposition of the great vessels with extracorporeal circuit.' *Surgery*, **36**, 39-51.

40 Mustard WT, Sapirstein W, Pav D. (1958). 'Cardiac bypass without artificial oxygenation.' *Journal of Thoracic Surgery*, **36**, 479-87.

41 Bailey CP. In discussion following: Mustard WT, Sapirstein W, Pav D. (1958). (Ref. 40 above, p.531.)

42 Andreasen AT, Watson F. (1952). 'Experimental cardiovascular surgery.' *British Journal of Surgery*, **39**, 548-51.

43 Andreasen AT, Watson F. (1953). 'Experimental cardiovascular surgery: discussion of results so far obtained and reports on experiments concerning a donor circulation.' *British Journal of Surgery*, **41**, 195-206.

44 Cohen M, Lillehei CW. (1953). 'Autologous lung oxygenator with total cardiac bypass for intracardiac surgery.' *Surgical Forum*, **4**, 34-40.

45 Warden HE, Cohen M, Read RC, Lillehei CW. (1954). 'Controlled cross circulation for open intracardiac surgery. Physiologic studies and results of creation and closure of ventricular septal defects.' *Journal of Thoracic Surgery*, **28**, 331-41

46 Lillehei CW, Cohen M, Warden HE, Varco RL. (1955). 'The direct-vision intracardiac correction of congenital anomalies by controlled cross circulation. Results in thirty-two patients with ventricular septal defects, tetralogy of Fallot, and atrioventricularis communis defects.' *Surgery*, **38**, 11-29.

47 Lillehei CW, Warden HE, DeWall R, Stanley P, Varco RL. (1957). 'Cardiopulmonary by-pass in surgical treatment of congenital or acquired cardiac disease.' *Archives of Surgery*, **75**, 928-45.

48 Campbell GS, Crisp NW Jr, Brown EB Jr. (1955). 'Maintenance of respiratory function with isolated lung lobes during cardiac inflow occlusion.' *Proceedings of the Society for Experimental Biology and Medicine*, **88**, 390-3.

CHAPTER 25: HYPERBARIC OXYGEN AND EXTRACORPOREAL COOLING

1 Bureau of Investigation (1928). 'The Cunningham "tank treatment". The alleged value of compressed air in the treatment of diabetes mellitus, pernicious anaemia

and carcinoma.' *Journal of the American Medical Association*, **90**, 1494-6.

2   Boerema I, Kroll JA, Meijne NG, Lokin E, Kroon B, Huiskes JW. (1956). 'High atmospheric pressure as an aid to cardiac surgery.' *Archivum Chirurgicum Neerlandicum*, **8**, 193-211.

3   Boerema I, Meijne NG, Vermeulen-Cranch DME. (1962). 'Observations during operation on deeply cyanotic young children breathing oxygen at three atmospheres absolute.' *Surgery*, **52**, 796-9.

4   Barclay RS, Ledingham I McA, Norman JN. (1964). 'Experimental and human cardiac surgery with hyperbaric oxygen.' In: *Clinical Application of Hyperbaric Oxygen. Proceedings of the First International Congress, Amsterdam, September 1963*, ed. Boerema I, Brummelkamp WH, Meijne NG. Amsterdam,London, New York; Elsevier.

5   Bernard WF, Tank ES, Frittelli G, Gross RE. (1963). 'The feasability of hypothermic perfusion under hyperbaric conditions in the surgical management of infants with cyanotic congenital heart disease.' *Journal of Thoracic and Cardiovascular Surgery*, **46**, 651-64.

6   Giaja J. (1940). 'Léthargie obtenue chez le rat par la dépression barometrique.' *Comptes Rendus Hebdomadaires des Séances de l'Académie des Sciences*, **210**, 80-2.

7   Barbour JH, Seevers MH. (1943). 'Narcosis induced by carbon dioxide at low environmental temperatures.' *Journal of Pharmacology and Experimental Therapeutics*, **78**, 296-303.

8   Andjus R. (1951). 'Sur la possibilité de ranimer le rat adulte refroidi jusqu'à proximité du point de congélation.' *Comptes Rendus Hebdomadaires des Séances de l'Académie des Sciences*, **232**, 1591-3.

9   Juvenelle AA, Citret C, Wiles CE, Stewart JO. (1951). 'Pneumonectomy with replantation of the lung in the dog for physiologic study.' *Journal of Thoracic Surgery*, **21**, 111-5.

10 Demikhov VP. (1962). *Experimental transplantation of vital organs*, ch. 3, pp.129-35. Translated by B Haigh. New York; Consultants Bureau.

11 Juvenelle A, Lind J, Wegelius. (1952). 'Quelques possibilités offertes par l'hypothermie générale profonde provoquée. Une étude expérimentale chez le chien.' *Presse Médicale*, **60**, 973-8.

12 Juvenelle AA, Lind J, Wegelius C. (1954). 'A new method of extracorporeal circulation. Deep hypothermia combined with artificial circulation.' *American Heart Journal*, **47**, 692-736.

13 Cookson BA, Costas-Durieux J. (1954). 'The use of arterial transfusion as an adjunct to hypothermia in the repair of septal defects.' *Annals of Surgery*, **140**, 100-6.

14 Gollan F, Blos P, Schuman H. (1952). 'Exclusion of heart and lungs from circulation in the hypothermic, closed-chest dog by means of a pump-oxygenator.' *Journal of Applied Physiology*, **5**, 180-90.

15 Heymans J-F. (1919). 'Iso-hyper- et hypothermisation des mammifères par calorification et frigorification du sang de la circulation carotido-jugulaire anastomosée.' *Archives Internationales de Pharmacodynamie et de Thérapie*, **25**, 1-215.

16 Gollan F, Grace JT, Schell MW, Tysinger DS, Feaster LB. (1955). 'Left heart surgery in dogs during respiratory and cardiac arrest at body temperatures below 10°C.' *Surgery*, **38**, 363-72.

17 Gollan F. (1959). 'Physiology of deep hypothermia by total body perfusion.' *Annals of the New York Academy of Sciences*, **80**, 301-14.

18 Sealy WC, Brown IW Jr, Young WG Jr, Stephen CR, Harris JS, Merritt D. (1957). 'Hypothermia, low flow extracorporeal circulation and controlled cardiac arrest for open heart surgery.' *Surgery, Gynecology and Obstetrics*, **104**, 441-50.

19 Sealy WC, Brown IW Jr, Young WG Jr. (1958). 'A report on the use of both extra-corporeal circulation and hypothermia for open heart surgery.' *Annals of Surgery*, **147**, 603-13.

20 Gollan F. (1959). *Physiology of cardiac surgery*. Springfield, Ill.; Thomas.

21 Shields TW, Lewis FJ. (1959). 'Rapid cooling and surgery at temperatures below 20°C.' *Surgery*, **46**, 164-74.

22 Drew CE, Keen G, Benazon DB. (1959). 'Profound hypothermia.' *Lancet*, **1**, 745-7.

23 Drew CE, Anderson IM. (1959). 'Profound hypothermia in cardiac surgery. Report of three cases.' *Lancet*, **1**, 748-50.

24 Drew CE. (1960). 'Profound hypothermia in cardiac surgery.' In: *Modern trends in cardiac surgery*, ed. Harley HRS, ch. 21, pp.273-8. London; Butterworths.

CHAPTER 26: TRANSPOSITION OF THE GREAT VESSELS

1   Hanlon CR, Blalock A. (1948). 'Complete transposition of the aorta and pulmonary artery. Experimental observations on venous shunts as corrective procedures.' *Annals of Surgery*, **127**, 385-97.

2   Blalock A, Hanlon CR. (1950). 'The surgical treatment of complete transposition of the aorta and the pulmonary artery.' *Surgery, Gynecology and Obstetrics*, **90**, 1-15.

3   Mustard WT, Chute AL, Keith JD, Sirek A, Rowe RD, Vlad P. (1954). 'A surgical approach to transposition of the great vessels with extracorporeal circuit.' *Surgery*, **36**, 39-51.

4   Bailey CP, Cookson BA, Downing DF, Neptune WB. (1954). 'Cardiac surgery under hypothermia.' *Journal of Thoracic Surgery*, **27**, 73-95.

5   Lillehei CW, Varco RL. (1953). 'Certain physiologic, pathologic, and surgical features of complete transposition of the great vessels.' *Surgery*, **34**, 376-400.

6   Murphy TO, Gott V, Lillehei CW, Varco RL. (1955). 'The results of surgical palliation in 32 patients with transposition of the great vessels.' *Surgery, Gynecology and Obstetrics*, **101**, 541-4.

7   Björk VO, Bouckaert L. (1954). 'Complete transposition of the aorta and pulmonary artery.' *Journal of Thoracic Surgery*, **28**, 632-5.

8   Cross FS, Kay EB, Jones RD. (1954). 'A simple shunting technique for surgery of the aortic and pulmonary valves and proximal great vessels. An experimental study.' *Journal of Thoracic Surgery*, **28**, 229-34.

9   Kay EB, Cross FS. (1955). 'Surgical treatment of transposition of the great vessels.' *Surgery*, **38**, 712-6.

10 Senning Å. (1959). 'Surgical correction of transposition of the great vessels.' *Surgery*, **45**, 966-80.

11 Crafoord C. (1955). In discussion of: Mustard WT. (1955). 'Evaluation of transposition operations.' *Cardiovascular Surgery; Proceedings of the Symposium held at Henry Ford Hospital*. Ed. Lam CR. Philadelphia and London; Saunders.

12 Baffes TG. (1956). 'A new method for surgical correction of transposition of the aorta and pulmonary artery.' *Surgery, Gynecology and Obstetrics*, **102**, 227-33.

13 Baffes TG, Riker WL, De Boer A, Potts WJ. (1957). 'Surgical correction of transposition of the aorta and the pulmonary artery.' *Journal of Thoracic Surgery*, **34**, 469-84.

14 Kay EB, Cross FS. (1957). 'Transposition of the great vessels corrected by means of atrial transposition.' *Surgery*, **41**, 938-42.

15 Merendino KA, Jesseph JE, Herron PW, Thomas GI, Vetto RR. (1957). 'Interatrial venous transposition.' *Surgery*, **42**, 898-909.

16 Kirklin JW, Devloo RA, Weidman WH. (1961). 'Open intracardiac repair for transposition of the great vessels: 11 cases.' *Surgery*, **50**, 58-66.

17 Barnard CN, Schrire V, Beck W. (1962). 'Complete transposition of the great vessels: a successful complete correction.' *Journal of Thoracic and Cardiovascular Surgery*, **43**, 769-79.

18 Mustard WT. (1964). 'Successful two-stage correction of transposition of the great vessels.' *Surgery*, **55**, 469-72.

19 Kidd L, Mustard WT. (1966). 'Hemodynamic effects of a totally corrective procedure in transposition of the great vessels.' *Circulation*, **33**, suppl. 1, 29-33.

CHAPTER 27: VALVE REPLACEMENT

1 Murray G. (1956). 'Homologous aortic-valve-segment transplants as surgical treatment for aortic and mitral insufficiency.' *Angiology*, **7**, 466-71.

2 Hufnagel CA, Harvey WP, Rabil PJ, McDermott TF. (1954). 'Surgical treatment of aortic insufficiency.' *Surgery*, **35**, 673-83.

3 Lillehei CW, Gott VL, DeWall RA, Varco RL. (1958). 'The surgical treatment of stenotic or regurgitant lesions of the mitral and aortic valves by direct vision utilizing a pump-oxygenator.' *Journal of Thoracic Surgery*, **35**, 154-91.

4 Denton GR. (1950). 'A plastic prosthesis (without moving parts) for the atrio-ventricular valves.' *Surgical Forum*, **1**, 239-45.

5 Hufnagel CA. (1959). 'Direct approaches for the treatment of aortic insufficiency.' *American Surgeon*, **25**, 321-7.

6 Hufnagel CA. (1961). 'Aortic insufficiency.' *Progress in Cardiovascular Diseases*, **4**, 278-84.

7 McGoon DC. (1961). 'Prosthetic reconstruction of the aortic valve.' *Proceedings of the Staff Meetings of the Mayo Clinic*, **36**, 88-96.

8 Braunwald NS, Cooper T, Morrow AG. (1960). 'Complete replacement of the mitral valve. Successful clinical application of a flexible polyurethane prosthesis.' *Journal of Thoracic Surgery*, **40**, 1-11.

9 Ellis FH, Bulbulian AH. (1958). 'Prosthetic replacement of the mitral valve. I. Preliminary experimental observations.' *Proceedings of the Staff Meetings of the Mayo Clinic*, **33**, 532-4a.

10 Doumanian AV, Ellis FH Jr. (1961). 'Prolonged survival after total replacement of the mitral valve in dogs.' *Journal of Thoracic Surgery*, **42**, 683-95.

11 Harken DE, Soroff HS, Taylor WJ, Lefemine AA, Gupta SK, Lunzer S. (1960). 'Partial and complete prostheses in aortic insufficiency.' *Journal of Thoracic Surgery*, **40**, 744-62.

12 Harken DE, Taylor WJ, Lefemine AA, Lunzer S, Low HBC, Cohen ML, Jacobey JA. (1962). 'Aortic valve replacement with a caged ball valve.' *American Journal of Cardiology*, **9**, 292-9.

13 Starr A, Edwards ML. (1961). 'Mitral replacement: clinical experience with a ball-valve prosthesis.' *Annals of Surgery*, **154**, 726-40.

14 Cartwright RS, Palich WE, Ford WB, Giacobine JW, Zubritzky SA, Ratan RS. (1962). 'Combined replacement of aortic and mitral valves. An original transatrial approach to the aortic valve.' *Journal of the American Medical Association*, **180**, 6-10.

15 Brock RC. (1950). 'The arterial route to the aortic and pulmonary valves. The mitral route to the aortic valve.' *Guy's Hospital Reports*, **99**, 236-46.

16 Starr A, Edwards ML, McCord CW, Wood J, Herr R, Griswold HE. (1964). 'Multiple-valve replacement.' *Circulation*, **29**, suppl. 1, 30-5.

17 Litwak RS, Gadboys HL, Scott GB, Ferrara JF. (1952). 'Surgical approach for stenotic lesions of the semilunar valves by excision and cusp replacement under direct vision.' *Journal of Thoracic Surgery*, **24**, 165-89.

18 Beall AC, Morris GC, Cooley DA, De Bakey ME. (1961). 'Homotransplantation of the aortic valve.' *Journal of Thoracic and Cardiovascular Surgery*, **42**, 497-506.

19 Beall AC, Morris GC, Cooley DA, De Bakey ME. (1964). In: discussion of Bigelow WG, Yao JK, Aldridge HE, Heimbecker RO, Murray GDW. (1964). (Ref. 22 below.)

20 Kerwin AJ, Lenkei SC, Wilson DR. (1962). 'Aortic-valve homograft in the treatment of aortic insufficiency. Report of nine cases, with one followed for six years.' *New England Journal of Medicine*, **266**, 852-7. [The six-year follow-up was of Murray's patient.]

21 Heimbecker RO, Baird RJ, Lajos TZ, Varga AT, Greenwood WF. (1962). 'Homograft replacement of the human mitral valve. A preliminary report.' *Canadian Medical Association Journal*, **86**, 805-9.

22 Bigelow WG, Yao JK, Aldridge HE, Heimbecker RO, Murray GDW. (1964). 'Clinical homograft valve transplantation.' *Journal of Thoracic and Cardiovascular Surgery*, **48**, 333-45.

23 Duran CG, Gunning AJ. (1962). 'A method for placing a total homologous aortic valve in the subcoronary position.' *Lancet*, **2**, 488-9.

24 Ross D. (1964). 'Homotransplantation of the aortic valve in the subcoronary position.' *Journal of Thoracic and Cardiovascular Surgery*, **47**, 713-9.

25 Ross DN. (1962). 'Homograft replacement of the aortic valve.' *Lancet*, **2**, 487.

26 Barratt-Boyes BG. (1964). 'Homograft aortic valve replacement in aortic incompetence and stenosis.' *Thorax*, **19**, 131-50.

27 Hurley PJ, Lowe JB, Barratt-Boyes BG. (1967). 'Débridement-valvotomy for aortic stenosis in adults. A follow-up of 76 patients.' *Thorax*, **22**, 314-9.

28 Duran CG, Gunning AJ. (1965). 'Heterologous aortic-valve transplants in the dog.' *Lancet*, **2**, 114-5.

29 Binet JP, Duran CG, Carpentier A, Langlois J. (1965). 'Heterologous aortic valve transplantation.' *Lancet*, **2**, 1275.

30 Hoeksema TD, Titus JL, Guiliani ER, Kirklin JW. (1967). 'Early results of use of homografts for replacement of the aortic valve in man.' *Circulation*, **35**, suppl. 1, 9-14.

31 Hubka M, Šiška K, Holec V. (1967). 'Replacement of the mitral valve with an aortic valve homograft implanted into the left atrium.' *Journal of Thoracic and Cardiovascular Surgery*, **53**, 260-7.

32 Ionescu MI, Wooler GH, Smith DR, Grimshaw VA. (1967). 'Mitral valve replacement with aortic heterografts in humans.' *Thorax*, **22**, 305-13.

33 Ross DN. (1967). 'Replacement of aortic and mitral valves with a pulmonary autograft.' *Lancet*, **2**, 956-8.

34 Ross D. (1968). Report of the Sixteenth Biennial Congress of the International College of Surgeons, held in Tokyo, in: *Medical News*, November 1, 1968, p.8.

CHAPTER 28: ARTIFICIAL HEARTS AND SUPPORT OF THE CIRCULATION

1 Newman MH, Stuckey JH, Levowitz BS, Young LA, Dennis C, Fries C, Gorayeb EH, Zuhdi M, Karlson KE, Adler S, Gliedman M. (1955). 'Complete and partial perfusion of animal and human subjects with the pump oxygenator. A study of factors yielding consistent survival. Successful application to one case.' *Surgery*, **38**, 30-7.

2 Stuckey JH, Newman MM, Dennis C, Berg E, Goodman SE, Fries CC, Karlson KE, Blumenfeld M, Weitzner SW, Binder LS, Winston A. (1957). 'Partial perfusion in the treatment of selected cases of myocardial infarction.' *Transactions. American Society for Artificial Internal Organs*, **3**, 30-2.

3 Dennis C, Hall DP, Moreno JR, Senning Å. (1962). 'Left atrial cannulation without

Sources

thoracotomy for total left heart bypass.' *Acta Chirurgica Scandinavica*, **123**, 267-79.

4   Liotta D, Hall CW, Henly WS, Beall AC Jr, Cooley DA, De Bakey ME. (1963). 'Prolonged assisted circulation during and after heart or aortic surgery.' *Transactions. American Society for Artificial Internal Organs*, **9**, 182-5.

5   Liotta D, Hall CW, Henly WS, Cooley DA, Crawford ES, De Bakey ME. (1963). 'Prolonged assisted circulation during and after cardiac or aortic surgery. Prolonged partial left ventricular bypass by means of intracorporeal circulation.' *American Journal of Cardiology*, **12**, 399-405.

6   Clauss RH, Birtwell C, Albertal G, Lunzer S, Taylor WJ, Fosberg AM, Harken DE. (1961). 'Assisted circulation. I. The arterial counterpulsator.' *Journal of Thoracic and Cardiovascular Surgery*, **41**, 447-58.

7   De Bakey ME. (1968). 'Indirizzi attuali nel programma del cuore artificiale.' *Gazzetta Sanitaria*, **39**, 313-23.

8   De Bakey ME. (1967-68). In: *The year book of general surgery*, p.46. Chicago; Year Book Medical Publishers.

9   Kantrowitz A, Akutsu T, Chaptal P-A, Krakauer J, Kantrowitz AR, Jones RT. (1966). 'Clinical experience with an implanted mechanical auxiliary ventricle.' *Journal of the American Medical Association*, **197**, 525-9.

10 Kantrowitz A, Tjønneland S, Freed PS, Phillips SJ, Butner AN, Sherman JL Jr. (1968). 'Initial clinical experience with intraaortic balloon pumping in cardiogenic shock.' *Journal of the American Medical Association*, **203**, 113-8.

11 Kantrowitz A, Tjønneland S, Krakauer J, Butner AN, Phillips SJ, Yahr WZ, Shapiro M, Freed PS, Jaron D, Sherman JL Jr. (1968). 'Clinical experience with cardiac assistance by means of intraaortic phase-shift balloon pumping.' *Transactions. American Society for Artificial Organs*, **14**, 344-8.

12 Haiderer D, Kennedy JH. (1968). 'Assisted circulation: a comparison of three methods of circulatory bypass of the left heart.' *Diseases of the Chest*, **54**, 44-9.

13 Kennedy JH. (1969). 'Assisted circulation: an extended concept of cardiopulmonary resuscitation.' *Journal of Thoracic and Cardiovascular Surgery*, **57**, 688-701.

14 Landé AJ, Dos SJ, Carlson RG, Perschau RA, Lange RP, Sonstegard LJ, Lillehei CW. (1967). 'A new membrane oxygen-dialyzer.' *Surgical Clinics of North America*, **47**, 1461-70.

15 Mantini E, Tanaka S, Horta-DaSilva P, Lillehei CW. (1967). 'Some aspects of altered physiology during partial right and left ventricular bypass.' *Transactions. American Society for Artificial Organs*, **13**, 288-92.

16 Demikhov VP. (1962). *Experimental transplantation of vital organs*, ch. 5, pp.212-3. Translated by B Haigh. New York; Consultants Bureau.

17 Atsumi K, Hori M, Ikeda S, Sakurai Y, Fujimori Y, Kimoto S. (1963). 'Artificial heart incorporated in the chest.' *Transactions. American Society for Artificial Organs*, **9**, 292-8.

18 Atsumi K. (1967). Personal communication.

19 Houston CS, Akutsu T, Kolff WJ. (1960). 'Pendulum type of artificial heart within the chest: preliminary report.' *American Heart Journal*, **59**, 723-30.

20 Akutsu T, Houston CS, Kolff WJ. (1960). 'Roller type of artificial heart within the chest: preliminary report.' *American heart Journal*, **59**, 731-6.

21 Nosé Y, Topaz S, SenGupta A, Tretbar LL, Kolff WJ. (1965). 'Artificial hearts inside the pericardial sac in calves.' *Transactions. American Society for Artificial Organs*, **11**, 255-62.

22 'Nuclear energy for mechanical heart.' *Medical World News*, June 14, 1968, p.18.

CHAPTER 29: TRANSPLANTATION OF THE HEART – THE BACKGROUND

1 Guthrie CC. (1912). *Blood-vessel surgery and its applications*. London: Arnold.

2 Carrel A, Guthrie CC. (1906). 'Anastomoses des vaisseaux sanguins.' *XV Congrès International de Médecin* (Lisbon, April 1906). Section de Chirurgie, 238-49.

3 Carrel A, Guthrie CC. (1906). 'Unilateral and biterminal venous transplantations.' *Surgery, Gynecology and Obstetrics*, **2**, 266-86.

4 Carrel A. (1906). 'Surgery of the blood-vessels and its application to the changes of circulation and transplantation of organs.' *Bulletin of the Johns Hopkins Hospital*, **17**, 236-7.

5 Carrel A. (1907). 'The surgery of the blood vessels etc.' *Bulletin of the Johns Hopkins Hospital*, **18**, 18-28.

6 Morris RT. (1906). 'A case of heteroplastic ovarian grafting, followed by pregnancy, and the delivery of a living child.' *Medical Record*, **69**, 697-8.

7 Kolff WJ, Berk HTJ, ter Welle M, van der Ley AJW, van Dijk EC, van Noordwijk J. (1944). 'The artificial kidney: a dialyser with a great area.' *Acta Medica Scandinavica*, **117**, 121-34.

8 Kolff WJ. (1944). *The artificial kidney*. Kampen; Kok.

9 Medawar PB. (1945). 'The behaviour and fate of skin autografts and skin homografts in rabbits.' *Journal of Anatomy*, **78**, 176-99.

10 Medawar PB. (1945). 'A second study of the behaviour and fate of skin homografts in rabbits.' *Journal of Anatomy*, **79**, 157-76.

11 Mann FC, Priestley JT, Markowitz J, Yater WM. (1933). 'Transplantation of the intact mammalian heart.' *Archives of Surgery*, **26**, 219-24.

12 Demikhov VP. (1962). *Experimental transplantation of vital organs*, ch.3, pp.49-182. Translated by B Haigh. New York; Consultants Bureau.

13 Sinitsyn NP. Cited by Demikhov VP. (1962). (Ref. 12 above, ch. 1, p.3.)

14 Ognev BV. Cited by Demikhov VP. (1962). (Ref. 12 above, ch. 3, p.52.)

15 Marcus E, Wong SNT, Luisada AA. (1951). 'Homologous heart grafts: transplantation of the heart in dogs.' *Surgical Forum*, **2**, 212-7.

16 Marcus E, Wong SNT, Luisada AA. (1953). 'Homologous heart grafts.' *Archives of Surgery*, **66**, 179-91.

17 Luisada AA, Marcus E. (1954). 'The behavior of a transplanted heart.' *Cardiologia*, **25**, 197-211.

18 Cookson BA, Neptune WE, Bailey CP. (1952). 'Hypothermia as a means of performing intracardiac surgery under direct vision.' *Diseases of the Chest*, **22**, 245-60.

19 Neptune WB, Cookson BA, Bailey CP, Appler R, Rajkowski F. (1953). 'Complete homologous heart transplantation.' *Archives of Surgery*, **66**, 174-8. [This is the paper that irked Demikov: see the footnote on p.107 of his book – ref. 12, above – although he cited the journal incorrectly as *Surgery*. His pique is understandable, since he listed 167 non-Russian references in his bibliography in addition to 700 or so Russian ones.]

20 Blanco G, Adam A, Rodriguez-Perez D, Fernandez A. (1958). 'Complete homotransplantation of canine heart and lungs.' *Archives of Surgery*, **76**, 20-3.

21 Willman VL, Cooper T, Cian LG, Hanlon CR. (1962). 'Autotransplantation of the canine heart.' *Surgery, Gynecology and Obstetrics*, **115**, 299-302.

22 Hurley EJ, Dong E Jr, Stofer RC, Shumway NE. (1962). 'Isotopic replacement of the totally excised canine heart.' *Journal of Surgical Research*, **2**, 90-4.

23 Goldberg, Berman EF, Akman LC. (1958). 'Homologous transplantation of the canine heart.' *Journal of the International College of Surgeons*, **30**, 575-86.

24 Cass MH, Brock R. (1959). 'Heart excision and replacement.' *Guy's Hospital Reports*,

108, 285-90.

25 Lower RR, Shumway NE. (1960). 'Studies on orthotopic homotransplantation of the heart.' *Surgical Forum*, **11**, 18-9.

26 Lower RR, Stofer RC, Shumway NE. (1961). 'Homovital transplantation of the heart.' *Journal of Thoracic and Cardiovascular Surgery*, **41**, 196-204.

27 Reemtsma K, Williamson WE Jr, Iglesias F, Pena E, Sayegh SF, Creech O Jr. (1962). 'Studies in homologous canine heart transplantation: prolongation of survival with a folic acid antagonist.' *Surgery*, **52**, 127-33.

28 Reemtsma K. (1964). 'The heart as a test organ in transplantation studies.' *Annals of the New York Academy of Sciences*, **120**, 778-85.

29 Blumenstock DA, Hechtman HB, Collins JA, Jaretzki A III, Hosbein JD, Zingg W, Powers JH. (1963). 'Prolonged survival of orthotopic homotransplants of the heart in animals treated with methotrexate.' *Journal of Thoracic and Cardiovascular Surgery*, **46**, 616-28.

30 Kondo Y, Grädel F, Kantrowitz A. (1965). 'Homotransplantation of the heart in puppies under profound hypothermia: long survival without immunosuppressive treatment.' *Annals of Surgery*, **162**, 837-48.

31 Shumway NE, Lower RR. (1964). 'Special problems in transplantation of the heart.' *Annals of the New York Academy of Sciences*, **120**, 773-7.

CHAPTER 30: TRANSPLANTATION OF THE HEART – THE ACHIEVEMENT

1 Webb WR, Howard HS. (1957). 'Cardiopulmonary transplantation.' *Surgical Forum*, **8**, 313-7.

2 Lower RR, Stofer RC, Hurley EJ, Shumway NE. (1961) 'Complete homograft replacement of the heart and both lungs.' *Surgery*, **50**, 842-5.

3 Webb WR, Howard HS, Neely WA. (1959). 'Practical methods of homologous cardiac transplantation.' *Journal of Thoracic Surgery*, **37**, 361-6.

4 Hardy JD, Webb WR, Dalton ML Jr, Walker GR. (1963). 'Lung homotransplantation in man. Report of the initial case.' *Journal of the American Medical Association*, **186**, 1065-74.

5 Hardy JG, Chavez CM, Kurrus FD, Neely WA, Eraslan S, Turner MD, Fabian LW, Labecki TD. (1964). 'Heart transplantation in man. Developmental studies and report of a case.' *Journal of the American Medical Association*, **188**, 1132-40.

6 Reemtsma K, McCracken BH, Schlegel JU, Pearl MA, DeWitt CW, Creech O Jr. (1964). 'Reversal of early graft rejection after renal heterotransplantation in man.' *Journal of the American Medical Association*, **187**, 691-6.

7 Schrire V, Barnard CN. (1966). 'An analysis of cardiac surgery at Groote Schuur Hospital, Cape Town, for the 14 years April 1951-April 1965.' *South African Medical Journal*, **40**, 279-84, 461-7.

8 Barnard MS. (1967). 'Heart transplantation: an experimental review and preliminary research.' *South African Medical Journal* **41**, 1260-2.

9 Barnard CN. (1967). 'A human cardiac transplant: an interim report of a successful operation performed at Groote Schuur Hospital, Cape Town.' *South African Medical Journal*, **41**, 1271-4.

10 Thompson JG. (1968). 'Heart transplantation in man – necropsy findings.' *British Medical Journal*, **2**, 511-7.

11 Kantrowitz A, Haller JD, Joos H, Cerruti MM, Carstensen HE. (1968). 'Transplantation of the heart in an infant and an adult.' *American Journal of Cardiology*, **22**, 782-90.

12 Barnard CN. (1968). 'Human cardiac transplantation. An evaluation of the first two operations performed at the Groote Schuur Hospital, Cape Town.' *American Journal*

of Cardiology, **22**, 584-96.

13   Stinson EB, Dong E Jr, Schroeder JS, Harrison DC, Shumway NE. (1968). 'Initial clinical experience with heart transplantation.' *American Journal of Cardiology,* **22**, 791-803.

14   Cost of Kasperak's operation. Reported in: *Medical World News,* June 28, 1968, p.28.

15   Cost of Cooley's operations reported by: Rusk HA. (1968). 'Behind the news. Point of no return.' *Medical World News,* September 27, 1968, p.84.

16   Cooley DA. (1968). Quotations from an Exclusive Tribune Interview. *Medical Tribune,* June 20, 1968, pp.1, 18.

17   Cooley DA, Bloodwell RD, Hallman GL, Nora JJ. (1968). 'Transplantation of the human heart. Report of four cases.' *Journal of the American Medical Association,* **205**, 479-86.

18   Cooley DA, Bloodwell RD, Hallman GL, Leachman RD, Nora JJ, Rochelle DG, Milam JD. (1969). 'Human cardiac transplantation.' *Circulation,* **39**, suppl. 1, 3-12.

19   Ross D. (1968). 'Report of a heart transplant operation.' *American Journal of Cardiology,* **22**, 838-9.

20   Paget S. (1896). *The surgery of the chest.* Bristol; Wright. London; Simpkin, Marshall, Hamilton, Kent.

INDEX OF PERSONAL NAMES

SUBJECT INDEX